PALLIATIVE
TOUCH

of related interest

Hands in Health Care, Second Edition
Massage Therapy for the Adult Hospital Patient
Gayle MacDonald and Carolyn Tague
Forewords by Ruth Werner and Wolf E. Mehling
ISBN 978 1 91208 554 5
eISBN 978 1 91208 555 2

Oncology Massage
An Integrative Approach to Cancer Care
Janet Penny and Rebecca Sturgeon
Foreword by Cal Cates
ISBN 978 1 91208 575 0
eISBN 978 1 91208 576 7

Integrative Pain Management
Massage, Movement, and Mindfulness Based Approaches
Diana Thompson and Marissa Brooks
Forewords by Wayne Jonas and John Weeks
ISBN 978 1 90914 126 1
eISBN 978 1 91208 521 7

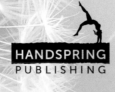

HANDSPRING
PUBLISHING

Cynthia Heep Spence

PALLIATIVE TOUCH

Massage for people at the end of life

Forewords
Gayle MacDonald
Madeleine Kerkhof

First published in Great Britain in 2023 by Handspring Publishing, an imprint of Jessica Kingsley Publishers
An imprint of Hodder & Stoughton Ltd
An Hachette UK Company

1

A CIP catalogue record for this title is available from the British Library and the Library of Congress

ISBN 978 1 91342 619 4
eISBN 978 1 91342 620 0

Printed and bound in China by RR Donnelley

Jessica Kingsley Publishers' policy is to use papers that are natural, renewable and recyclable products and made from wood grown in sustainable forests. The logging and manufacturing processes are expected to conform to the environmental regulations of the country of origin.

Handspring Publishing
Carmelite House
50 Victoria Embankment
London EC4Y 0DZ

www.handspringpublishing.com

CONTENTS

Acknowledgments   vii

Foreword by Gayle MacDonald   viii

Foreword by Madeleine Kerkhof   ix

Preface   x

Introduction   xii

PART 1 Solid ground

1   Defining this work   3

2   Preparing and sustaining yourself, with Ronna Moore   17

3   Skills, safety, and supplies   29

4   The session   51

5   Stages of dying   75

PART 2 Diving deeper

6   Common symptoms at the end of life   95

7   Common conditions   117

8   Medications in end-of-life care   145

9   Equipment, devices, and procedures   165

PART 3 An expanded view

10   Therapies to complement massage   185

11   Providing inclusive care   199

Epilogue: Parting lessons   213

Appendix: Patient assessment   215

Appendix: Simplified assessment tool   217

Resources   218

Index   223

*This book is dedicated to my father-in-law, Dr Wayman R. Spence,
whose dying wish for gentle touch inspired my vocation.*

*And to my dad, Robert W. Heep, who told me I could do
anything I set my mind to, even write a book.*

ACKNOWLEDGMENTS

This book would not have been written without Gayle MacDonald and Valerie Hartman. Valerie's teachings were the beginning of my hospice education, and her wise and gentle ways inspire me to this day. Gayle has likewise been a fundamental influence on my work and on the book you are holding. She reviewed and helped make every word better.

Susan Gee is my ever-steady teaching partner and co-founder of Final Touch Training, the 20-hour class that spawned this book. She is *always* the calm one in the room.

My kindred spirit and new best friend from across the ocean, Ronna Moore, created Chapter 2 with me and provided brilliant input on the remaining chapters. I'll always be grateful to Cal Cates for introducing Ronna and me, and for their generous sharing of Healwell resources.

Candice White is the extraordinary photographer who captured most of the images in this book. Her skill as an artist is equaled by her ability to walk softly through the delicate world in which these photographs were taken.

Others provided crucial direction, input, feedback, and encouragement, especially Deb Rice, Steve Hines, Jeanna Thompson, Catherine Kannenberg, and Madeleine Kerkhof. My teammates at Faith Hospice are family to me; I love them all. Special thanks to my massage therapy pals, Glo Umphress and Lisa Castillo, who helped care for our patients so that I could be a part-time writer.

My spouse and children cheered me on, kept my world spinning, and endured an appalling mess on every surface of our home. Thanks to David, Parker, and Sarah; I can't imagine my life without you.

My extended tribe includes healers of every stripe – LVNs, RNs, PTs, OTs, a veterinarian, and an acupuncturist. My sister, Debbie, has been a nurse to many, including me. My mother, Mary Frances, was the first hospice social worker I ever met. They are my roots.

Uncle Larry, thank you for proofreading this manuscript! You are among a large group of dearly beloved humans and one canine who are always there for me, enriching my life and reminding me not to take myself too seriously.

But there are no greater thanks I owe than to the thousands of people who have shared their lives and deaths with me, and to their loved ones who have allowed me to share their stories. I bow to them, and to the fearless pioneers of this work, and to every unknown person who has ever gently touched another person in distress. You are the heart and soul of these pages.

FOREWORD *by Gayle MacDonald*

Cindy Spence is a humanitarian with a humble heart. She is also a very rare combination of deeply skilled massage practitioner and beautiful writer. Her wisdom and skill don't come from book learning but from having her hands on thousands of people who were at the end of their lives, people to whom she is devoted.

Writing a book is a daunting task that requires sacrifice. Everyone around the writer – spouse, friends, and family – must share the author for a prolonged period of time with "the calling." This is true during normal times, but when the writing had to occur as this did, during the COVID pandemic, the sacrifice and focus needed were amplified many times over. Everyone had their own challenges to carry during the pandemic. Cindy's were to organize her life around protecting the patients under her care and to write this book.

This book is not just for professional touch practitioners; it is for everyone. Massage and touch belong to all of us, and at some point we will all have the experience of attending a friend, family member, patient, or client who is on this "once in a lifetime adventure," as the author refers to it. This stage is not just about the final breaths; it includes the months and maybe years in which the patient needs this specialized care. However, because of fear or discomfort, many people don't know what to do for others during this time. *Palliative Touch: Massage for People at the End of Life* presents information that is accessible to anyone, from uncomplicated suggestions to more clinical knowledge.

Often, when something such as touch therapy becomes professionalized, it evolves to be surrounded by regulations, protocols, and training requirements. As professionals we have to navigate our way through these hindrances to find our way into the middle, the core, the heart and soul of the matter. This book boils the topic down to its essence. You will feel as if you are touching the marrow and be inspired or reminded once again of why you went to massage or nursing school, or studied Reiki, aromatherapy, or another helping vocation.

It is with honor and privilege that I walked this writing path with Cindy. When it comes time for me to leave this life, Cindy is one of the people I would want to be at my bedside.

Gayle MacDonald, MS, LMT

Author of *Hands in Health Care: Massage Therapy for the Adult Hospital Patient* (Handspring Publishing, 2021); *Medicine Hands: Massage Therapy for People with Cancer* (Findhorn Press, 2014)

Portland, Oregon
March 2022

FOREWORD *by Madeleine Kerkhof*

When I received this book, I was immediately impressed by Cindy Spence's wonderful fusion of talents, love, and passion. Cindy offers tools for compassionate touch in some of the most impactful times of anyone's life.

Cindy offers such a wealth of information, from helpful practical tips, such as suggestions on positioning and what kind of supplies are suitable for particular situations, to insights into symptoms, medications, commonly used equipment, and medical and nursing procedures in end-of-life care. These insights make it easier for touch practitioners and others around the patient to just focus on the essence: to be there for the patient and their loved ones. I also appreciate her attention to those therapies that may complement massage, such as music, energy work, and essential oils, for which I was honored to stand beside her.

Her devotion to patient and practitioner well-being is in every chapter, every quote, and every technique and piece of advice. She has a wonderful talent for describing her work, backed by science and thorough experience, in a way that all those involved in the care of the patient can resonate with.

I highly recommend this book, where she so empathetically describes the stages of progression towards the end of life, demonstrating her attention to every detail and, most of all, her dedication to the well-being of patients and their loved ones.

Madeleine Kerkhof, RNret, CA, MT, ACS

Global Director, Kicozo – Knowledge Institute for Integrative & Complementary (Nursing) Care

Wernhout, The Netherlands
May 2022

PREFACE

The news was not good. The cancer was widespread. All my father-in-law asked of me was to locate a therapist who could provide massage for him. It sounded so simple. But it was not.

Phone call after phone call, I was told no. No because he was "too sick." No because "massage is contraindicated for people with cancer." No because "that's not the kind of massage I do." With a heavy heart, I called to let Wayman know that I was unable to meet his request.

A year later, still grieving Wayman's death, I could not shake the feeling that I was meant to do more. So I did the only thing I could think of: I signed up for massage therapy school.

That was in 1999, and it would have been a very lonely time for me had it not been for the release of Gayle MacDonald's first edition of *Medicine Hands: Massage Therapy for People with Cancer*. Gayle's book affirmed my belief that people with serious illness should not be deprived of massage. Indeed, I knew from my father-in-law's experience that sick people sometimes need skilled touch more than ever.

A lot has changed since that time. Oncology massage is a recognized specialty in most parts of the world. There are wonderful books and trainings about massage for people living with cancer. But there are not many resources for those who wish to provide massage for people who are dying.

Palliative Touch: Massage for People at the End of Life is the book I wish I'd had in 1999. In a sense, it has taken more than two decades to write it. In that time, I've provided more than 6,000 massages for people at the end of life. These sessions have occurred in home settings, hospitals, nursing homes, and hospice inpatient units. I have grown from each encounter, painfully at times, joyfully at times, and often without realizing it until much later. My goal is to share as freely with you as so many others have shared with me.

Three experiences weighed on my mind and heart as I wrote this book. The first was my awareness that the content of these pages is limited to the experience of dying in a resource-rich country. Though wealth in the US does not translate to equity of care for all our people, there is much greater potential for this dream to be realized where I live and work than in Guatemala, for example, where I served as a Peace Corps volunteer in the 1980s. I often think about the millions of people around the world who live and die without access to basic healthcare.

A second source of emotion as I worked on this project was the COVID-19 virus. I was blessed to be employed by a hospice agency that welcomed properly screened loved ones and massage therapists at the bedside throughout the pandemic. But my colleagues and I have also been privy to heartbreaking stories of deaths that occurred in isolation. We observed tearful reunions that were all too short, following separations that were all too long. We assisted people to die comfortably as they were withdrawn from mechanical ventilation which did not bring the recoveries that they and their families hoped for. And we coped, as the rest of the world coped, with scarce supplies, along with staffing shortages as some of our own became ill. At the time of this writing, the COVID story is not yet finished.

The final experience which shaped the following pages was the unexpected death of my father on October 9, 2021. For nine soul-stirring days, my siblings and I provided care for him at home. Dad's last gift to me was a deeper, more personal understanding of the power of touch to ease the dying process. His death, described in my epilogue, served as a bookend for this project.

Perhaps because of these tender realities that tapped at my heart while I tapped at my keyboard, I felt with great clarity the importance of doing what we can, where we can. If enough of us respond to this urge, the world will surely be better for it.

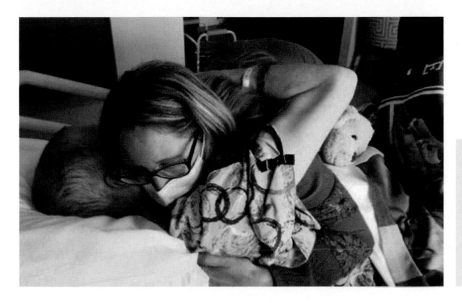

A reunion of childhood friends at the T. Boone Pickens Hospice Center, following months of separation due to COVID-19.

(Photo courtesy of Amy Nader and Margot Bleyen.)

A word about the title of this book

The word "palliate" comes from the Medieval Latin "palliare," meaning to conceal, or to cover with a cloak (Moore, 2017). In the context of healthcare, a palliative approach is one that alleviates symptoms without curing disease. *Palliative Touch*, then, describes a form of touch that relieves suffering without fixing the cause.

Now an emerging specialty, palliative care is broadening the hospice ideal of symptom management not just for people at the end of life, but for anyone suffering from serious disease, as early in the disease process as possible, and whether the diagnosed individual is receiving curative treatment or comfort care only. The World Health Organization describes this care as a basic human right, a global ideal that has yet to be met, though many are working to achieve it. Touch therapists have a crucial role to play in these efforts.

What is this book about?

Mark Twain famously said to "write what you know." What I have known for more than two decades is the world of hospice care for adults in the United States, care that is focused on comfort during the last six months of life when curative treatments have been discontinued. Touch therapists working in palliative care settings where active treatment is provided will need to develop knowledge of these treatments and the accommodations they require. The principles in this book will provide a solid foundation from which to build.

Who is this book for?

This book is for any allied health professional who has ever desired to comfort a dying person with gentle touch. You may be a massage therapist or other complementary care provider, an energy worker, end-of-life doula, nurse, nurse assistant, home health aide, or other helper. *Palliative Touch* is for you, *all* of you. The terms "therapist" and "touch therapist" will be used throughout this book in an effort to be inclusive and welcoming.

How the book is organized

This book is divided into three parts, and readers are encouraged to access the information at whatever level speaks to their needs. Part 1, Solid ground (Chapters 1–5), contains the basic information required to provide a safe, effective massage for a dying person.

Part 2, Diving deeper (Chapters 6–9), provides more in-depth information for therapists who practice in clinical settings, or those who simply wish to know more about common symptoms, terminal diseases and their complications, medications, and other interventions that may be initiated or discontinued during the dying process.

Part 3, An expanded view (Chapters 10 and 11, the Epilogue, and the Appendix), offers a broader perspective of the work, along with tools and resources that any therapist might find helpful.

Some readers may wonder why this book is so clinical. Others may feel it is not clinical enough. I endeavored throughout the writing to find balance between the simplicity of gentle touch for dying people and the more clinical information that is included in some of these pages. It is often said that death has become a medicalized experience, and I do not want to contribute to that inclination.

But palliative care is medical care, and people with advanced illness are often encountered in medical settings. A growing number of hospice agencies and palliative care departments are adding complementary therapists to their care teams. Therapists need to be literate in these cultures so that we can step into the roles that are being created for us. For these reasons, *Palliative Touch* includes chapters on clinical topics. If you are a nonmedical person trying to read a medical chart, you may be as lost as I was. I hope this book will shed some light where you might need it.

To that end, one of the recurring features of this book is *chart talk*, which clarifies terminology that may be new to you. Other features include *touching stories*, *personal notes to the reader*, *tips*, and *heads ups*. Names and details of patients have been altered to protect privacy unless families requested that I use their loved one's actual name. Therapists and colleagues have been credited for tips and stories with their permission. I will be eternally grateful to the village that it took to write this book.

A personal note to the reader

To quote Meg Ryan in the movie *You've Got Mail*, "Whatever else anything is, it ought to begin by being personal." I have sought wherever possible in this book to use the personal "I" to address the personal "you." If you are reading this, we are already connected by this material and our interest in it. People who work in end-of-life care often speak of *being called* to the work and finding kindred spirits among our colleagues. Work with dying individuals and their families is an intimate experience, and it ought to begin by being personal.

I invite you to read as much of this book as you find useful, and to pursue further study with qualified teachers. I have personally found it fascinating and enriching to know this work deeply; it is my passion and my purpose. But the truth is that much of what we need to know cannot be taught in a book; it can only be learned at the bedside. My hope is that *Palliative Touch* will open your heart, your mind, and your hands to the extraordinary gift of providing gentle touch for people at the end of life.

Reference

Moore, R., 2017. Strengthening the presence of massage therapy in palliative care. *Massage & Myotherapy Journal*, [e-journal] (1), pp. 14–19. Available at: <https://www.oncologymassagetraining.com.au/userfiles/Strengthening%20the%20Presence%20of%20Massage%20Therapy%20in%20Palliative%20Care%20-%20Ronna%20Moore.pdf>.

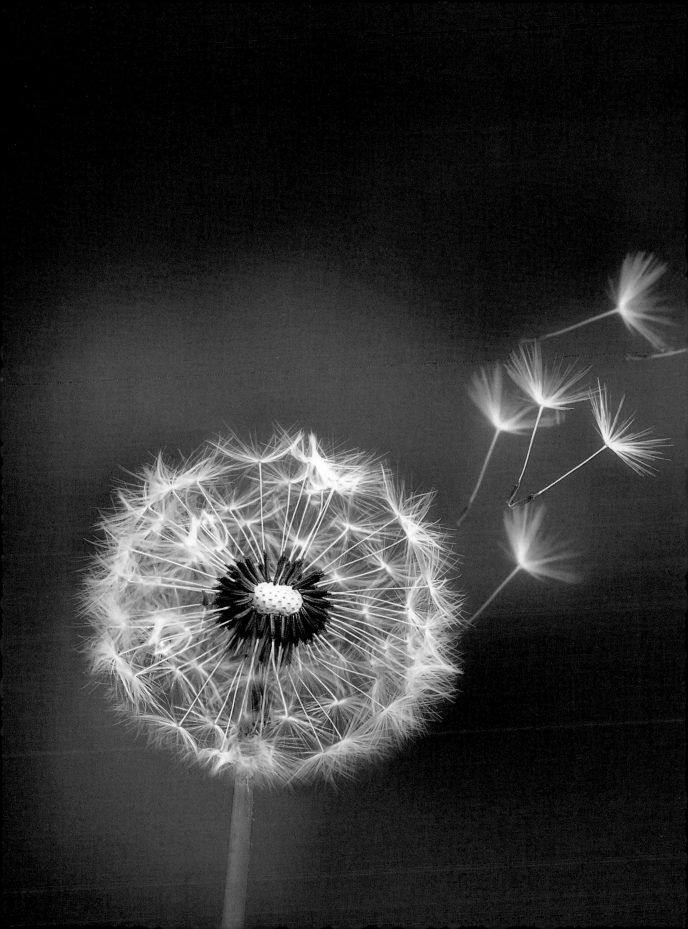

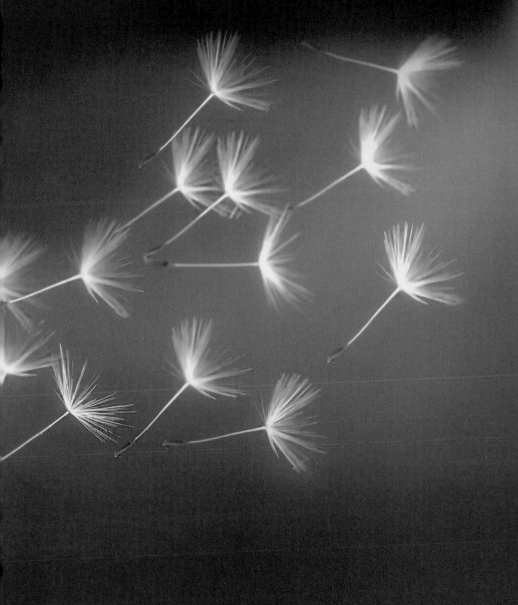

Solid ground *1*

Defining this work 3

Preparing and sustaining yourself, with Ronna Moore 17

Skills, safety, and supplies 29

The session 51

Stages of dying 75

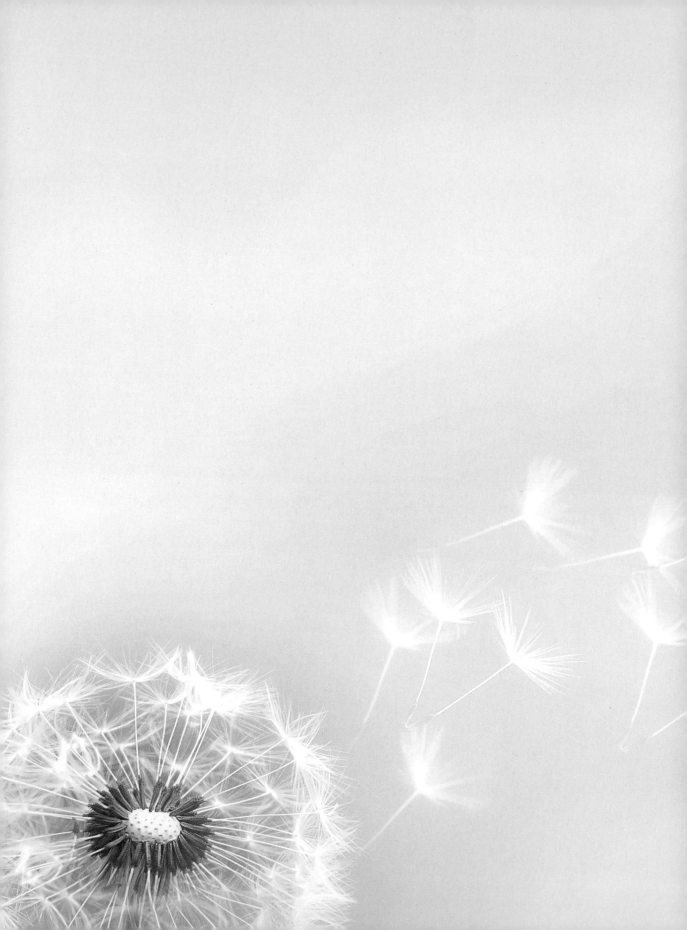

Like any intense trip, things may not always go as planned.

–Andrew Holecek

The work of dying from a terminal illness involves a long dance between the inhalation and the exhalation, a dialogue between holding on and letting go. The dance has patterns that become familiar to observers. But each dance has its own tempo, rhythm, and energy. "Nothing can we call our own but death," said Shakespeare. This means that every client, every family, every death is a new story to be witnessed with fresh eyes and unvarnished humility.

What it means to accompany someone on this once-in-a-lifetime adventure is hard to define, despite the ambitious title of this chapter. Yet it seems helpful to begin the journey with an attempt to describe the landscape. Chapter 1 will introduce the spectrum of end-of-life care during the last six months of life, including hospice and palliative care, and how massage can contribute to these approaches. The settings in which death occurs (private homes, group homes, and inpatient environments) will be explored, as well as the ways that each of these settings impacts the work of the touch therapist. While the dying person is at the heart of our work, this chapter will introduce other people we are likely to encounter at the bedside, including patients' families and members of the palliative or hospice care team. The chapter will conclude with practical ideas for connecting with this work.

My hope is that Chapter 1 will inspire you to follow whatever impulse prompted you to pick up this book. But before you read further, a word of warning. Touching a dying person can be a profound experience for both the receiver and the giver. If you choose this experience, you will never be the same. The job is not easy. You *will* change, though I can't say how. I only know that, for me, there is nothing I'd rather do with my remaining time on the planet.

The spectrum of end-of-life care

Even at the end of life, people hope for many things. They may hope for a peaceful death, a miracle, or time to reach an important milestone such as a holiday or anniversary. Some people hope for the relief of pain, a bowel movement, or to have their hair washed prior to a loved one's visit. As touch therapists working in end-of-life care, you will meet people across a spectrum of shifting hopes that determine many of the choices they make, including whether to continue or stop treatment. People often move back and forth on this spectrum, talking about funeral services one day and miracles the next. Our job is to follow their lead, remembering that the journey belongs to them.

Touching story 1.1. Meeting patients where they are

Jennifer was my friend, not my client, though I did occasionally provide massage for her. We became mothers around the same time and were both diagnosed with cancer when our children were young. I got well, but Jen did not. Her breast cancer was treated aggressively, but to no avail. I last saw her when I accompanied her to a medical consult in Houston, Texas, where we were shown her latest MRI scan. The cancer was everywhere, the doctor said; there was nothing more they could offer. We took a taxi back to the hotel, stopping on the way to buy a bottle of wine.

Jen returned home to North Carolina, but she did not give up on treatment. She was in a clinical trial for a short time but was unable to tolerate the drugs in her weakened condition. She sought alternative healers, and took large doses of experimental supplements, which she ordered online. One night, unable to breathe, she called 911. She had a neighbor come over to stay with her sleeping children.

When Jen's partner called me the next morning, she told me the story of the previous night. Jen was fighting to catch her breath while quizzing the ER doctor about the possibility of metabolic therapy when her cancer-riddled body gave out midsentence, likely from a pulmonary embolism. She died in the emergency room despite lengthy efforts at resuscitation. Jennifer never once spoke to me about dying. She never had a conversation with her children that I know of. I still feel emotional when I think of Jennifer's mother, who had to wake her grandchildren and tell them their mother had died.

People who remain in treatment at the end of life do so at a cost, and each patient gets to balance that cost with the benefit they hope to achieve. For a young mother hoping to buy more time with her children, the cost of ongoing treatment, however difficult, may outweigh the cost of stopping. Another who has grown exhausted with the effort to stay alive may place more hope in the quality of her remaining time than the number of days. The decisions are personal and difficult.

Had I been with Jen in the ER, or had you been with her, what could we have done? In the chaos of what turned out to be her final hours, it seems clear that our goal would not have been to fix this scared, hurting person with a 60-minute session of advanced massage techniques. Had we been there, we might have held Jen's hand. We might have gently brushed the hair from her face or stroked her furrowed brow. We might have found another pillow to place behind her back or offered to massage her feet with a calming oil. This is palliative touch, meeting the patient where they are.

Jennifer's story provides an instructive template for informing the work we do with *all* patients at the end of life, regardless of where they are on the spectrum of hope. Terminal illness can be akin to a long emergency, in which massage can offer a safe resting place. Indeed, the concept of safe haven is how hospice care began.

The beginnings of hospice

The word hospice comes from the Latin word *hospitium*, meaning hospitality. The first hospice houses offered sanctuary to pilgrims making their way to and from the Holy Land during the Middle Ages. As many of these weary travelers fell sick, a tradition of caring for "incurables" developed. This care was nonmedical and comfort-oriented, including "the finest foods and linens" that could be offered (Connor, 2018). The Catholic Sisters of Charity took up the cause in seventeenth-century France, followed by Irish nuns a century later in Dublin and later still in London. It was a passionate and ambitious young woman at a London hospice house who expanded the concept of hospice into end-of-life care as we know it.

Dame Cicely Saunders, cross-trained as a nurse, social worker, and physician, was the first to declare that doctors should care for the dying, rather than nuns and volunteers (Adrien, 2016). Saunders founded St. Christopher's hospice of London in 1967, providing an unprecedented level of patient care and groundbreaking research to perfect methods of symptom relief. For the first time, medicine became a central component of end-of-life care. But Saunders recognized that dying was more than a physical process. She encouraged patients at St. Christopher's to sit in the garden, drink sherry or scotch if they wished, and spend time with their families and pets.

As the world took notice of Saunders's novel approach, other healthcare professionals flocked to St. Christopher's to study her work. Two of those visitors were Florence Wald, an American nurse who brought the hospice movement to the United States, and Balfour Mount, a Canadian surgeon who established the first palliative care unit in Montreal. It was Mount who coined the term "palliative care," the name later adopted by the World Health Organization (WHO) to denote the specialty of relief of suffering for people with serious illness.

Hospice today

In some parts of the world, hospice is still a term that describes a place where people go to be cared for as they die. In other countries, including the US, hospice is a philosophy and a set of services that are provided wherever the patient is located, whether home, group home, or inpatient facility. Hospice teams, working under the supervision of a doctor, include nurses, social workers, chaplains, nurse aides, and potentially other disciplines. The purpose of this interdisciplinary approach is to provide care for the *whole* person – body, mind, and spirit. Services include support for the loved ones of the dying person and bereavement care following the patient's death.

Known as "terminal care" in some places, hospice was designed from inception to be provided during the last months of life, though this period is defined differently around the world. Hospice is provided during the last six months of life in the US, the last three months in the Netherlands (Kerkhof, 2013), and the last 12 months in Australia (Australian Institute, 2016). Life expectancy is, of course, an inexact science. People who outlive their hospice benefits are reassessed at regular intervals to determine whether they still qualify for services. If death remains likely during the specified time frame, the patient is recertified. If prognosis improves, the patient may be discharged from hospice care but can recertify at a future date when their health declines.

Regardless of timing, a defining feature of hospice is that care is focused on comfort, not a cure. Patients must choose to forego or stop curative treatment prior to hospice enrollment. Hospice should never be equated with "no care," however. Symptoms are treated by the hospice team, aggressively if necessary, so that patients can live their remaining days to the fullest. This singular focus on quality of life resulted in unparalleled expertise at symptom management that eventually begged the question: why must people be dying in order to be comfortable?

The emergence of palliative care

Palliative care has expanded over time as a response to this question. In 1990, the WHO formally declared palliative care as the global standard for people with life-limiting illness. Unlike hospice or terminal care that is confined to the end of life, palliative care is "applicable early in the course of illness, in conjunction with other therapies . . . such as chemotherapy or radiation therapy" (Radbruch et al., 2020). Other than this key difference, palliative care emulates the hospice model in its dedication to the following principles:

- A focus on quality of life, supporting patients to live as actively and comfortably as possible.

- An interdisciplinary approach that includes physical, emotional, and spiritual care.

- Relief of pain and other distressing symptoms of serious illness.

- A commitment to neither hastening nor postponing death.

- Support for families during the patient's illness and following the patient's death (WHO, 2020).

Palliative care has been declared a human right by the WHO, but the ideal of global access to this young specialty is far from realized. Integration of palliative care into existing healthcare systems is inconsistent, particularly in low- and middle-income countries, but also in wealthy countries with fragmented healthcare. In the US, for example, public and private pay structures have made hospice readily available, but palliative medicine has yet to receive this same support. It is likely that hospice and palliative care practices will continue to be shaped by the societies in which they function.

Touching story 1.2. Palliative care and hospice as a continuum

I met Ronald in the chemotherapy infusion room of a local hospital, where I provided foot massage with a volunteer organization. Ronald was a dapper dresser and relentlessly playful, teasing his nurses with gusto and affection. His gastrointestinal cancer required him to use a feeding tube, and he frequently bragged about his low grocery bill.

We had a cold, wet winter that year, and Ronald was in and out of the hospital with pneumonia. He told me by telephone that he felt "puny." He developed left hip pain that was determined to be metastatic cancer. Ron's oncologist referred him to the palliative care team at the hospital. The palliative team met with Ron and his family to clarify his goals of care, which were to continue treatment while addressing his pain. The team recommended palliative radiation and ibuprofen. Ron's pain immediately improved, and his condition stabilized for several months. He continued to enjoy weekly massage during his chemo infusions.

Late that summer, Ron's hip pain returned, and it was determined that chemotherapy and radiation were no longer helping. With his family's blessing and the support of the palliative care team, he signed on to home hospice. Home health aides visited three times per week, helping Ron to maintain his impeccable appearance. His nurse started him on a low dose of steroids that helped his breathing and put "pep in his step" (his words). His family and friends threw him a huge birthday party in August at which he enjoyed a few bites of cake and ice cream.

Ron declined quickly after his birthday. He became confined to bed and needed more medication for pain and shortness of breath. His family took turns caring for him at home, heartbroken but faithful to his wishes for comfort only. The hospice team provided education and emotional support, along with medical care and equipment, including oxygen to keep Ronald comfortable. Ron enjoyed talks with the chaplain, who shared his love of golf. The family placed Ron's hospital bed in the center of the living room, where he slept an increasing number of hours. I continued to provide massage for him, sometimes assisted by a family member.

Late one night, Ronald developed severe agitation, crying out to his deceased wife, and attempting to climb out of bed. After a distraught call from Ron's daughter, a hospice nurse arrived at the home, adjusting Ron's medications, and providing calm reassurance to his loved ones. Shortly after dawn the next morning, Ronald became quiet. His breaths grew farther apart, and he died peacefully, surrounded by his family.

Massage as a palliative discipline

Massage is a natural fit for the comfort-oriented goals of hospice and palliative care. Once taught as a core skill for hospital nurses, massage can be provided in a variety of care settings and adjusted to patient needs, preferences, and safety. The remaining chapters of this book are devoted to describing these adjustments.

While some studies on massage efficacy are faulted for small sample size and poor design, there is compelling evidence to endorse the benefits of massage for people with advanced disease. Results from a recent pilot study (Havyer et al., 2022) report a 40% improvement in patient pain scores and a 54.5% improvement in anxiety, results comparable to earlier research conducted at Suncoast, one of the largest nonprofit providers of hospice care in the US. The Suncoast study, while also small, revealed a 52% improvement in pain and a 53% improvement in anxiety (Polubinski and West, 2005). These numbers echo the findings of a large three-year study of 1,290 patients at Memorial Sloan-Kettering Cancer Center in which patients reported a 40.2% improvement in pain scores and a 52.2% improvement in anxiety. The MSKCC study found that benefits were achieved after just 20 minutes of massage with results lasting up to 48 hours, even when symptoms were described by patients as moderate to severe. These findings were declared "major" and "clinically relevant" by the researchers (Cassileth and Vickers, 2004). Gayle MacDonald, in the first edition of *Medicine Hands*, put it like this: "If a drug were discovered that provided the many benefits [of] massage, pharmaceutical companies would be falling all over themselves to bottle it" (MacDonald, 1999).

Research has primarily focused on interventions provided by massage therapists, but there is evidence to suggest that massage by other healthcare professionals can achieve favorable results, even on a limited area of the body. Hospitalized cancer patients who received 10-minute foot massages by nurses on three consecutive nights reported significant improvements in pain, nausea, and relaxation (Grealish et al., 2000). Another study revealed "meaningful relief of suffering" following light strokes for 20 minutes of either hand and arm or foot and leg by healthcare workers with just one day of training (Billhult and Dahlberg, 2001).

My personal experience is that gentle touch provided by any number of caring individuals can be a positive experience, including a certified nursing assistant (CNA) applying lotion after a bath or a family member caressing a loved one's face. With information, training, and practice, the potential increases for massage to achieve benefits such as those cited in the literature. Massage is noninvasive and has no side effects when performed appropriately. In light of these benefits, a growing number of hospice agencies and palliative care providers worldwide are seeking to add massage therapy to their services. A list of ideas for getting connected with this work is offered on p. 12.

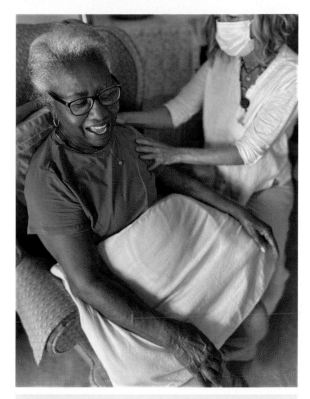

Figure 1.1
Massage can promote a greater sense of well-being and comfort at the end of life, goals that are consistent with the values of palliative care. A number of studies cite significant improvements in pain and anxiety.

(Photo by Candice White.)

The location of care at the end of life

Touch therapists seeking roles in end-of-life care will find themselves working wherever patients live and die. This can be a private home, assisted living facility, skilled nursing home, inpatient hospice unit, hospital, or any combination of these settings. One hope that people frequently express is the wish to die at home. Hospice provides support to accomplish this goal. Palliative care programs, traditionally hospital-based, are making efforts to extend their reach through outpatient clinics and home services.

But neither hospice nor palliative care provides full-time help. The majority of day-to-day caretaking is provided by the family or privately hired caretakers. Hospice does offer occasional respite care, typically five days at a time, for home caregivers to have periodic breaks from the demands of patient care. Caregivers can schedule this time to rest, travel, or take care of their own healthcare needs.

If symptoms warrant, a more intensive level of care can be provided by hospice. This may be offered on a short-term basis until symptoms are stabilized in the home (called *continuous care* in the US). If symptoms cannot be managed at home, patients may qualify for the most intensive level of hospice care, which is *general inpatient care (GIP)*. GIP care is provided in an inpatient setting, most often a designated area of an existing hospital or in a freestanding hospice facility. Strict criteria must be met for each level of care. Examples of qualifying symptoms include uncontrolled pain, vomiting, seizures, extreme agitation, and respiratory distress. *Triage* and telephone support are available 24/7 to address urgent needs, and to facilitate changes in level of care when appropriate.

It must be acknowledged that dying at home is labor-intensive and requires help, ideally from multiple people who are willing to provide intensely personal care such as bathing. Carers may face scenarios that can feel frightening or overwhelming, particularly when symptoms are hard to manage or dying occurs over a long period of time. I have heard family members express relief when their loved one is brought to our hospice inpatient unit after caring for them at home became untenable. Other deaths, such as my father's, are manageable with hospice support at home. A palliative and hospice care continuum is ideal, with a range of locations and levels of care that can be accessed as needed. Descriptions of these locations are offered in the following pages, from the touch therapist's point of view.

Working in the patient's home

I loved my years of field work, traveling across North Texas to provide massage for hospice patients in their homes.

I found it fascinating and enjoyed the independence, flexibility, and variety of experiences. There is an opportunity for resourcefulness and creativity in designing a session that meets the patient's needs with the environment and materials at hand. The corresponding drawback is lack of control. The home environment may be quiet or noisy, calm or chaotic, clean or messy. The ergonomics can be challenging if there is clutter or if the patient does not have an adjustable hospital bed. Some of these issues will be discussed in Chapter 3, along with tips for on-the-go hygiene and a list of supplies to take with you. Chapter 3 will also address the subject of pets, who often play a significant role in home visits.

Depending on distances covered, there can be considerable wear and tear on your vehicle. It is wise to invest in good maintenance of engine and tires. Some people find driving to be difficult; others use the time for quiet reflection, podcasts, or soothing music. Over the years, my car choices have revolved around gas mileage and dependability (in my area, weather performance is not an issue). But I've found that comfort, room for supplies, an outlet for charging my devices, cupholders, and heated seats are all indulgences that make the hours on the road more pleasant. It is not unusual for home-based therapists to spend more time in their cars than with clients.

Perhaps the biggest emotional impact of field work is that patients in the home setting are likely to be more stable. There's an opportunity to build rapport over time, and some of these relationships will last for months, a year, or longer. Getting to know a patient and family over time can add real depth to the therapeutic relationship. It can also bring real grief when that patient dies. Spending time in someone's home is a very intimate experience. The boundaries we learned for traditional massage therapy practice may or may not apply. What is clearly inappropriate in a typical client relationship may be acceptable or even comical in end-of-life home care (see more on the topic of boundaries in Chapter 2). Field work requires flexibility, a sense of adventure, and grit. You either love it or you don't.

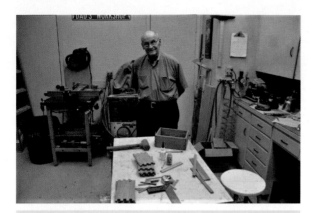

Figure 1.2
Home visits are an illuminating experience that reveal things about the dying person. This patient showed me the workshop where he handcrafted beautiful boxes for all his favorite people. I will treasure forever the box he made for me, which has his initials burned into the bottom.

(Photo by David Spence.)

Working in facilities

Many patients reside in some type of group setting at the end of life, including assisted living facilities and skilled nursing homes. Working in these environments requires compliance with regulations for parking, entering and exiting the building, checking in and checking out, documenting the visit, and other policies. In one elegant high rise I visited, all healthcare providers were instructed to use the service elevator. Group settings also require that massage be scheduled around meals and group activities. Massage might take place in the patient's room (which may or may not be private), a quiet corner of the facility, or in the midst of a lively group sing-along. Therapists may find themselves interacting with other residents who are curious about their presence.

Each facility has its own "vibe." Therapists must be able to move in and out of these different environments, adapting to various staff and protocols. There can be a bit of dreariness in some of these settings, which can make massage a most welcome gift. The opportunity to provide this care, along with the potential to see a larger number of people with reduced time on the road, make this work worthwhile.

Working in inpatient settings

The inpatient environment (hospital or hospice) can be an intense place. People typically arrive in crisis with severe symptoms and anxious family members. The therapist must be able to remain calm in these scenarios where calm is needed most. Depending on the size of the unit, the therapist may be expected to see large numbers of patients in a day. There can be high patient turnover, with numerous deaths in a short period. It is more likely that the therapist will observe active dying and may even be present at the moment of death. In this accelerated environment, it is extremely important to move slowly and to bring a sense of composure and ease into the patient rooms. The highest compliment I ever received was one particularly busy day when a family member joked that I moved "like a sloth."

Therapists working in inpatient settings must adapt to the inpatient culture. Gayle MacDonald describes this environment as "standardized, hierarchical and complicated" (MacDonald and Tague, 2021). Some of us take to this setting more easily than others. There may be less independence than in field work, with expectations of set hours of availability. You will have more contact with other team members and may benefit from the support, comradery, and stimulation that comes from this contact. Learning opportunities include team rounds and interdisciplinary team meetings. Teamwork is valued and it can feel at times like "all hands on deck" to meet patient needs. Answering the telephone, responding to a call light, and fetching a blanket or snack are all within the possible realm of a therapist's role in the inpatient setting.

Inpatient settings are clean, controlled environments, with the support of housekeeping staff who are important members of the team. Hospital beds are more ergonomic for therapists, though working around family members at the bedside can be a challenge, as discussed in Chapter 4.

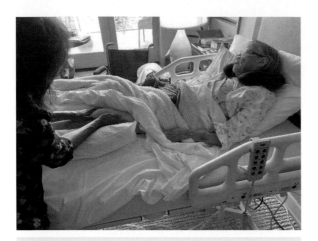

Figure 1.3
Massage in the hospice inpatient setting.
(Photo by author.)

these facilities are still sometimes referred to as "hospice houses." I would describe the unit where I work as a hybrid. The building was beautifully designed with rooms that open to waterfront patios. But we have been described as the "ICU of hospice," in that we are able to provide a higher level of comfort care than is typically offered in noninstitutional settings. Our inpatient unit also houses residential patients, who live at the unit as an alternative to a skilled nursing home.

There may be interruptions to the session, with visitors and care staff coming in and out of the room. There will likely be more medical paraphernalia to work around and more etiquette to adhere to. But the rewards of working with patients, families, and colleagues in the inpatient setting can also be extraordinary.

Personal note to the reader 1.1

Just as home environments vary greatly, so do inpatient environments. When located inside an existing hospital, the feel is much more clinical. Efforts may be made to soften the setting with home furniture, candescent lighting, and inviting spaces for family. But the floorplan and access to the unit are undeniable reminders that the patient is in a hospital.

The advantage of a freestanding inpatient unit (IPU) is that the atmosphere can more closely resemble a home experience; in fact,

Scope of practice

Touch therapists must be constantly on guard to maintain integrity in terms of scope of practice. Patients will often ask questions that we don't know the answers to, or questions that we might *think* we know the answers to but don't have the credentials to discuss. The benefit of working with a hospice or palliative care team is that other team members will have expertise that we don't have, and vice versa. It is completely acceptable (in fact, it is preferable) to say, "I don't know, but that would be a great question for your nurse."

At the end of life, there are things that *no one* knows. I have observed seasoned hospice doctors and nurses decline to give an estimate of how long a patient has to live, for example. As death draws near and the signs become more distinct, the medical team might give a range of possibilities. But they will typically add that "no one really knows." This is an excellent example of unvarnished humility. It can also keep us out of trouble by avoiding an expectation that may not be met.

Scope of practice is defined by the regulatory and licensing requirements of each profession or discipline, subject to location. If circumstances arise where scope is unclear, it is better to err on the side of caution and refrain from overextending ourselves.

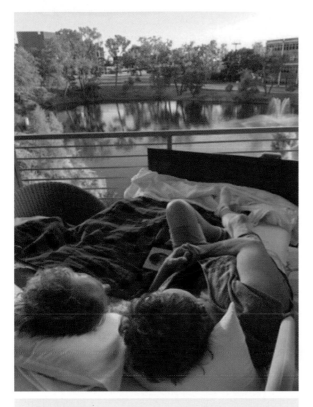

Figure 1.4
Patients and families alike benefit from spending time outdoors at the T. Boone Pickens Center for Hospice and Palliative Care. The doors are designed such that the hospital beds can be pushed onto the patio.

(Photo courtesy of patient's family.)

The people you may meet

A description of the landscape would be incomplete without addressing the fellow humans with whom we are privileged and sometimes challenged to work. While the dying person is at the center of the care we provide, that person is typically surrounded by a constellation of others, including family by birth or choice and other healthcare providers. Meeting patients where they are often includes meeting the people who accompany them.

Family as the unit of care

End-of-life services, both palliative care and hospice, consider the family to be the unit of care. Family is defined by the patient, and may involve parents, siblings, children, a spouse or partner, and extended family including in-laws. Sometimes an ex-spouse will return to the relationship to provide end-of-life care. "Family" may also include friends, professional caretakers, colleagues, and groups such as fellow church members, fellow AA members, and business associates. I cared for one young woman with Huntington's Disease who had been a firefighter; her entire squad set up camp in her home, rotating in and out on a 24-hour basis. They referred to her, and she to them, as "family," and behaved as such.

While a variable number of people may play a role in the patient's life and death, hospice encourages the patient to designate a primary caregiver (PCG). The PCG may also serve as the patient's medical power of attorney (MPOA), or healthcare power of attorney (HPOA), endowed with the right to speak on the patient's behalf when the patient becomes unable to speak for themselves. Ideally, the PCG and others come together in a supportive and cooperative manner to assist the dying process. It's rarely a seamless experience, however. Just as the patient is adjusting to changes that can feel catastrophic, the loved ones of that patient are facing their own fears, anxieties, grief, and uncertainties. Such challenges are unsettling and can bring out both the best and worst in all of us.

As touch therapists in end-of-life care, we may find ourselves in the midst of complex relationships undergoing extreme transition. It is not unusual to observe power struggles and conflict at the bedside. But it is just as common to witness extraordinary courage, grace, and tenderness. There can be heartrending reconciliation, quiet selflessness, noisy drama, or a mystifying absence of family members. Suggestions for communicating with and supporting families will be offered in the coming chapters. For now, it is enough to say that working with family can be messy, but also deeply moving.

The care team

To a greater or lesser degree, touch therapists will also interact with the palliative or hospice team members who provide care for the patient. These relationships will vary depending on where the care is provided (private home or facility) and whether the therapist is an independent provider or a fellow employee. Greater interaction requires time, energy, and diplomacy. But the quality of our care is unquestionably better when it is provided in the context of a team approach.

The opportunity to consult with an interdisciplinary group of individuals contributes to a more informed care plan. The ideal scenario is a mutual exchange in which the touch therapist plays an active role, with an opportunity to educate others about our work and how it can support the patient's goals. We must be careful as we educate others not to "oversell" the work we do. A humble approach based on a growing body of evidence that gentle touch is helpful to many people is often enough to soften skeptics; once we are allowed access to the bedside, the work generally speaks for itself.

In addition to humility, we are called to adapt ourselves to the team cultures in which we work. This is of course much easier when the culture is a healthy one, with positive leadership that supports and values the contributions of each team member. There is much to be gained if we can resonate with the highest frequency possible in any given dynamic, including the opportunity to share the joys and sorrows of this work. Being open to the perspectives and suggestions of others and aware of each team member's priorities and burdens can go a long way in building bridges with others who share a common goal. Our patients will benefit from this kind of teamwork, as will our ongoing development as professionals and human beings.

Getting connected with the work

If you are feeling drawn to this work and wondering how to begin, the following paragraphs will offer some ideas.

Private practice

It takes a while to build any type of private practice. Specializing in oncology massage, manual lymphatic drainage, geriatric massage, massage for Veterans, or a specific chronic disease (Parkinson's or dementia, for example) will help you develop targeted skills and a clientele who will need end-of-life services in the future. Outpatient support groups often welcome guest presenters to speak about the benefits of massage, especially when accompanied by demos or freebies. Something as simple as a zip-lock baggie with Epsom salt and a few drops of essential oil can be a vehicle for a label with your contact information. Death doula programs offer another model for private practice. The *Doula Business Guide* is an excellent resource with suggestions that can be applied to a variety of complementary therapy practices, including massage (Brennan, 2019).

My personal experience as a massage therapist has been that word of mouth from satisfied clients is the single most powerful tool for growing a business. As you acquire expertise, word gets out and people do find you. A website and inexpensive business card can advertise your interest and training in palliative or hospice massage. While there is currently no hospice massage "certification" that can be claimed in most countries, listing completed coursework is a way to communicate your knowledge and skills.

Agency and facility work

Hospice and palliative care agencies, assisted living facilities, and nursing homes are interfaces where touch therapists can access clients, and where clients can access therapists. One obvious strategy is to identify and investigate local agencies and facilities to see if they currently offer or might *want to offer* massage for their patients or residents. Healthcare is a competitive commodity, and many organizations look for ways to distinguish themselves from other providers in the area. One hospice I worked with offered massage, aromatherapy, and cosmetology services that they marketed as a "pampered patient" program. Be prepared that you will likely be required to complete an orientation, drug screening, tuberculosis (TB) test, criminal background check, and possibly other protocols.

Volunteering

Many of us started this work when complementary therapies were not widely accepted practice. We felt that we had to offer our services free of charge as volunteers. The disadvantage of this scenario is that agencies may be reluctant to pay for massage that they have previously gotten for free. Some therapists have come to feel that working without pay undermines the value of our work. That said, volunteering has some benefits.

If you have never had contact with the dying experience, volunteering is a great way to explore whether the work will be a good fit for you. Hospices generally require volunteers to participate in an orientation, which can be valuable training. Some agencies use "eleventh hour volunteers," who sit vigil with a patient who would otherwise die alone.

But be clear if it's patients you want to work with. I completed orientation for the first hospice I attempted to volunteer with, only to learn that what the director really wanted was massage for the staff. They certainly deserved it, but that wasn't the work I wanted to do. Some hospice agencies, in fact, have rules prohibiting volunteers from touching patients, even if the volunteer is a licensed massage therapist (LMT). Open communication will clarify whether your goals are a good fit for the agency, and vice versa.

Contracting

Smaller hospices with a patient census of 100 or fewer may be more likely to enter a contract arrangement with a therapist for services as needed, rather than a commitment of employment. An advantage of independent contract work is that the therapist may get to set the fee. Contract therapists can often designate a geographical area they are willing to service, something to consider since agencies may not reimburse contractors for travel time or mileage.

Payment typically requires the therapist to submit an invoice for service, and payment delays can occur, especially if the agency is headquartered elsewhere.

The biggest drawback to contract work is that collaboration with other team members may be limited. Contract therapists typically do not have access to the patient's medical record and communication can suffer. Pitfalls include not being advised of changes in patient status, including change of location from home to the inpatient unit, or even the patient's death. One possible way to improve communication is to ask if you might attend a team meeting to introduce yourself, inform others of your work, and exchange contact information.

For therapists who are eager to get started, it can be tempting to contract with a third-party agency. A third-party agency provides services for hospice and other healthcare providers, using a work force of contract therapists. These agencies typically keep a large percentage of the fee that is earned by the contracted care provider. They may also have a strict noncompete clause, which means that a therapist may be unable to work directly with contracted hospice or palliative care agencies for up to a year after terminating the contract. It pays to read the fine print carefully!

Employment

Hospice agencies with a census of more than 100 patients are sometimes able to hire PRN (*pro re nata*, Latin for "as needed"), part-time, or even full-time therapists. In the case of employment, the agency typically sets the pay scale, which can appear to be significantly lower than contract work. Therapists may have to drive where needed and distances can be quite long. Agencies do reimburse employees for travel time and mileage, however, so wages can end up comparing favorably to contract pay.

Employed therapists are generally supplied with the means to communicate electronically, via agency-issued cell phone or laptop. But by far the biggest advantage of employment is that employees are more embedded in the hospice or palliative care team, increasing contact, collaboration, and communication. There may be more opportunities for ongoing training, either in house or at hospice and palliative care conferences. Employed therapists are typically welcome or required to attend team meetings and will have the credibility of agency affiliation, including a name badge that bears the agency logo. This can facilitate trust with a patient or family, assuming their agency experience has been positive.

Dual roles

Some people feel called to more than one helping role and have expanded their knowledge and skills to include a second credential. I know several nurses who have Reiki or massage therapy training, for example. There are massage therapists who pursue training as end-of-life doulas, and doulas who practice massage or energy work. If you are trained in more than one area of expertise, you will likely encounter situations that require you to adhere to one role at a time. A massage therapist with a nursing background would not administer medications or provide medical advice while functioning in the role of massage therapist, for example.

But there may also be times when an expanded understanding can be beneficial for a touch therapist. Touching story 1.3 describes the experience of one LMT with doula training who has found a way to embrace her roles as complementary rather than separate.

Touching story 1.3. The ultimate couple's massage

Massage therapist and end-of-life doula Melanie Eggleston describes her dual expertise as "tightly woven worlds" which are blended in her private practice. The arc of care she is able to provide is beautifully illustrated in her relationship with two clients, Claire and Joseph.

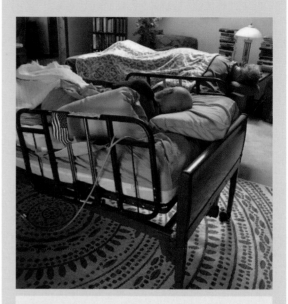

Figure 1.5
Claire deemed this session with Joseph to be "the ultimate couple's massage."
(Photo courtesy of Melanie Eggleston.)

Melanie began providing massage for Claire after Claire was diagnosed with cancer. The two bonded quickly and massage became an integral part of Claire's treatment and recovery. Years later, while Claire remained a faithful client, Melanie met and began providing massage for Claire's husband, Joseph, after he too was diagnosed with cancer. Melanie massaged Joseph's feet during his chemotherapy infusions, which helped him to relax. Despite a year of aggressive treatment, Joseph's cancer progressed, and he eventually chose hospice care. Melanie's role then expanded to providing biweekly home sessions for this "wonderful, kind couple."

Melanie's training as a doula gave her the confidence to accept Claire's invitation to help her bathe Joseph's body following his death. Having shared this intimate continuum of life and death with these two special clients, Melanie continues to provide massage for Claire as she grieves the loss of her partner.

EOL Doula, LMT Melanie Eggleston, US

Conclusion

In Chapter 1, we laid the groundwork for a common understanding of hospice and palliative care. We considered ways to meet patients where they are on the spectrum of care, whether at home, in a group home, or in an inpatient setting. Each environment has a particular flavor, and some of us will be drawn or more temperamentally suited to one setting compared to another. Regardless of the settings in which we work, we will likely meet other professionals and family members who are important to the patients we serve. Touch therapists have much to offer, and much to receive.

Ronna Moore writes that there is an "amplifying quality" to end-of-life work, "which renders the palliative landscape a particularly intense one for its inhabitants" (Moore, 2017). Like any big journey, the work calls us to be prepared. The following chapters will show you how.

References

Adrien, C., 2016. *A history of hospice: a timeline of one of medicine's oldest disciplines.* [online] Available at: <https://www.1800hospice.com/end-of-life-care/history-hospice>.

Australian Institute of Health and Welfare, 2016. *End-of-life care.* [pdf] Available at: <https://www.aihw.gov.au/getmedia/68ed1246-886e-43ff-af35-d52db9a9600c/ah16-6-18-end-of-life-care.pdf.aspx>.

Billhult, A. and Dahlberg, K., 2001. Meaningful relief from suffering. *Cancer Nursing.,* [e-journal] 24(3), pp. 180–184. Available at: Cancer Nursing website <https://journals.lww.com/cancernursingonline/pages/default.aspx>.

Brennan, P., 2019. *The doula business guide: how to succeed as a birth, postpartum or end-of-life doula.* 3rd ed. Ann Arbor, MI: DreamStreet Press.

Cassileth, B. R. and Vickers, A. J., 2004. Massage therapy for symptom control: outcome study at a major cancer center. *Journal of Pain and Symptom Management,* [e-journal] 28(3), pp. 244–249. Available at: <http://doi.org/10.1016/j.jpainsymman.2003.12.016>.

Connor, S. R., 2018. *Hospice and palliative care: the essential guide.* 3rd ed. New York: Routledge.

Grealish, L. et al., 2000. Foot massage. A nursing intervention to modify the distressing symptoms of pain and nausea in patients hospitalized with cancer. *Cancer Nursing,* [e-journal] 23(3), pp. 237–243. Available at: <http://doi: 10.1097/00002820-200006000-00012>.

Havyer, R. D. et al., 2022. Impact of massage therapy on the quality of life of hospice patients and their caregivers: a pilot study. *Journal of Palliative Care,* [e-journal] 37(1), pp. 41–47. Available at: <https://pubmed.ncbi.nlm.nih.gov/33213233>.

Kerkhof, M., 2013. *Complementary nursing in end of life care: integrative care in palliative care.* Wernhout, The Netherlands: Kicozo.

MacDonald, G., 1999. *Medicine hands: massage therapy for people with cancer.* Forres, Scotland: Findhorn Press.

MacDonald, G. and Tague, C., 2021. *Hands in health care: massage therapy for the adult hospital patient.* 2nd ed. Edinburgh: Handspring Publishing.

Moore, R., 2017. Strengthening the presence of massage therapy in palliative care. *Massage & Myotherapy Journal,* [e-journal] 15(1), pp. 14-19. Available at: <https://www.oncologymassagetraining.com.au/userfiles/Strengthening%20the%20Presence%20of%20Massage%20Therapy%20in%20Palliative%20Care%20-%20Ronna%20Moore.pdf>.

Polubinski, J. P. and West, L., 2005. Implementation of a massage therapy program in the home hospice setting.

Journal of Pain and Symptom Management, [e-journal] 30(1), pp. 104–106. Available at: <https://www.jpsmjournal.com/article/S0885-3924(05)00245-9/pdf>.

Radbruch, L. et al., 2020. Redefining palliative care – a new consensus-based definition. *Journal of Pain and Symptom Management,* [e-journal] 60(4), pp. 754–764. Available at: <http://doi.org/10.1016/j.jpainsymman.2020.04.027>.

WHO, 2020. *Palliative care: key facts.* Available at: <https://www.who.int/news-room/fact-sheets/detail/palliative-care>.

Additional resources

Blaisdell, C. and Westman, K. F., 2016. Many benefits, little risk: the use of massage in nursing practice. *American Journal of Nursing,* [e-journal] 116(1), pp. 34–39. Available at: <https://nursing.ceconnection.com/ovidfiles/00000446-201601000-00021.pdf>.

Cherny, N. et al., 2015. *Oxford textbook of palliative medicine.* 5th ed. Oxford: Oxford University Press.

CHPCA, n.d. *Dr. Balfour Mount.* [online] Available at: <https://www.chpca.ca/award-recipient/balfour-mount>.

GMC, 2010. *Treatment and care towards the end of life: good practice in decision making.* [pdf] Available at: <https://www.gmc-uk.org/-/media/documents/treatment-and-care-towards-the-end-of-life---english-1015_pdf-48902105.pdf>.

St. Christopher's Hospice: Available at: <https://www.stchristophers.org.uk>.

And when they played, they really played.
And when they worked, they really worked.
                                    –Dr. Seuss

To care for a terminally ill person is to enter a tender and sometimes mysterious space. Many palliative care professionals experience satisfaction in their vocation, finding purpose, joy, and gratitude in their roles, and deeper connections with life and living. There are undeniable challenges, however. The most obvious, perhaps, is the continual loss of people we come to care about. Intimate engagement with the suffering and grief of others invites a range of intense experiences into our lives. "You will witness everything imaginable," says Jack Kornfield. "Your only job is to stay in your seat" (Kornfield, 1993).

Chapter 2 seeks to illuminate a path for therapists who are considering or already engaged in this field as a career choice, to identify practices and skills for staying in one's seat, and to encourage habits that support long-term personal and occupational well-being. This chapter is written in the voice of the collective "we." With a combined 60 years as massage therapists engaged in end-of-life care, we present strategies drawn from our own experience, blended with evidence-based practices and the wise guidance of our many teachers. Our approach represents a departure from commonly endorsed self-care endeavors such as yoga, adequate rest, and social connection. While these habits are beneficial and encouraged, our path involves a more interior and integrated process. Across three domains, we offer a reflective model of self-care, exploring the thoughts, feelings, attitudes, beliefs, and behaviors that can be both challenged and strengthened by the caregiving experience.

In the first domain, *preparing* to do the work, readers will be guided through a process of self-reflection to assess whether end-of-life work might be a good fit for them. In the second, *being with* the work, a menu of mobile self-care practices will be offered, any of which can be incorporated into the workday. The third and final domain, *staying with* the work, identifies activities to cultivate enduring resilience and joy as healthcare workers and human beings.

Both of us share a conviction that the subject of caring for oneself belongs at the *front* of this book rather than the *back*. While there are aspects of caring for dying patients and families that will test our coping skills, we believe that burnout is largely preventable. The key, in our experience, is a contemplative approach to caregiving which does not shield us from suffering but allows us to sit in its presence without being overwhelmed. We write this as seasoned but humble therapists, your fellow sojourners in the daily endeavor of caring for ourselves so that we can care for others.

The complex nature of caring

There is no light without corresponding darkness, a theme that has been explored in sacred texts, Greek mythology, and writings by Carl Jung and countless others. There is even a dark side that accompanies our most noble impulses and gifts, shadows that remain "untamed, unexplored territory to most of us" (Zweig and Abrams, 1991). A willingness to traverse this territory can help us to address imbalances that might otherwise lead to vicarious trauma, compassion fatigue, burnout, and other consequences commonly attributed to the cost of caring (Maslach, 2003). A "right relationship" with shadows can, in fact, offer us a great gift. "We can achieve a more genuine self-acceptance, based on a more complete knowledge of who we are" (Zweig and Abrams, 1991). This is a gift that we can, in turn, extend to those we touch.

Chapter 2

The shadow side of altruism

Many of us are drawn to helping professions, including nursing, doula work, and massage therapy, by a sincere desire to alleviate suffering. Altruism is often understood to include an element of self-sacrifice for the giver. A less frequently acknowledged truth is that the feel-good hormone, oxytocin, is experienced by both giver and receiver in a helping interaction; thus *both* parties benefit from the exchange. The notion of healthcare workers as "angels" or "special" is inaccurate and unhelpful, leading to distortions in the caregiving dynamic and unrealistic expectations of ourselves. The seat we occupy at the bedside should never be a pedestal.

Pathological altruism is a term that describes a shadow side of helping, when the role of helper becomes essential to our self-worth, personal validation, or desire for social approval. It is not that such yearnings are wrong; indeed, they are part of being human. We are simply called to be aware of these needs and to guard against reliance on our work to meet them. Striving to save or fix others, or helping to the point of ignoring our own needs, can result in "help that harms" both therapist and client (Halifax, 2018). A more balanced approach is one that creates the potential to connect with another human being as an equal, neither denying our own needs, nor viewing the other as broken.

Wounded healers

Many people find the means to metabolize personal trauma into positive contributions to the well-being of others. "It is our wounds," says Rachel Naomi Remen, "that enable us to be compassionate with the wounds of others" (Remen, 2006). There is a risk, however, in failing to recognize that one's drive to care may be coming from unprocessed or unhealed personal pain. Caregiving from this source can be detrimental to the "wounded healer" and can degrade the integrity and quality of care that the healer is able to provide. Some palliative care agencies and hospices attempt to mitigate this risk by requiring a waiting period between any significant loss and commencement of employment. This strategy may be helpful in some cases, but it fails to address the variability of human experience when it comes to defining, processing, and coping with trauma and grief. The fact is that personal pain, recent or long past, may be triggered *or* healed by this work. Self-awareness helps us to determine the impact of our wounds on our work, and vice versa.

The shadow side of empathy

Empathy is the capacity to be aware of another person's experience. Compassion is empathy combined with a desire to ease another's suffering. Together, empathy and compassion transform the therapist's skills of touch into trust, connection, and healing presence. Yet there is a shadow even to these affirming aspects of being human. When we identify *too* closely with another person's suffering, we risk the phenomenon of emotional contagion in which we assume emotional burdens that are not ours to carry. Our inability to separate ourselves from the suffering of another can become so debilitating that we cannot be helpful to anyone. The development and maintenance of new tools and skills will allow us to walk *alongside* another person without losing ourselves in the process.

Tools for finding balance

Shadows can become activated in the hospice or palliative care environment where the emotional demands of the work are sometimes compounded by understaffing, inadequate resources, and lack of administrative support. But the good news is that the cost of caring can be managed in a way that fosters well-being for both therapist and client. The middle ground is a space that allows us to be present for others, while also being present to ourselves. Self-awareness, self-compassion, self-regulation, and boundaries are the pillars of our approach to self-care. Each requires ongoing maintenance and honing as the work *shows us* where we need to develop strength. Our primary challenge is remembering that we have these tools and using them consistently.

Self-awareness

Self-awareness is the capacity to turn our attention inward, to notice and honor our own body, thoughts, and emotions. This allows us to be simultaneously aware of our internal reality and the external reality in which we are functioning. Self-awareness manifests as a constant low-volume monitoring of how we are in the world, alerting us to moments of vulnerability or overwhelm whenever they arise. This practice enables us to engage protective measures such as self-regulation or boundaries as we need them.

Self-compassion

It is often easier for us to be kind to others than to be kind to ourselves. We can be prone to self-criticism, speaking to ourselves in harsh or unforgiving ways that we would never use with another person. Self-compassion asks us to extend to ourselves the same empathy and kindness that we extend to others, treating ourselves as if we were "our own best friend" (Otis-Green, 2011). How we talk to ourselves and how we create space and permission to be fully human, with strengths *and* weaknesses, is the starting point from which we can be a healing presence to other people.

Self-regulation

Self-regulation refers to the process of managing our thoughts, emotions, and energy states in a way that leads to well-being and positive engagement with others. The science of self-regulation largely revolves around our understanding of the nervous system and how this system operates in response to real or perceived danger. The Window of Tolerance developed by Dan Siegel and Polyvagal Theory by Steve Porges are two models that describe these responses. One response is *hyper*arousal, the sympathetic state of "fight or flight," in which we are highly activated, tense, anxious, and mobilized for action. Another is *hypo*arousal, a state of parasympathetic "freeze," in which we are immobilized, shut down, withdrawn, and disconnected (known as the dorsal vagal response in Polyvagal Theory). The optimal arousal zone, known as the window of tolerance (or ventral vagal response), is a state in which we feel safe, calm, open, and curious.

The constant surveillance of our environment for signs of safety or danger occurs below our level of awareness. But we can bring attention to these responses, using the skill of self-awareness to notice when we are highly activated or defensively shut down. Self-regulation allows us to settle our nervous system, using the simple practices described in this chapter to return as needed to a sense of ease in the present moment. This ease, mindfully cultivated and faithfully tended, has profound potential to ease the suffering of others.

Boundary awareness

The profound intimacy that is often at the heart of palliative care requires that we manage the therapeutic relationship with sensitivity. Boundaries should not be so rigid that they cannot accommodate the fullness and ambiguity of human experience at the end of life. Nor should they be so porous that they cannot provide respectful space for patients, their loved ones, *and* therapists. The ideal balance is found in boundaries that protect and flex, forming and safely softening by just the right amount at just the right time. Professionalism and tender human care can thus co-exist (Byock, 2013).

End-of-life care may pose dilemmas beyond the familiar boundaries that define most therapeutic relationships. Below are examples of transgressions that represent unethical, problematic, or potentially harmful behavior:

- Unsanctioned sharing of a patient's protected information, or inappropriate sharing of our own.

- Stepping outside our scope of practice, such as giving medical advice.

- Receiving significant gifts from patients or families.

- Overpromising or overdoing, such as offering visits outside of work hours or setting unrealistic frequencies for visits.

- Assuming the problems or suffering of others as if they are our own.

- Yielding to a request from a patient, family member, or colleague that makes us feel uncomfortable. Examples include the use of inappropriate massage pressure or agreeing to be responsible for a dependent home patient while the caregiver runs errands.

- Inserting ourselves into a dynamic in which we have no legitimate role, such as failing to respect a family's need for privacy.

Each tool for finding balance informs and enables the next tool. Self-awareness allows us to become cognizant of our own needs and vulnerabilities. A compassionate response to these is a desire to soothe ourselves with practices of self-regulation so that we can feel safe. From a place of safety, we can navigate delicate but necessary boundaries in our relationships. The formula is not so much linear as circular, each practice facilitating the next as we engage in the daily work and play of being human.

The first domain: Preparing to do the work

"Before I can tell my life what I want to do with it," says Parker Palmer, "I must listen to my life telling me who I am" (Palmer, 2000). Given that end-of-life care requires so much of its practitioners, it is wise to consider thoughtfully one's motivations and capacity. Honest self-appraisal is a fundamental aspect of caring for one's future self. When you listen to your life, is it telling you that caring for people at the end of life is in alignment with your desires and abilities?

Why are you here?

People drawn to end-of-life care cite many reasons for choosing this work. A significant loss of someone close – parent, grandparent, sibling, or friend – may ignite an interest in a caregiving role, sometimes inspired by observations of caregivers at the bedside. Any motive can be worthy and viable, so long as our desire to be of service is mined for insight. The following questions can provide clarity:

- What is it that draws me here?

- What do I have to offer?

- What am I hoping to gain?

- Why do I find myself here *now*?

- What are my thoughts or fears about death, dying, and the meaning of life?

- What is my definition of a "good death" or a "bad death"?

- How might my beliefs and feelings color my responses to others?

- Can I be unconditionally supportive of others who look, feel, think, sound, and behave differently than I do?

- What are the other demands in my life at present?

- How will these demands accommodate this work?

- What is my capacity? How many hours per week do I feel I can devote to this work?

- What is the state of my physical, mental, and emotional health at present?

- Do I have any losses or traumas that need more time or further attention?

- How solid is my commitment to caring for my own needs?

Does the job fit?

Some people seem temperamentally suited to this work. Others grow into their roles over time, developing attributes that allow them to function with more ease. But end-of-life caregiving is clearly not for everyone. Acknowledging this can, in itself, be a courageous act of self-care. The following may be helpful indicators of the "goodness of fit" for this job (Maslach, 2003):

- Comfort with ambiguity and ambivalence.

- The ability to "go with the flow" without needing to control things.

- Appreciation for the diversity of human experience.

- The ability to be nonjudgmental.

- A willingness to meet people where they are without needing to change them.

- The ability to balance confidence and independence with humility and teamwork.

- Being reconciled to the inevitability of suffering and death and willing to be present with both.

- A tolerance for the "messy side" of being human, including sights, sounds, and smells that might disturb others.

- A firm commitment to self-care.

Personal preference will best guide how this introspection might occur – in discussion with friends, family, or colleagues; learning from the experiences of others or texts such as this; through journaling and reflective writing; or perhaps in meditation, prayer, or contemplation. Insights will help clarify your purpose, capacity, and suitability for the task of caring for the dying, serving as a baseline for future reflective practice.

The second domain: Being with the work

Many recommendations for self-care involve actions to be undertaken after the workday is done. We wholeheartedly encourage participation in activities that restore and maintain any dimension of well-being. However, our intention is to identify approaches to self-care that take place while actively engaged in the work of caring for another. Roshi Joan Halifax describes a kind of rest found in the experience of being at ease *in the midst of things*, even difficult situations. This ease, she says, "is about having a lack of resistance to what is before me, and being present and steady" (Halifax, 2018).

If you are a therapist, you may have incorporated strategies into your day which prepare you for each patient visit, keep you grounded while the session unfolds, and enable you to move from one encounter to the next. We wish to encourage and amplify such approaches by sharing a number of ideas which we ourselves have found helpful. Many of our suggestions draw on evidence-based practices of mindfulness which foster self-awareness, self-compassion, self-regulation, and healthy boundaries. Collectively, these habits bring our inner world into focus, allowing us to make more insightful choices in our responses to the external world and others in it. We believe these practices are both self-protective and a reliable means of delivering exemplary care.

One of the most profound gifts of this work is that much of our time at the bedside is spent in silence. This provides a sense of spaciousness and stillness in which it feels quite natural to focus on the breath. Resting in this opportunity, the therapist retains the capacity to reorient, refocus, and respond as needed. When these moments present themselves, our bedside care becomes a contemplative practice benefitting both therapist and patient. The following questions, hovering at the periphery of our awareness, may be helpful.

Noticing the breath

- Am I holding my breath?

- Is my breathing fast and shallow, or is it slow, steady, regular, and deep?

- Is my inhalation equal in length to my exhalation?

Noticing the body

- Am I physically comfortable?

- Am I grounded and centered in my body?

- Do I feel light or heavy? Hot or cold?

- Is there stress, strain, or pain in my body?

- Are my hands soft, relaxed, connected, and present?

Noticing thoughts

- Am I here in the present moment, or am I elsewhere, lost in thought?

- Is my mind racing or distracted?

- Am I judging?

- Do I have an agenda?

- Am I open?

- Am I curious?

Noticing feelings

- How am I feeling?

- Am I sad, angry, irritated, worried, or hurried, or am I calm and serene?

- Am I distressed about something, either in the here and now or outside of this experience?

- Is there peace in this room, within me?

Breathing and grounding exercises

Resmaa Menakem notes that "when one unsettled body encounters another, the unsettledness tends to compound in both bodies" (Menakem, 2017). It is not surprising that patients and their loved ones, grappling with the trauma of life-threatening illness, often embody highly activated nervous systems. This presents for caregivers, especially touch therapists, the potential for another form of "contagion." The most caring thing we can do for ourselves *and* for others is to stabilize our own nervous systems. The breath is a powerful tool for this, reliable and readily available. Simply bringing the attention to the inhalation and the exhalation, even briefly, may calm an unsettled mind and body. Extending the out-breath to become longer than the in-breath enhances this effect. Additional ideas include the following:

- SLOW DOWN. There is no emergency.

- Mindfully take one breath for yourself ("one breath for me"), then one for the other person ("and one for you"). Or perhaps two breaths for you, and one for the other (Neff and Germer, 2018). Allow the nourishment of oxygen to ground and strengthen you.

- Ground yourself by bringing awareness to your feet. Feel them firmly planted on the ground (Kerr, 2015).

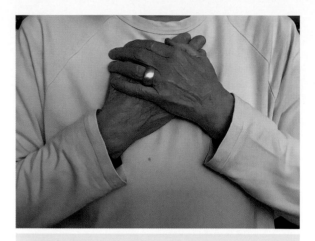

Figure 2.1
Mindful attention to the breath and the heart are simple but effective self-care techniques to regulate the nervous system, helping us find rest in the middle of things.

(Photo courtesy of Ronna Moore.)

- Set an intention for the session, focusing on the process of caring rather than outcome ("may I be a calm, caring presence").

- Invoke the Anchoring Heart Technique (Opus Peace, 2020). Place a hand firmly and tenderly over your heart and breathe deeply. Sit quietly with any discomfort that appears, even if only for a few seconds. Be curious about the place inside you that can be strong enough to hold whatever arises.

- Carry or wear a protective talisman, or recite a helpful mantra or prayer to focus your thoughts and energy.

Recognizing and responding to discomfort

Self-awareness may reveal discomforts that require action and others that do not. One of the most common categories of discomfort known to massage therapists is that of one's own body. Positioning and body mechanics are fundamental to this work, and yet they are often compromised by "what we're doing to our bodies to take care of other people's bodies" (Wolf et al., 2016).

Ask yourself the following questions:

- Do I need to adjust the bed height or other furniture so that I'm not leaning?

- Do I need to move, sit, or use a pillow for support?

- Can the client be brought closer to my hands so that I'm not reaching?

Self-awareness also attunes us to our emotional well-being, especially in response to intense or triggering events. Something may be said, seen, or evoked during a session which challenges or distresses us. Equanimity – the state of being calm and composed, especially when stressed – is a highly desirable quality that allows us to recognize, make space for, and stabilize emotions without being overwhelmed. Questions to elicit equanimity might include the following:

- What is the kindest thing I can do for myself right now?

- Can I notice and silently name uncomfortable feelings, allowing them to be present and trusting they will pass?

- Can I offer words of silent comfort to myself?

- Can I summon the imagined presence of a friend, mentor, religious figure, angel, guide, animal, or bright light to imbue a sense of safety or protection?

John Baugher observes that in doing this work, we are likely from time to time to come up against the limits of our compassion (Baugher, 2019). It is rare but may happen that the wisest and most compassionate action is to acknowledge that the degree of one's own discomfort warrants bringing the session, as mindfully and gently as one can, to an end. This is an entirely valid and acceptable choice. Any adverse experience of this magnitude merits careful follow-up with an appropriate supervisor or mentor.

Taking in the good

Self-care in the midst of things is not only about recognizing the challenges, but also about noticing the deeply rewarding experiences. Moments of humor, connection,

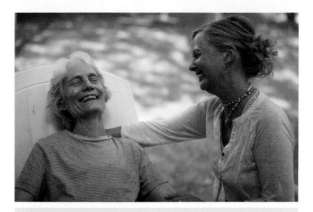

Figure 2.2
Even in the midst of suffering, patients, families, and care staff often share moments of lightness and humor. Savoring these is a way to take in the good.
(Photo by Candice White.)

and wonder provide affirmation and nourishment. As Rick Hanson reminds us, "taking in the good" is both how and why we stay with the work (Hanson and Mendius, 2009). Therapists can be receptive to these moments by showing up to each encounter with a "playfully receptive spirit" and a willingness to be surprised (Baugher, 2019). Small pleasures and beauty that might otherwise go unnoticed rise to the surface of attuned awareness.

The third domain: Staying with the work

The practices described in the preceding pages will carry us a long way in our self-care efforts. Our third domain speaks to the broader context of our work, with ideas to foster long-term resilience and contentment. Resilience is more than bouncing back after a hard day. It reflects healthy coping over time and integration of work as one dimension of our lives which sits alongside others: family and friends, interests, leisure activities, and our own healthcare needs. Staying with the work requires the cultivation of habits that form a bridge between each day and the next, month after month and year after year. In our experience, there is no other way to sustain a rewarding career in end-of-life care.

At day's end

Establishing a routine of reflective inquiry, however brief, can serve to process the events of the day, allowing some to be savored and others to be released. The following are questions to inspire this process:

- Am I satisfied with how things went? If not, why?
- What touched, inspired, or moved me? What made me laugh?
- Is anything unresolved from the day?
- Are there ways that I could have responded more wisely or more compassionately toward another person or toward myself?
- Do I need to do anything more to allow myself to move on in a healthy way?

Self-reflective journaling is one recommended means of capturing thoughts, processing events, refining meaning, and clarifying values. This can be a solitary process in which we become our primary resource for self-knowledge, or shared with others in formal or informal reflective practices. Remember to take care in written and verbal communications to protect patient privacy.

Supervision

Many organizations provide or recommend clinical supervision for their employees. Regular support from a trusted supervisor, coach, mentor, or peer can provide rich opportunities for new perspectives. It can be profoundly enlightening and reassuring to "debrief" a difficult experience with someone who can relate to the nature of the work we do. As a means of self-care, seeking supervision or professional help is essential and urgent if we feel ourselves suffering from significant costs of caring.

Professional and personal development

Ongoing learning facilitates mastery and competence, resulting in increased confidence and job satisfaction. It can be energizing to engage with others in the acquisition of new skills and knowledge, whether through online or in-person events. Relevant training for touch therapists can be sourced from a wide range of related disciplines such as nursing, end-of-life (EOL) doula programs, grief and bereavement, hospice and palliative care agencies and associations, oncology or elder massage, and other bodywork modalities, such as Reiki or Therapeutic Touch. Training in communication skills, mindfulness and meditation, and spiritual retreats also offer the potential for meaningful development, serving to strengthen personal resources for both working and living.

Leaving work behind

Balancing the weight of this work presents an ongoing quest for a lightness of being in other dimensions. Sharon Salzberg views balance as "being with pain and pleasure, joy and sorrow in such a way that our hearts are fully open and also whole and intact" (Salzberg, 2021). How that is achieved will be different for each of us, determined by our preferences and resources. Emerging from the writings of wise teachers, including Joan Halifax, Resmaa Menakem, and Andrew Weil, are consistent themes and specific recommendations for creating protective sanctuary and healing rituals.

Creating sanctuary

Sanctuary is a place of refuge where the body, mind, and heart can rest and play. It offers not only self-*preservation*, but self-*expansion* (Baugher, 2019). In our own version of this personal sanctum, we can choose experiences that help us to feel cared for, nourished, and joyful. We can also choose to be mindful of exposures that place additional demands on our internal resources. Our four pillars of self-care – self-awareness, self-compassion, self-regulation, and boundaries – are the tools we use to build and maintain this sacred space. Below are ideas for inspiration:

- Create a home environment that gives you a sense of well-being, with dedicated indoor or outdoor space.

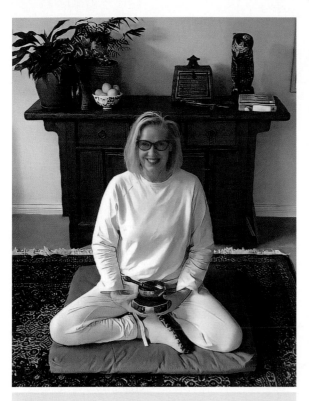

Figure 2.3
A small corner of a room can be devoted to self-care practices which promote well-being.
(Photo courtesy of Ronna Moore.)

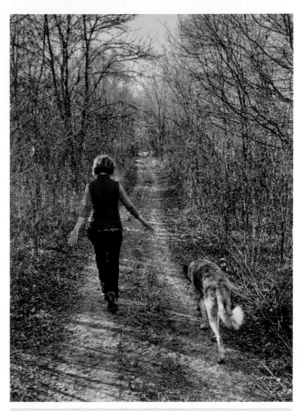

Figure 2.4
Nature can provide a sense of deeply restorative sanctuary.
(Photo by David Spence.)

- Bring small touches of beauty into your space: a potted plant, wildflowers, herbs, fragrance, a wind chime, a soft shawl, crystals, feathers, or a beautiful teacup.

- Connect regularly with activities that bring you pleasure. Music, art, cooking, reading, pets, being with nature, travel, and recreation are all potential sources of delight and sustenance for body, mind, and spirit.

- Choose to step back from overcommitting, overreaching, and overexposure to events, people, and activities that are not restorative. This could include social media and the news cycle.

- There may be times in life when personal losses, family crises, and our own health issues strain our capacity to be present for the suffering of others. Temporary breaks in our professional caregiving may be necessary to sustain our well-being and long-term commitment.

Creating rituals

Rituals can be any series of steps, thoughts, or activities that entail the elements of intention, attention, and repetition to give meaning to our lives (Ter Kuile, 2019). They can be private or communal, as simple as removing one's name badge to mark the transition from work to home at day's end, or as reverential as planting a garden to commemorate one's patients. Rituals invite us to slow down and connect with something larger than ourselves,

Chapter 2

allowing us to acknowledge and process celebrations *and* losses. Below are some examples:

- Last holidays, birthdays, anniversaries, and other milestones can be extremely important to the families we care for. Touch therapists can participate by offering massage, with or without the addition of one of the complementary therapies described in Chapter 10, to make the occasion special.

- Many agencies and individuals send sympathy cards after a death. One hospice we work with hosts an annual "grief camp" for youth, at which young artists who have lost family members create handmade cards for this purpose.

- Some agencies offer a seasonal ceremony to which families and staff are invited. The program might include special music, candles, or shared reflections.

- Handwashing provides frequent opportunities for private rituals of gratitude for the work of one's hands.

- One inpatient unit makes beautiful wreaths out of ribbons on which the first names of patients who have died are written. The wreaths are hung throughout the building.

Lessons are everywhere

Being human, we are bound to forget ourselves, get distracted, or otherwise not be present. "Practice is beginning. Again, and again" (Cook, 2019). As the following story illustrates, lessons may appear out of nowhere, just when we need them most. Self-awareness can be a form of listening for these experiences.

Personal story from Cindy 2.1. The parable of the rock in my shoe

One morning as I rushed to my car, a piece of gravel from my driveway made its way into my shoe. I was late to work and didn't want to stop. I drove to the inpatient unit and stepped out of my car. The rock had shifted, nestling itself under the curve of my toes. It wasn't too uncomfortable, and I was in a hurry. So, I ignored the rock.

Throughout the day, I was aware of the rock as it moved around in my shoe. Whenever it caused discomfort, I tapped my toes on the ground until the rock moved to a more convenient spot. I grew so accustomed that I forgot about it as I saw patients, did my charting, and attended a staff meeting. I drove home and took off my shoes, leaving them at the back door as I always do.

The next morning, I picked up my shoes to put them on and heard the rock roll around. Dumping it out on the ground, I thought to myself how great to be so adaptable. How useful to be able to compartmentalize a minor irritation like a rock in one's shoe. I actually felt a pang of pride. And then I stopped myself. Because pride is always my red flag to have a little talk with myself.

How often do we go about the day with a proverbial rock in our shoe? We deny ourselves some basic comfort in the name of service to others, until denying our own needs and comfort becomes habitual behavior. Examples include:

- Skipping or delaying meals or eating junk food because it's quicker.
- Delaying urination.
- Saying yes to another obligation when you don't know where you'll put it on your calendar.
- Staying late at the end of a long day to see one or more additional patients.
- Working in an uncomfortable position at the bedside.

- Skipping routine care such as doctor, dentist, and haircuts.
- Never finding time to receive bodywork, go the gym, or take a walk.
- Letting household chores go undone until the mess causes distress for you.
- Neglecting friendships or family.
- Failing to take paid time off (PTO) or vacation.

If you recognize yourself in any of the above, I invite you, as I continually invite myself, to slow down. Take a minute to assess your own needs. The work will wait while you address the rock in your shoe.

Conclusion

Those who choose to work with people at the end of life will be privy to both extraordinary sweetness and extraordinary suffering. Few of us are prepared or equipped for the intensity of this experience. This chapter has outlined an approach to choosing, carrying out, and maintaining this work in a sustainable way that allows touch therapists to be of service to others and to thrive in the process. Self-awareness, self-compassion, self-regulation, and boundaries are tools that will increase both the tenure and effectiveness of our caregiving. Someone asked palliative care physician James L. Hallenbeck what it takes to do this job well. "More than anything else," he said, "it is the ability to enter deeply into the pain, suffering, and sadness that are a part of living and dying, and then emerge on the other side into peace and joy" (Hallenbeck, 2003). With mindful attention and practice, we emerge with a deeper capacity for life.

References

Baugher, J., 2019. *Contemplative caregiving: finding healing, compassion, and spiritual growth through end-of-life care.* Boulder, CO: Shambhala Publications, Inc.

Byock, I., 2013. *The best care possible: a physician's guide to transform care through the end of life.* New York: Penguin Group.

Cook, D., 2019. *Practice is beginning. Again.* [online] Available at: <https://deeppeacepractice.com/2019/01/17/practice-is-beginning>.

Halifax, J., 2018. *Standing at the edge: finding freedom where fear and courage meet.* New York: Flatiron Books.

Hallenbeck, J., 2003. *Palliative care perspectives.* New York: Oxford University Press.

Hanson, R. and Mendius, R., 2009. *Buddha's brain: the practical neuroscience of happiness, love and wisdom.* Oakland, CA: New Harbinger Publications.

Kerr, L., 2015. *Living within the window of tolerance: the different zones of arousal.* [pdf] Available at: <https://www.complextrauma.uk/uploads/2/3/9/4/23949705/tolerance_window_short_wot_handout.pdf>.

Kornfield, J., 1993. *A path with heart: a guide through the perils and promises of spiritual life.* New York: Bantam Books.

Maslach, C., 2003. *The cost of caring.* Englewood Cliffs, NJ: Prentice-Hall.

Menakem, R., 2017. *My grandmother's hands: racialized trauma and the pathway to mending our hearts and bodies.* Las Vegas: Central Recovery Press.

Neff, K. and Germer, C., 2018. *The mindful self-compassion workbook: a proven way to accept yourself, build inner strength, and thrive.* New York: Guildford Press.

Opus Peace, 2020. *Anchoring heart technique.* [online] Available at: <https://opuspeace.org/soul-injury-inventory/soul-restoring-resources/anchoring-heart>.

Otis-Green, S., 2011. Embracing the existential invitation to examine care at the end of life. In: Qualls, S. and Kasl-Godley, J., eds. 2011. *End-of-life issues, grief, and bereavement.* Hoboken, NJ: John Wiley & Sons, Inc. Ch. 17.

Palmer, P., 2000. *Let your life speak: listening for the voice of vocation.* San Francisco: Jossey-Bass.

Remen, R. N., 2006. *Kitchen table wisdom: stories that heal.* New York: Penguin Publishing Group.

Salzberg, S., 2021. *Calm in the midst of chaos.* [online] Available at: <https://www.lionsroar.com/calm-in-the-midst-of-chaos>.

Ter Kuile, C., 2019. *The power of ritual: turning every-day activities into soulful practices.* Sydney: HarperCollins Publishers.

Wolf, L. et al., 2016. It's a burden you carry: describing moral distress in emergency nursing. *Journal of Emergency Nursing,* [e-journal] 42(1), pp. 37–46. Available at: <http://dx.doi.org/10.1016/j.jen.2015.08.008>.

Zweig, C. and Abrams, J., 1991. *Meeting the shadow: the hidden power of the dark side of human nature.* New York: Penguin Publishing Group.

Some assembly required.

−Author

In many ways, massage at the end of life is extraordinarily simple. The basics include a space that will accommodate a minimum of two people, positioning that is comfortable for both parties, and gentle touch that feels good to the recipient. Humans are wired to touch one another this way.

Those who choose this kind of touch as a profession will build on these basics to create a skill set of distinct value to patients, families, and the interdisciplinary team. We begin with a few techniques to help us get started, along with a working knowledge of infection control and what pressure to use under which conditions. Supplies are required, including functional work clothes, suitable lotion, and a tool for collecting and recording necessary information about the patient. Chapter 3 will address skills, safety and supplies, all precursors to the actual session.

An underlying premise of a safe approach to massage for people at the end of life is that a dying body is not a stable body. Organs that normally work in concert to maintain homeostasis are not functioning as they usually do. Filtration, metabolism, and elimination are slowing down, shifting the balance between fluids and electrolytes. Blood sugar, blood pressure, and blood oxygen levels are fluctuating. These changes, monumental but largely invisible, place tremendous demands on the body, and are experienced with mounting intensity by the dying person. The massage we provide must not add to these demands.

A second premise is that the changes described above are part of a natural process that can rarely be halted or reversed by artificial means. The body, brilliantly designed, labors to survive for as long as it can, functioning on reduced oxygen, holding on to scarce resources, and routing fluid away from vital organs. It is an arduous process, during which massage can offer moments of deep rest. But attempts to *override* the process, while well intentioned, can create new burdens that are ultimately not helpful to the dying person. An example of this might be a session aimed at moving fluid out of the legs when they are swollen with edema. This fluid, moved from the lower extremities into the torso, may complicate breathing in a patient whose heart and kidneys are already overwhelmed. Any massage with an agenda to "fix" the dying person can produce unintended results.

These realities need not create fear for us as touch therapists. On the contrary, they allow us to surrender our ambitions and relax into simply *being* with another person. This is the framework from which to approach Chapter 3. Training, preparation, and informed judgment are vital for professionals working with vulnerable people. But our expertise is always secondary to our humanity. Every dying person deserves to be seen as a *whole* person, rather than the sum of their broken parts.

Skills

Massage techniques

If you are a massage therapist, you have already learned the basic strokes, including effleurage, petrissage, and compression. Any technique in your toolbox can likely be adapted to provide massage at the end of life. Effleurage will be the primary stroke used over exposed skin. Light petrissage and gentle compression will fill in the gaps when working over clothing or in tight spaces on the body where bandages, medical devices, or extreme weight loss prevent a long, gliding stroke. Holds can be used to begin and end the session, and to signal transitions from one body part to another.

If you are not a massage therapist, be assured that these techniques can be mastered with practice. Effleurage (from the French *effleurer*, meaning "to skim" or "to touch lightly") is a smooth, gliding stroke with one or two hands, typically applied over bare skin with lotion or oil. Petrissage (from the French *pétrir*, meaning "to knead") describes use of the fingers to gently lift and lightly roll the tissue, as if kneading a soft dough. Compression is what it sounds like, applying gentle pressure with a full hand, or lightly pressing the skin with the tips or flat surfaces of the fingers. Compressions can be static or involve some circular movement.

Regardless of the stroke used, a slow rhythmic pressure is ideal. Repetition, predictability, and an unhurried speed are soothing to the nervous system. A study of pleasure-sensing nerves found that gentle strokes at a rate of 3 centimeters (or about 1 inch) per second reduce heart rate and are perceived as more pleasant than faster strokes (McGlone et al., 2014). The direction of our strokes also matters. Strokes toward the heart support venous return, the flow of blood back to the heart and lungs for reoxygenation. One or both of the therapist's hands may be moving at any time, or one or both hands may be stationary. The power of holding is elaborated in Chapter 4.

Part of what feels good to be on the receiving end of massage is not the depth but the *breadth* of the contact. The hands of the therapist remain soft enough to meld and conform to the contours of the recipient's body. This results in full-handed contact that says, "I am here, I am with you, I am *all* with you." A relaxed hand is also better for the therapist, in that the muscles of the hand are not working harder than they need to. Beyond this basic principle, every massage is a once-in-a-lifetime experience, influenced by the giver, the receiver, and the unique chemistry between the two. At times, it can feel that everything else falls away, except the present moment.

If you are a bodyworker, your focus will be adaptation of techniques for end-of-life work by applying the modifications described in the following pages. If massage is new to you, I highly recommend that you *receive* massage from several different therapists who specialize in gentle work. Being on the receiving end of touch is always a learning experience, not to mention a great form of self-care.

Massage is a skill that improves with practice. Pair up with a partner and ask for honest feedback. Imagine how you would want to be touched if you were sick or in pain. In-person training is highly recommended if you are able. There really is no substitute for hands-on learning.

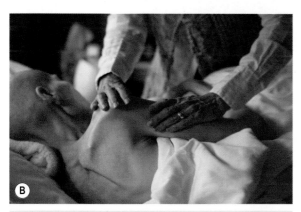

Figure 3.1

Two of the basic massage strokes. (A) Effleurage is a long stroke typically applied over bare skin with lotion or oil. (B) Petrissage involves lifting and gently kneading the tissue with the hands or fingers. The third basic stroke, compression, is demonstrated in Figure 3.2.

(Photos by Candice White.)

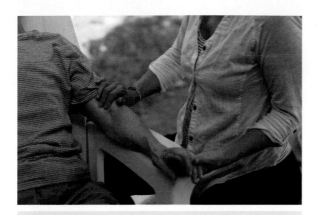

Figure 3.2
Demonstration of a comforting technique which Valerie Hartman calls the "mother hand." The therapist's right hand in this photo is providing slow, gentle compressions on the upper arm, while the left hand is stationary, simply holding.

(Photo by Candice White.)

Massage dose

Limiting the dose, or duration, of the session is one way to control the demand placed on the recipient's body. While a 60-minute session is standard in the massage industry, an hour of massage is nearly always too much at the end of life. A patient who is in early decline and having a good day might tolerate a 45- or 50-minute session, while a patient in late decline having a hard day might tolerate 20 minutes or less. Massage therapists at M. D. Anderson Cancer Center in Houston have observed that a 20-minute massage is adequate to achieve relaxation and satisfaction in most patients (Walton, 2013). References to specific adjustments in session length will be made as they correspond to each stage of dying in Chapter 5.

Massage pressure

No question gets asked with greater frequency or more concern than what pressure to use when providing massage for people at the end of life. Some people are surprised by the extreme tenderness of this work. Others can't believe that gentle pressure applied with grounded

fullness can *feel* so powerful. It is not deep pressure but deep *presence* that is our goal. The challenge in addressing this topic is that pressure is a subjective experience which is difficult to measure and convey to others. A common reference point is needed.

Fortunately, the field of oncology massage has yielded a five-point scale to quantify and communicate massage pressure. Massage at the end of life makes liberal use of the two lightest pressures on the scale, levels 1 and 2. The third level of pressure, level 3, is used rarely and then only selectively as described in the following pages. The two deepest pressures, levels 4 and 5, are never appropriate for massage at the end of life. A description of pressure guidelines and their indicated uses is summarized in Table 3.1.

Level 1 pressure, for active dying or severe symptoms

Level 1 is the lightest pressure, described as "light lotioning," or the minimum pressure needed to spread lotion across the skin (Walton, 2011). Level 1 pressure is limited to surface contact. There is no engagement or displacement of underlying tissue. Gayle MacDonald suggests that level 1 pressure is what a person might use to handle a ripe peach (MacDonald, 2014). I have personally found this analogy to be useful, as the human tissues at the end of life can feel spongy and saturated, covered by a thin membrane that bruises and breaks easily.

Level 1 pressure is used for severe symptoms at the end of life, which are indicated in Table 3.1; they include advanced age, widespread bruising, high risk of bleeding, severe edema or lymphedema, fever, and extreme fatigue. These are examples of scenarios when the greatest care must be taken to avoid causing harm.

Many massage therapists find level 1 to be the most difficult pressure to master, as it can feel like they are "holding back." A good beginning is to simply rest the hands on the patient's body. Take a few deep breaths in this resting position and check in with yourself. Are your hands relaxed and truly resting? Is every surface of your hand soft, so that your palm and fingers conform to the shape of the client's body? Are your shoulders relaxed in a neutral position? Level 1 is easiest and most effective when it is effortless. Tip 3.1 offers additional suggestions that learners may find helpful.

Tip 3.1. Mastering level 1 pressure

- Adjust your working position. The therapist should be positioned at the height of the patient's body so that there is no leaning. If the therapist is standing at the bedside, the bed will need to be raised to meet the hands. If the bed cannot be raised or if the patient is seated in a wheelchair or recliner, it may be necessary for the therapist to sit.

- Adjust the consistency and amount of lotion. When working over skin, level 1 will be easier if you use plenty of lubrication. Beginners might find that a thinner lotion (versus a thicker cream) will facilitate lighter pressure. Remember you are applying the lightest pressure needed to spread the lotion across the skin. If too much lotion remains on the skin at the end of the session, a hand towel or washcloth can be used to gently remove the excess.

- Most touch therapists position themselves facing the head of the patient, providing pushing strokes. If level 1 pressure feels difficult, try repositioning yourself so that your hands can pull the skin toward you rather than pushing it away (see Figure 3.3B). This pulling technique also seems to work well for therapists with larger hands.

- Anxiety can create difficulty in attempting to use level 1 pressure. If the hands are not relaxed, ask yourself if you are feeling anxious. If the answer is yes, acknowledge

this feeling by breathing into it. On the exhalation, see if you can soften the anxiety by surrounding it with loving compassion for yourself and for the person you are touching. There is nothing to fix here, no brokenness to correct. The only goal is connection. Return to Chapter 2 as needed for ideas to cultivate a settled nervous system.

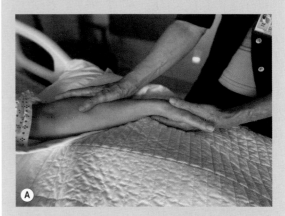

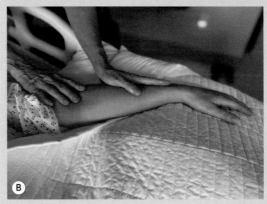

Figure 3.3
Two different ways to apply effleurage. In (A) the therapist is pushing strokes toward the heart. In (B) strokes are pulled toward the heart. Touch therapists can choose the method that feels most comfortable and that facilitates control over their pressure.

(Photos by Candice White.)

Chart talk 3.1. Cachexia and temporal wasting

One of the conditions listed for level 1 pressure is cachexia with temporal wasting, pictured below. Cachexia is defined as a state of severe muscle wasting which can occur in the late stages of serious illnesses (Medical Dictionary for the Health Professions and Nursing, 2012). It is described further on p. 95.

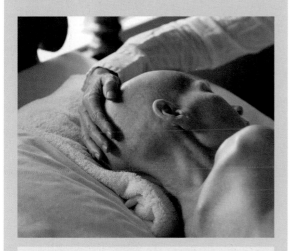

Figure 3.4
Severe cachexia, an indication for level 1 massage pressure, is indicated by temporal wasting, visible as a shadow or indentation of the patient's temple area.

(Photo by Candice White.)

Heads up 3.1. The concept of "reddening" the skin

Reddening of the skin is sometimes used as an indicator that massage pressure is too deep. This outcome is more obvious on fair-skinned people than darker-skinned people. Therapists should therefore not depend on this benchmark when providing massage over skin that has more pigmentation.

joints or deeper muscles. MacDonald describes level 2 as the pressure one might use to wash a plum.

Level 3 pressure, used selectively on limited areas of the body and under limited conditions

Level 3 pressure is a "medium pressure" and might be used for an entire massage on a healthy client. Level 3 pressure is slightly firm, with some mild displacement of surrounding tissues. Level 3 is used very selectively in end-of-life care and never for an entire massage.

In the absence of conditions warranting level 1 or level 2 as described in Table 3.1, level 3 pressure might be applied with the fingertips to a limited area of the body. Use of level 3 is mindfully targeted and brief. It can be a way of responding to a patient's request for deeper pressure in a way that is focused and safe. An example of this might be the plantar aspect (or bottom) of the feet in an individual who is still ambulatory.

There is still no leaning or use of the therapist's body weight when using level 3 pressure on a person at the end of life. Sitting to work, or standing parallel while working, helps the therapist to stay mindful that level 3 pressure should be a nurturing, nondemanding experience for the receiver. There should be no reddening of the skin, and no attempt to be ambitious (MacDonald and Tague, 2021). Relying on arm or hand strength rather than body weight will require enough effort from the therapist that level 3

Level 2 pressure, for most conditions and most parts of the body

While it's important for touch therapists to master level 1 pressure for situations where it's needed, level 2 is the baseline pressure I use most often in my work. Level 2 pressure is described as "heavy lotioning," which is "a shade deeper than light lotioning" (Walton, 2011). This is the amount of pressure needed to rub lotion *into* the skin, involving slight displacement of superficial muscle, but no displacement of

Table 3.1 Pressure guidelines for massage therapy at the end of life

Pressure	Type of touch	Suggested technique	Suggested uses	Appropriate for these conditions
1	Light touch or holds	Energy technique or light lotioning Nurturing Slow or still Full hand As if handling a ripe peach	Active dying, severe symptoms, high-risk scenarios	Advanced age Limbs with medical devices Site of known or suspected deep vein thrombosis (DVT) Widespread bruising High risk of bleeding Severe edema/lymphedema Extreme fatigue Cachexia with temporal wasting Fractures (entire quadrant) Other acute injuries Fragile skin Fever/sepsis Severe pain
2	Superficial muscle	Contact with superficial muscle Nurturing Slow Full-handed As if gently washing a ripe plum	Safe for most conditions and parts of the body	Lower extremities Ascites Bone metastases Osteoporosis Limited bruising Mild edema/lymphedema Fatigue Cachexia without temporal wasting Neuropathy
3	Slightly firm	Slightly firm muscle contact Not forceful Not ambitious No reddening of skin As if massaging a tangerine	Limited conditions and limited area of the body	Never with above conditions Never with impaired feedback Patient alert and verbal Patient ambulatory or active Limited surface area Limited duration of time

Heavy, forceful massage is never appropriate for people at the end of life.

Table adapted for Final Touch Training, with permission from Gayle MacDonald, author of *Medicine Hands* (2014, Findhorn Press).

will more likely be confined appropriately: to a small area of the body, for a short period of time, in a select group of patients.

Safety

Massage precautions

When appropriate adjustments are made in dose and pressure, most concerns about safety will have been addressed. Many of the conditions that are listed in Table 3.1 are self-evident and will be obvious to the therapist. Other conditions are underlying or less obvious, and warrant some explanation before proceeding further. The following paragraphs are intended to provide the rationale for use of conservative pressure at the end of life, even in the absence of obvious debility.

Impaired sensation and feedback

Due to changes in the brain, medications, and reduced level of arousal during the dying process, people at the end of life experience changes in physical perception and the ability to communicate with others. This means that the typical question from massage therapists ("How is the pressure?") is not an accurate gauge for determining comfort *or* safety. Clients may experience massage pressure as enjoyable while they are medicated, but later feel adverse effects. Therapists must therefore rely on their own learning rather than patient input to confine massage dose and pressure appropriately.

Adapting the massage session

- Level 1 and level 2 pressures are generally safe. Level 3 pressure should *never* be used on any patient with impaired sensation or feedback.

- If a patient requests deeper pressure, briefly explain the rationale for level 1 or level 2. In short, deep pressure can create demands that the body cannot presently handle. The explanation can be tailored to the patient's specific issues, based on information in this book.

- Reassure the patient that you are hearing their request and that you will provide "focused attention" to the area of concern.

Loss of skin integrity

Skin, the largest organ of the body, bears much of the brunt of the dying experience. One of the most common issues at the end of life is dehydration of the dermis, a problem which massage can help address. But therapists must be mindful of the extreme fragility of the skin and how easily it can be damaged. Once damaged, healing can be slow or impossible. A tear in the skin can result in infection that causes severe pain and can hasten death.

Massage should always be confined to intact skin. At the end of life, this often requires a customized session built around areas to be avoided. A massage of a single area of the body (the head and neck or a foot massage), provided with focused attention and mindful care, can feel profound and complete.

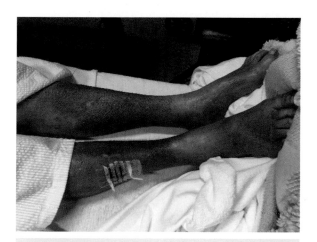

Figure 3.5

An example of impaired skin integrity in a patient with advanced lung disease. It is common to see changes in skin color and texture, thinning of the skin, and chronic wounds in patients with poor circulation.

(Photo by author.)

Chart talk 3.2. Terminology for bedsores

A pressure injury (known previously as a bedsore, decubitus ulcer, or pressure ulcer) is the current term for skin breakdown that occurs over a bony prominence or under a medical device, due to prolonged pressure on the area. The term was changed to reflect the finding that breakdown begins in the tissue prior to these changes becoming visible as an ulcer. Pressure injuries are rated with a numeric system using numbers 1–4, with stage 1 describing soft tissue damage that has not yet resulted in ulceration (Edsberg et al., 2016).

Adapting the massage session

- Level 1 and level 2 pressures are generally safe for intact skin. A moisturizing lotion applied during light massage can help maintain skin health.

- Avoid any area where the skin is broken, including skin tears, cracks in the skin, scabs, rashes, and tumors that break the skin.

- Avoid areas with devices such as intravenous (IV) devices, catheters, dialysis access sites, feeding tubes, and tracheostomies.

- Be mindful when working over bony areas that maintain prolonged contact with a bed or chair, as these areas are at risk of a pressure injury.

Blood clots and bleeding risk

In healthy people, the body maintains an optimal balance between clotting and bleeding. Many conditions at the end of life can disrupt this balance. Too much clotting can lead to a thrombus, the clinical term for a blood clot, which is a solid clump of cells, protein, and debris. A thrombus that occurs in a large vein is called a deep vein thrombosis, or DVT. DVTs can form in any vein of the body but are most common in the pelvic veins and lower extremities. Any vein that houses a foreign object, such as an IV device or port, is at increased risk for DVT. Additional risk factors include advanced age, congestive heart failure, stroke, organ failure, recent surgery, infection, prolonged inactivity, paralysis of an extremity, and cancer. While DVTs can sometimes cause symptoms such as pain, warmth, swelling, and redness, half or more of all cases are "clinically silent" (Walton, 2011).

Massage therapists have long been advised to avoid deep pressure or "circulatory massage" (vigorous strokes that increase circulation) in people at risk of DVT. The concern is that massage might cause a clot to detach from the vein wall and travel through the bloodstream to the lung, resulting in a pulmonary embolism (PE). A PE can block a pulmonary artery, causing severe shortness of breath, chest pain, and risk of sudden death.

While DVT and PE represent one extreme of the clotting spectrum, bleeding at the opposite extreme warrants equal caution from the therapist. Bruising and bleeding are very common at the end of life. Risk factors include age over 65 years, cancer, liver failure, kidney failure, and the use of certain drugs, such as anticoagulants, aspirin, or nonsteroidal anti-inflammatory drugs (NSAIDs). Bleeding is elaborated on p. 121.

Adapting the massage session

Due to numerous risk factors for DVT and bleeding, the following precautions are indicated for *all* patients at the end of life:

- Maximum of level 2 pressure in the lower extremities.

- Level 1 pressure, holds, or avoidance of areas of the body with a known DVT, treated or untreated.

- Level 1 pressure in an area of the body with an IV or other medical device.

- Level 1 pressure or holds in patients with widespread bruising or known bleeding risk.

Loss of bone strength

Bones can be weakened by numerous conditions at the end of life, including age, poor nutritional status, atrophy, previous fracture, osteoarthritis, osteoporosis, HIV infection, and cancer. Particularly in the case of cancer, the disease or radiation to treat the disease can render bones so fragile that they break from minimal exertion such as leaning on an elbow or rolling over in bed. These changes may occur long *before* symptoms appear. In fact, spontaneous fractures (also known as pathological fractures) are often the first sign that cancer has spread to bones. A spinal fracture may be referred to as a compression fracture, or a vertebral compression fracture.

If a bone is so delicate that it can break while rolling over in bed, it is not difficult to imagine that use of the therapist's body weight, leaning on the client, or applying deep pressure could be disastrous. Massage therapists are trained to avoid applying pressure directly over the spine even in healthy clients. When our clients have advanced disease, we must *assume* that bone health may be compromised and adjust our pressure accordingly.

Adapting the massage session

- Due to risk of bone fragility, light pressure is indicated (no greater than level 2) in patients with end-stage cancer, advanced age, poor nutrition, previous fracture, osteoarthritis, osteoporosis, or HIV infection.

- In case of existing fracture, use holds or no touch at all to the area, depending on patient tolerance.

- Care must be taken when performing range of motion (see p. 193).

Lymphedema and lymphedema risk

Lymphedema, localized swelling from accumulation of lymphatic fluid, is a risk that primarily pertains to people with cancer and those with a history of cancer. This represents a large number of people at the end of life, including those for whom cancer is the terminal diagnosis and many others who are dying of other diseases but have cancer in their medical histories. Anyone who has *ever had* cancer is at lifelong risk for lymphedema if lymph nodes have been damaged by disease, radiation, or surgery.

Lymphedema can have a significant impact on quality of life, causing discomfort, impaired wound healing, and increased risk of infection. It is imperative for touch therapists working in end-of-life care to be knowledgeable about this risk because massage that is too forceful or too ambitious can trigger or worsen lymphedema. Once the condition is activated, it never completely resolves. The resulting distress for the patient is an outcome that no therapist wants to be responsible for.

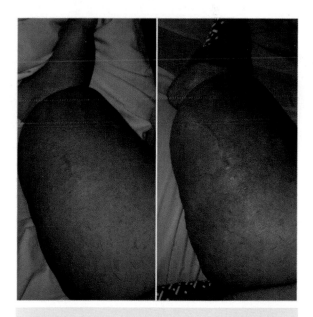

Figure 3.6
A limb with lymphedema is prone to infection, and infection can likewise trigger or worsen lymphedema. These photos demonstrate progress in a hospital patient being treated for infection under the skin, also known as cellulitis. While the photo on the left shows improvement, a touch therapist should avoid this limb until the infection is fully resolved. The patient in the photo, four days into IV antibiotics, enjoyed a 15-minute level 2 head, neck, and shoulder massage.

(Photo courtesy of Devora Herskovits.)

A maximum pressure of level 2 is generally safe for people with mild lymphedema or those at risk. When lymphedema is more severe, level 1 pressure, light holds, or avoidance of the area may be necessary. Lymphedema can be so extreme that the lymphatic fluid seeps through the pores of the skin, a phenomenon known as weeping, or lymphorrhea. A weeping limb is extremely prone to infection.

Adapting the massage session

Due to the risks described above, the following precautions are indicated for people with cancer *or* cancer history.

- No touch to any limb with weeping or active infection.

- For an area of the body with severe lymphedema but no weeping, holds or level 1 compressions may be used. Touch to the area should be brief in duration.

- For mild lymphedema, level 1 or level 2 pressure is generally safe. While strokes toward the heart are advised, the intention is *not* to move fluid, only to provide comfort. Duration of massage to the area should be brief.

- Any therapist who is new to the issue of lymphedema is urged to pursue additional training. In the absence of a deeper understanding of this condition, the most conservative approach should be taken.

Standard precautions

Standard precautions are practices used with every patient that protect patients and healthcare workers from the spread of infection. These practices include hand hygiene and the use of personal protective equipment (PPE) when appropriate. Standard precautions are based on the assumption that *any* fluid from *any* person may be infectious, including blood, excretions (except sweat), nonintact skin, and mucous membranes (CDC, 2016). Tracy Walton introduced me to a pithy summary of this guideline, the "body fluid principle" borrowed from emergency medicine: *If it's wet, and it's not yours, don't touch it* (Walton, 2011). This principle also applies to fluids that appear to

be dry, including scabs, soiled bedding or clothing, used bandages, and potentially contaminated surfaces.

Hand hygiene

Therapists employed or contracted to work in hospice and palliative care settings are required to complete annual hand hygiene training and to utilize this competency during every patient encounter. Upon entering *and* exiting the patient's home or room, hands should be washed thoroughly with soap and water, regardless of whether gloves are used. Liberal use of a liquid soap is required, rubbed over every surface and in between each finger, the hands, wrists, and arms up to the elbows for a minimum of 20 seconds. Nails, which should be kept short, will need to be cleaned by scratching the fingertips across the soapy palm of the opposite hand. After a good rinse with running water, dry hands thoroughly with a single-use paper towel. An additional paper towel should be used to turn the faucet off and to open the door handle as you exit the room. These instructions will be easy to carry out in any facility where handwashing materials are readily available. Private homes can be a different matter.

Conditions for handwashing in home environments are quite variable. In some cases, the patient or family is able to offer a clean sink with liquid soap and paper towels. In other cases, what is available is a bar of soap and a communal towel, both sources of bacteria. I have visited homes where every sink was full of dirty dishes, soiled clothing, or contaminated medical supplies. I have visited homes where there was no running water. On these occasions, I've been glad to have hand sanitizer in my pocket, not as a substitute for handwashing, but as a measure of protection until soap and water can be accessed at the earliest opportunity.

Hand sanitizer is widely available and effective against nearly all pathogens, if used properly. The US Centers for Disease Control (CDC) recommend sanitizer with a minimum alcohol content of 60%. A generous amount of this solution should be applied in the same manner as soap: rubbed over every surface of each finger, the hands, and wrists until dry. Hand sanitizer, however, does not remove lotion or oil, and is therefore not an effective cleaner when there is massage lotion on the hands (Werner, 2019). Sanitizer is also not effective against *Clostridium difficile* (C. diff), a common diarrheal illness that is easily spread and potentially dangerous for immunocompromised people. For patients with known or suspected C. diff infection or diarrhea of unknown cause, soap and water (combined with gloves) are the only means of preventing spread.

Carrying your own liquid soap and paper towels is a good way to be prepared. I have used the contents of a water jug to clean my hands with soap on the side of the road, a crude but adequate "washroom" in a pinch. A hand hygiene kit is included in the supply lists on pp. 45–6.

Transmission-based precautions

Transmission-based precautions are used in addition to standard precautions whenever a patient is known or suspected to have a specific infection. These precautions are grouped according to how the infection is spread: through the air, via droplets, or by direct or indirect contact. Therapists who work in clinical settings where these infections are more common will need to be well versed in each set of precautions. The facility (hospital or inpatient unit) will likely require any therapist working onsite to participate in ongoing training to assure understanding and compliance. *Hands in health care: massage therapy for the adult hospital patient* by Gayle MacDonald and Carolyn Tague is an excellent resource for further study of this topic.

Airborne precautions

These practices are used for infections that spread through air or dust particles which may be contagious if inhaled by another person. An example is tuberculosis. Precautions include the use of a mask, gown, and gloves.

Droplet precautions

Some infections are spread through droplets when an infected person coughs, sneezes, or talks. Infected droplets can travel through the air and spread to another person in close proximity, typically 2 meters (6 feet) or less. COVID-19 is an example. A mask and goggles or mask and face shield are required PPE for droplet precautions.

Contact precautions

Some diseases are spread through direct or indirect contact. Direct contact occurs when one person touches another person's body, while indirect contact involves a contaminated surface or object that the infected person has touched. A number of infections require contact precautions, including vancomycin-resistant enterococcus

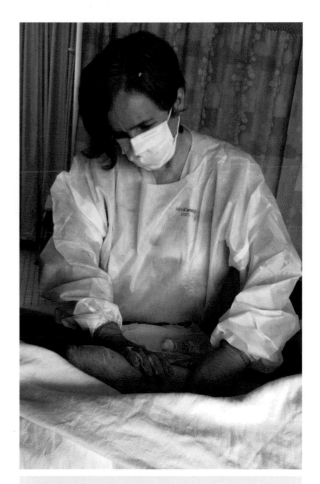

Figure 3.7
Touch therapists will be required to use a gown and gloves when providing massage for patients on contact precautions. PPE and related training are typically provided by the facility in which massage occurs.

(Photo by Gayle MacDonald, reprinted with permission from *Hands in health care.*)

(VRE) and methicillin-resistant *Staphylococcus aureus* (MRSA). Herpes simplex and C. diff are other examples of conditions requiring contact precautions.

Contact precautions involve thorough hand hygiene, gloving, and gowning prior to entering the patient's space. In inpatient or facility settings, a rack with these supplies is typically hung on the patient's door, with a designated container to dispose of used PPE inside the patient's room. In the home setting, you will know if you need a gown for contact precautions because a biohazard box will be on the patient's front porch for disposal on your way out of the home. There is a very specific sequence to donning (putting on) and doffing (taking off) PPE. Hospital, facility, and agency-based touch therapists will require training in these specific protocols. Private therapists should be aware of them and ask for clarification when needed.

Contraindications to massage: Is there anyone who should not receive massage?

This section will be short because there are so few circumstances in which a dying person cannot receive an adapted form of gentle touch, if they wish to. Many of the contraindications advised in massage school are irrelevant, given appropriate adjustments to dose and pressure, along with the fact that typical contraindications (including fever, diarrhea, DVT, and infection) are not managed as emergencies at the end of life. When the goal of care is comfort rather than cure, and when the definition of "massage" is expanded to include light caress and gentle holds, there is seldom a reason to withhold massage.

That said, there are times when our clinical team advises against massage. These include when the patient has any of the following:

- Scabies, lice, bed bugs, or ringworms, until resolved.
- Widespread skin disease or skin breakdown (from extensive burns, for example) that would make touch intolerable.

- A demonstrated aversion or intolerance to even very light touch.
- Seizures or agitation that are triggered by touch.

Gloves

When to glove

Gloving practices vary geographically, and from agency to agency. In some settings, gloves are worn by every staff member for every patient encounter. In these environments, touch therapists will be expected to follow suit. In other settings, staff are trained to use gloves only when clinically indicated. In their book on hospital massage, MacDonald and Tague cite a UK campaign in which selective gloving resulted in a reduction of skin-related problems for wearers, in addition to a significant decrease in environmental impact and expense. Of note, the study revealed *no* increase in the spread of infection when glove use is selective (NHS England, 2018).

The CDC recommends the use of gloves when it can be "reasonably anticipated" that contact with potentially infectious materials could occur, including body fluids, mucous membranes, nonintact or potentially contaminated skin, or contaminated equipment (CDC, 2019). MacDonald and Tague have clarified some of the situations in which bodyworkers should wear gloves for massage. Specific to end-of-life work, I would expand their guidelines regarding topical medications, and I would add that my own practice includes glove use with patients who have end-stage liver disease or HIV infection. These conditions are strongly linked to hepatitis B and C, which (like the HIV virus) are spread through blood and other body fluid. An infected person with intact skin poses little risk of transmission to healthcare workers. However, the end of life is characterized by progressive skin breakdown, presenting a scenario in which the CDC's threshold of reasonable anticipation of contact with infectious material could arguably be met.

Gloves are therefore recommended for any of the following circumstances when providing massage for people at the end of life:

- To touch any body part that poses a risk of contact with body fluids or nonintact skin, including scabs (MacDonald and Tague, 2021).

- To touch the patient's gown, clothing, or linen that has been contaminated by body fluid, even if the fluid has dried (MacDonald and Tague, 2021).

- When the therapist has open skin on the hands (hangnail, cut, scrape, burn, etc.), identified by any place that stings when antiseptic hand sanitizer is applied (MacDonald and Tague, 2021).

- Before touching a contaminated urinal, bedpan, or emesis bag or basin (MacDonald and Tague, 2021).

- When airborne or contact precautions are in effect, including infections with VRE, MRSA, *E. coli*, C. diff, or hepatitis A (MacDonald and Tague, 2021).

- When the patient has a contagious skin infection such as herpes simplex (MacDonald and Tague, 2021). Contagious fungal infections, such as toenail fungus, represent a site restriction to avoid during massage (Werner, 2019).

- When providing touch for patients who have received chemotherapy in the previous 72 hours or when steroidal cream has just been applied (MacDonald and Tague, 2021).

- When any other therapeutically active topical has just been applied, including analgesics or other drugs in gel, cream, or ointment form (NHS England, 2018).

- When the patient has compromised skin in combination with human immunodeficiency virus (HIV) infection or liver disease, including cirrhosis and primary liver cancer.

- Therapists working with patients who remain in active treatment may encounter additional scenarios that require glove use. An example is a blood cancer patient undergoing stem cell harvest or transplant who may be on contact precautions.

Types of gloves

The goal of medical gloves is to provide barrier protection without compromising hand function. Due to the potential for allergic reactions to latex, many medical providers have turned to latex alternatives, including vinyl and nitrile. Both vinyl and nitrile gloves can be used for massage, but nitrile gloves, though slightly more expensive, are highly recommended due to superior tactile sensitivity. Gloves should be stored in a cool environment, never over 90°F. However, my personal experience is that both vinyl and nitrile gloves hold up to 10–15 minutes of warming in an electric warmer (see Tip 3.3 and Figure 3.9).

It's important to know that gloves may impact the performance of massage lubricants. Thinner lubricants tend to perform better when gloves are used, as thicker creams may form clumps or take longer to absorb into the skin. Some lotions can have a detrimental effect on latex gloves, including those that contain petroleum, lanolin, mineral oil, palm oil, or coconut oil.

How to wear gloves

Hands should be washed before donning gloves. The fit should be snug and smooth. Gloves should be removed carefully to prevent hand contamination, and hands should be washed immediately after removing gloves. It goes without saying that a new pair of gloves must be worn for each patient. Gloves should be replaced *during* the session if they become damaged or soiled, with hand hygiene performed in between change of gloves.

Most patients in hospice care are accustomed to glove use by healthcare workers. It is likely that gloves will bother the uninitiated therapist more than they bother the patient. Over time, having identified personal preferences for glove type and lotion, the therapist will no longer be distracted by the use of gloves when they are needed. Patients, in my experience, seem not to notice at all.

Oxygen safety

Many people with advanced disease benefit from the use of supplemental oxygen. Oxygen by itself is a nonflammable gas, but it can cause a spark to ignite, or a flame to accelerate very rapidly. Oxygen can accumulate in materials such as clothing, hair, and bedding, causing them to burn more easily if they catch fire. Most fires from supplemental oxygen are caused by patients smoking while using oxygen therapy. E-cigarettes have also been implicated.

Home oxygen fires can result in serious injury or death, primarily for the oxygen user but also for others present in the home. These fires are entirely preventable. Patients who use oxygen in England are nearly 20 times less likely to die in a home oxygen fire than oxygen users in the US, due to safety measures to address this issue in the UK (Adderton, 2019). The following guidelines are recommended by the National Health Service (NHS) of England:

- People who use oxygen should not smoke, or let anyone near them smoke, when using their device.

- Keep oxygen at least 3 meters (10 feet) away from an open flame, such as a gas stove, heater, fireplace, lit candle, or cigarette lighter.

- Keep oxygen at least 1.5 meters (5 feet) away from electrical appliances that may produce a spark, such as a television, hair dryer, or electric heater. To this list from the NHS, I would add e-cigarettes, or "vapes."

- Avoid oil-based emollients such as Vaseline (NHS, 2020).

Supplies

Clothing and accessories

Our work clothes are often defined by the cultures in which we work, but also reflect personal preferences developed over time. I like to wear scrub bottoms for the pockets, but I prefer shirts and blouses that are less clinical. Another therapist at my agency prefers full scrubs. I sometimes lean into the patient's bed, so I often wear aprons that tie at the neck and waist as a physical barrier that can be changed between patients. I wear sleeves that end at the elbows so that my forearms can be thoroughly washed. Sturdy, comfortable shoes are worth the investment. Best practices regarding clothing and accessories include the following:

- Wear close-toed shoes.

- Secure hair away from the face.

- Avoid wearing rings and wrist jewelry.

- Avoid wearing long necklaces or lanyards that might fall into the patient's space.

- Be mindful that religious jewelry may be distracting or unsettling to some people. If worn, these might be tucked under clothing to project a neutral presence.

- Wear a name tag or badge, supplied by the agency or created by the therapist.

- Avoid wearing perfume or other scented products.

- Many agencies have specific guidelines regarding modest and neutral attire, nail polish, and nail extensions.

Lubricants

A quality lubricant is the central asset of the touch therapist's supplies. A number of factors contribute to a lubricant being a good choice for end-of-life massage. The product should be fragrance-free and moisturizing without leaving a greasy residue. Long-lasting moisture is preferred. For this reason, thicker massage creams often produce the best results in the last months of life. Lotions available in a pump bottle are typically thinner

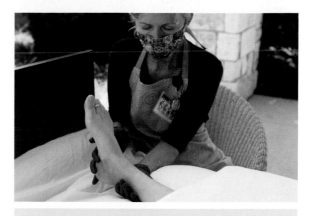

Figure 3.8
Sleeves should not extend beyond the elbows. Aprons (homemade or purchased online) are easy to change between patients and apron pockets can hold items to be carried into the home or room. My nurse's watch is visible in the photo. Shortly after this photo was taken, our inpatient unit added N95 masks and goggles to our required PPE as a COVID precaution.

(Photo by Pamela Robison.)

products, which also have advantages. Thinner products spread more easily across the skin and may work better when wearing gloves. Lotions provided by hospitals and nursing homes tend to be watered down and of inferior quality. Any lotion, cream, or oil thoughtfully chosen by the touch therapist is likely to be an improvement.

Many therapists prefer to avoid products with parabens, additives, and chemicals. Clean, organic products align with the organic nature of the dying process and are a way to honor the skin we care for (Hartman, 2009, 2012). Families often have questions about the products we use, so we should be prepared to speak knowledgeably about our choices. Some patients have sensitivities to common skin-care ingredients, so it is wise to keep a hypoallergenic option on hand.

Regardless of the lubricant chosen, single-serve containers are recommended. A 1-ounce (or 30-milliliter) container with lid (available from restaurant supply

---

Tip 3.2. On keeping time

I find a timepiece helpful for documenting the beginning and end of each session, recording the duration of periods of apnea, if present, and reporting time of last observed breath to the nurse who pronounces death. A nurse's watch can be worn on a lanyard, fob, or collar, designed to be hands-free and right-side-up when looking down from above. Some are made of silicone, which is ideal for cleaning. Watches are available for military or civilian time. Check reviews to find one that doesn't tick too loudly. Sound can feel magnified during a quiet massage session.

companies) is usually adequate for one to two sessions of partial-body massage; a larger person or a person with extremely dry skin will require more lotion. The container will be discarded if all lotion is used during the session or left behind with the patient or family if there is lotion remaining. I carry two containers into every session in case the family requests extra for later use.

A practical consideration when choosing a lubricant is cost. Price per ounce, shipping costs, the amount of product required to achieve results, and the ease of extracting every last ounce from the container are all part of the calculation.

Heads up 3.3. When patients provide their own products

Patients sometimes wish to provide their own products for massage, due to allergies, sentimental attachment to lotion that was a gift, or enduring habit. My approach is to accommodate these preferences and to be open to learning about them. Gloves can be worn if the therapist has sensitivities or concerns about exposures to these products.

A growing number of people are using marijuana-infused topicals that contain cannabidiol (CBD) or tetrahydrocannabinol (THC). Touch therapists should be prepared for clients to request the use of these products for massage. Laws and medical evidence are constantly changing, requiring therapists to stay abreast of accepted practices in their areas.

Managing supplies

Whether you work in homes, group homes, or inpatient settings, you'll need to divide your supplies into two sets. The first set is akin to a stationary or portable closet, containing bulk materials. The second is a small subset of the bulk materials which are needed to provide a

Tip 3.3. Warming lotion

There is nothing less soothing for someone who is sick than cold lotion! A single-serve lotion container can be warmed in the microwave with the lid off for a few seconds (start with 6 seconds, stir lotion with a coffee stirrer, and test the temperature on your inner arm). Another solution is an electric lunch kit or portable oven, such as the HOTLOGIC® Mini or RoadPro®. The Mini reaches a temperature of 165°F (74°C), which plastic cups can tolerate for a couple of hours (then they can be unplugged to "rest" for a little while). This product is also available with an adapter for use in the car. The cloth cover can be separated from the heating element for gentle washing as needed.

single session. The second set is what you'll carry into the patient's home or room.

Anything carried from one patient environment to another has the potential to transmit pathogens. Streamlining what you carry into each session can therefore mitigate risk of infection. It is better to put lotion or cream into a single-serve cup with a lid rather than a large pump bottle that is used for multiple patients. Any item carried between patients must be thoroughly sanitized.

Because material management varies from outpatient to inpatient settings, supplies are described below for each of these situations. If you work for an agency, many of the materials you need may be supplied for you. Items will vary according to local norms, along with the therapist's preferences and work habits. Therapists should tailor the lists below to their needs.

Supplies for home and group home visits

Your larger cache of materials will remain in your car, referred to in some agencies as "car stock." Car stock can

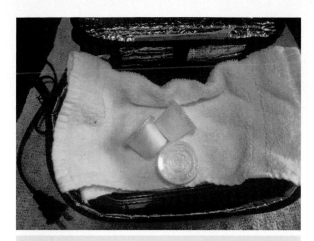

Figure 3.9
A folded washcloth is used above in the Mini portable oven to absorb and distribute heat. A thicker cream or oil will hold up better to warming than a thinner lotion, which may become watery.

(Photo by author.)

be placed in a bin or tub with a lid. You'll need a separate bin or bag for soiled materials. Soiled materials must be covered with a lid or clip that holds the top of the bag together. A prevailing principle is that *clean stays with clean* and *dirty stays with dirty*.

Suggested car-stock supplies

- Bulk lubricant.
- Topical analgesic, optional (see p. 110).
- Small collapsible stool and/or knee pad (such as gardeners use).
- Single-serve disposable containers with lids, available from restaurant supply companies.
- Long spatula, if needed, for transferring semisolid lubricant into single-serve containers.
- Gloves, facemasks, disposable gowns.
- Disposable shoe or foot covers, for homes that request shoes be covered or removed.

- Liquid soap for refilling travel-size bottle.
- Antiseptic gel for refilling travel-size bottle.
- Sanitizing wipes.
- Paper towels.
- Lint roller for pet hair.
- Aromatherapy supplies, optional (see Chapter 10).
- Nail clippers and file.
- Breath mints.
- Cough drops.
- Dryer sheets, dry shampoo, and/or change of clothing (see Tip 3.4).
- Chux, "blueys," or other waterproof pads (see Tip 3.5).
- Clean aprons, one per patient, optional.
- Self-heating glove pads or hand warmers, optional but nice in cold climates.
- Intake forms, brochures, and/or patient information, if used by your agency.
- Cell phone or tablet for entering data and/or connecting to the agency.

I also have the following items in my car:

- Note pad and pen to record mileage, time of arrival/departure, and brief notes.
- Water bottle (for drinking).
- Water jug with spout (for handwashing when needed).
- Snacks.
- Self-care items (see p. 47).

Carry-in items for home and group home visits

- 2 single-serve containers of lubricant.
- 1 single-serve container of topical analgesic, if using.
- 2 pairs of gloves.

- 1 facemask.

- 1 gown or apron, if needed.

- 1 folded waterproof pad.

- Small scissors (see Figure 4.1, p. 57).

- Hand hygiene kit in a plastic bag: 2 folded paper towels and a travel-size bottle of liquid soap.

- Travel-size bottle of antiseptic gel or foam.

- Single-use aromatherapy, optional (see Chapter 10).

- Small bottle of essential oil, if desired, to manage the presence of strong odors.

- Reading glasses if needed (see Heads up 8.3, p. 150).

- Cough drop.

- Cell phone in a plastic bag, to play music if desired or to place a call if needed.

How you carry these items needs to be considered carefully. A bag, purse, tote, or backpack that is set down while

---

Tip 3.4. Managing odors

It is not unusual to provide massage where odors are present from smoking, pets, or other sources, including patient wounds. One tip for managing these during the session is to place a few drops of essential oil directly under your nostrils or on the inside of a facemask. For lingering odors that might impact other patients on your schedule, weather permitting, roll down the windows while driving to your next client. Some therapists keep plant-based dryer sheets on hand, which can be rubbed over hair, clothing, and shoes. Even better is a fresh change of clothes. A quick application of an eco-friendly dry shampoo can help if odor clings to hair. Just beware of masking odors with another strong smell that might be just as offensive to your next patient.

---

you are working will be contaminated by the chair, bed, tray table, or floor. One solution is to use a disposable pad as a barrier; see Tip 3.5. Another option is to use a wearable bag, such as a fanny pack, waist pack, or HipKlip™ (which attaches to the waistband of any pant or skirt). A wearable bag prevents contamination because the bag remains on the body of the therapist rather than being set on a surface. A large HipKlip™ or fanny pack will easily hold sufficient carry-in items for a single session.

Dispose of or leave behind single-use items such as open lotion containers, used gloves, and/or disposable pads. Wash hands thoroughly if possible prior to leaving the patient's home, using your own supplies as needed; use hand sanitizer if immediate washing isn't possible. After you depart the home and arrive at your car, remove your dirty apron if wearing, folding dirty sides together, and place the soiled apron inside a bag or bin for dirty materials. Wipe down exposed items (your phone, if you took it out, stool or knee pad if used, and travel-size containers of soap or gel, if accessed inside the home). One more good squirt of hand sanitizer, record mileage and visit time, reload your carry-in supplies, and you're on your way to your next patient.

Supplies in the inpatient setting

Supplies are less complicated in an inpatient setting where materials are readily accessible. You will still need a cache of bulk materials to be stored in a designated space. Space is often at a premium in facilities, so you may have to be creative and flexible. A closet, cupboard, or locker will suffice.

Store bulk supplies in whatever container fits the available space: a bin, tub, or reusable shopping bag with handles. A clip can be used to keep the top of the bag closed so that contents are protected. You'll need a separate bin or bag for dirty aprons, if you use them, with a lid or clip to keep dirty laundry covered and isolated. A list of suggested bulk and carry-in items for inpatient settings appears below.

As with home visits, any items carried from one patient environment to another will need to be thoroughly cleaned.

It is therefore better to carry minimal items into each session. I confine a small number of carry-in items to pockets, since much of what I need is available in the patient's room. I don't carry my cell phone into the room since a call light is available for help if needed.

Locker/cupboard supplies for inpatient settings

- Bulk lubricant.
- Topical analgesic, optional (see p. 110).
- Single-serve disposable containers with lids.
- Long spatula, if needed for transferring semisolid lubricant into single-serve containers.
- Lint roller for pet hair, if pets are allowed in the setting.
- Aromatherapy supplies, optional.
- Nail clippers and file.
- Breath mints, cough drops.
- Clean aprons, one per patient, optional.
- Note pad and pen or pencil to record session times and brief notes.
- Self-care items (described below).

Carry-in items for inpatient visits

- 2 single-serve containers of lubricant.
- 1 single-serve container of topical analgesic, if desired.
- Gloves, if your preferred gloves aren't stocked in the patient's room.
- Small scissors (see Figure 4.1, p. 57).
- Single-dose aromatherapy, optional.

Supplies for self-care

Whether working in the field or onsite, I find it helpful to have access to spiritual-care items during my workday. By spiritual care, I mean the care of the spirit. What helps each of us to care for our spirits will vary, but I include here some ideas to help you begin to think about what

Tip 3.5. Tricks with "chux," also known as "blueys"

Chux was originally a brand name for disposable underpads developed in the early 1940s. The brand is not sold anymore, but the name "chux" is still commonly used in the US to refer to an absorbent sheet of fluff between two layers of waterproof material, often placed under patients with urinary or bowel incontinence. The equivalent term in Australia is "bluey." Nurses also use these pads at our IPU to loosely bandage a large wound or a weeping limb. Chux are one of my favorite multitasking tools because they can be used for the following purposes:

- To set underneath items carried into the patient's home or room. Once the session is done, pick up your belongings and remember to dispose of the pad onsite.

- As a barrier if you must lean into the patient's bed to reach them. This provides protection and a sense of boundary for the patient and reduces contamination from one setting to the next.

- Under a wet compress or other hydrotherapy to keep the bed dry (see Chapter 10).

- Underneath an area of the body on which you're working, to protect furniture from lotion.

Chux and blueys vary in quality. They are typically made from cellulose and bamboo and are considered to be biodegradable. A word of warning: one of our IPU nurses was shaking out a chux pad when it broke, releasing fibers that caused respiratory irritation. Handle these products gently so they remain intact.

might help you in those moments, in the midst of comforting others, when you might need to comfort your*self.*

I have a small but beautiful bag which I purchased while traveling many years ago. The bag is slightly tattered, but meaningful to me. I encourage you to think about the container in which you store your self-care supplies. These items are to be honored and treated with respect and gratitude.

My self-care bag includes bergamot and frankincense, two essential oils which are very calming to me. I carry mala beads, used in many traditions for meditative practices. Holding each bead, I inhale and exhale. There are 108 beads, and I find that it takes about 10 minutes to work my way around the string. I carry a small card with Frank Ostaseski's five precepts for work with the dying (2017), a beautiful handkerchief in case of tears, and a few facial towelettes to freshen up. When I'm on the road, my self-care occurs in the privacy of my car or whatever outdoor area I can access. At the IPU, I visit our beautiful chapel. I don't often need these supplies, but I find it's comforting just to know they are there.

Referral and intake

The relationship between a touch therapist and a client typically begins with an intake protocol in which the client provides a written or oral history, and the therapist has an opportunity to ask clarifying questions. This history often includes past injuries, surgeries, major illnesses, medications, and details regarding current complaints. The intake process may be lengthy, especially for clients with cancer and other medical conditions.

At the end of life, the intake process, like every other aspect of our care, must be adjusted for the dying person's energy level and capacity in the moment. The information acquired during intake remains important, but the details on which we focus are slightly different. Medical history tells the story of the patient's arrival at this moment, including the physical and emotional scars that may have a bearing on the session. But time is short, and

energy for communication may be waning or even impossible. In this context, history is often less relevant than what is happening today in this moment for this person.

That said, the touch therapist will require some information about the patient prior to a first session. This can be accomplished through access to the patient's medical chart, or a referral form that contains the most pertinent information. At the very least, a referral form should include the following:

- Patient's name, age, and date of birth.

- Patient's location and how best to reach the patient (address, phone number, and anything the therapist needs to know regarding particulars of the location).

- Primary caregiver's name, phone number, and relationship to the patient.

- Patient's primary diagnosis.

- Additional or secondary diagnoses, including history of cancer or other concurring conditions that might impact the touch session.

- Symptom(s), goals, or reasons for the massage referral.

- Psychosocial information, if available.

How this information is acquired will depend on your setting and whether you are a private therapist, a therapist contracted by an agency, or an employee. Who is it that initiates the referral? Is a doctor's order required, and if so, what is the process for obtaining the order? In many agencies, the nurse initiates the referral and acquires a doctor's order for a massage therapy assessment. The assessment is a first visit in which a trial of massage is provided, during which the therapist observes the patient's response and determines whether future visits are likely to be helpful. If the patient is determined to be a good candidate for ongoing service, you will likely need a protocol for advising the nurse or doctor of your intended care plan, including frequency of visits.

The intake process, like all aspects of the session, must be adjusted to the patient's energy level to avoid placing additional demand on the dying person. A primary care-giver or nurse may be able to provide useful information over the telephone, at the nurses' station, or at the bedside. Access to the patient's medical chart is extremely helpful, though its contents can seem like a foreign language for many of us (Chapters 6–9 offer some translation). The therapist must also become adept at eliciting information through observation, along with patient input, both verbal and nonverbal. This is all part of the patient assessment that begins with the first visit and continues at each visit thereafter.

Conclusion

Chapter 3 has focused on skills, safety, and supplies. Skills for end-of-life massage involve the informed application of massage techniques (effleurage, petrissage, compression, use of a comforting mother hand, and holds), all delivered with deep, caring presence. Massage pressure and duration of the session must be adapted so as not to place additional demand on the body which is engaged in the work of dying. Other safety measures include impeccable hand hygiene, and the possible use of gloves and other PPE. Adherence to airborne, droplet, and contact precautions is required when indicated. Touch therapists must become familiar with these practices in the specific settings where they work.

Functional work clothes and a quality lubricant are the mainstays of our supplies. Therapists will organize these and other items according to the setting in which they work, aiming to carry as little as possible into the patient environment. Good training, proper supplies, and key background on the patient will prepare touch therapists to arrive at the massage session with the "right stuff."

References

Adderton, J., 2019. *Home oxygen deaths higher in U.S.* Available at: <https://allnurses.com/home-oxygen-deaths-higher-u-t708668>.

Centers for Disease Control and Prevention (CDC), 2016. *Standard precautions for all patient care.* Available at: <https://www.cdc.gov/infectioncontrol/basics/standard-precautions.html>.

Centers for Disease Control and Prevention (CDC), 2019. *Guideline for isolation precautions: preventing transmission of infectious agents in healthcare settings.* [pdf] Available at: <https://www.cdc.gov/infectioncontrol/pdf/guidelines/isolation-guidelines-H.pdf>.

Edsberg, L. E. et al., 2016. Revised national pressure ulcer advisory panel: pressure injury staging system. *Journal of Wound, Ostomy, and Continence Nursing*, [e-journal] 43(6), pp. 585–597. Available at: <https://www.ncbi.nlm.nih.gov/pmc/articles/PMC5098472/pdf/wocn-43-585.pdf>.

Hartman, V., 2009, 2012. Circle of life: hospice and palliative massage workshops. Dallas training notes, Concord training notes.

MacDonald, G., 2014. *Medicine hands: massage therapy for people with cancer.* 3rd ed. Findhorn, Scotland: Findhorn Press.

MacDonald, G. and Tague, C., 2021. *Hands in health care: massage therapy for the adult hospital patient.* 2nd ed. Edinburgh: Handspring Publishing.

McGlone, F. et al., 2014. Discriminative and affective touch: sensing and feeling. *Neuron*, [e-journal] 82(4), pp. 737–755. Available at: <http://dx.doi.org/10.1016/j.neuron.2014.05.001>.

Medical Dictionary for the Health Professions and Nursing, 2012. *Cachexia.* [online] Available at: <https://medical-dictionary.thefreedictionary.com/cachexia>.

NHS, 2020. *Home oxygen therapy.* [online] Available at: <https://www.nhs.uk/conditions/home-oxygen-treatment>.

NHS England, 2018. *'The gloves are off' campaign.* [online] Available at: <https://www.england.nhs.uk/atlas_case_study/the-gloves-are-off-campaign>.

Ostaseski, F., 2017. *The five invitations: discovering what death can teach us about fully living.* New York: Flatiron Books.

Chapter 3

Tisserand Institute, n.d. *How to use essential oils safely.* [online] Available at: <https://tisserandinstitute.org/safety-guidelines>.

Walton, T., 2011. *Medical conditions and massage therapy: a decision tree approach.* Baltimore: Lippincott Williams & Wilkins.

Walton, T., 2013. *A healthy dose of hospital-based massage therapy.* [online] Available at: https://www.tracywalton.com/a-healthy-dose-of-massage-in-hospital-based-massage-therapy.

Werner, R., 2019. A massage therapist's guide to pathology: critical thinking and practical application. 7th ed. Boulder, CO: Books of Discovery.

Approach the dying person not with answers but with openness.

–Andrew Holecek

It's taken a lot of preparation and information to get to this point. We've acquired knowledge and skills, assembled supplies, and put thought into mundane details such as what to wear, what to carry, and where to set it down. We've received introductory data about a person with a serious illness, including a name, age, and terminal diagnosis. We may have access to this person's medical chart, potentially a long clinical story with details that must be sifted and sorted for our use. It can feel like a lot to hold.

I now invite you to take a deep breath. And as you exhale, I encourage you to *let go*. Let go of the facts and assumptions that might be churning in your brain, so that you can create space for the moment you are about to enter. It is not that skills or knowledge are unimportant, only that we must find a way to hold this information loosely in the back of our minds. For we are about to meet someone who will tell us what we *really* need to know. We must slow down, so that we can listen very carefully.

The kind of listening that we bring to the bedside of the dying involves all our senses, not just the ears. We are perceiving with our very being. If a common language is available, words can help. But we must also listen deeply for unspoken responses that transcend words. We are listening for receptivity to touch or lack thereof. Interpreting the input we receive to the best of our ability, we must determine how to proceed. And then we keep listening for input to guide our next step, and the next.

Chapter 4 will bring this process into focus, with practical suggestions for meeting the client and carrying out the session. Ideas for positioning clients comfortably will be presented, with photos to illustrate various possibilities. A tool for physical assessment of the patient is described, along with ideas regarding the massage sequence, care for caregivers, and tips for working in homes, group homes, and inpatient settings.

There is no one "right way" to do most of the above. After many years of practice, I am still learning and improving the way I do things. This process is delightfully nonlinear. Some of my evolution has been trial and error, such as the words I use to introduce the massage session to patients and families. Many lessons have been passed on to me by others, like the "Princess Leia" head scroll. And some of my learning has been serendipitous, such as the day I put my gloves in my lotion warmer to carry them upstairs and discovered that warm gloves are lovely for patients *and* for the therapist! Chapter 4 presents a collection of this wisdom, tried and true. You will no doubt make your own delightful discoveries, as you too listen and learn.

Meeting, greeting, and communicating with patients and families

Entering the space

Slowing down begins at the threshold of the dying person's space. Whether home, a room in a group home, or an inpatient hospice or hospital room, this space belongs to the patient and we are a guest. A deep breath helps us to cross this threshold with respect and mindful submission to the unknown. From a place of not knowing, we can enter the patient's environment with openness and curiosity. There is no room for an agenda or ego in this moment.

Irene Smith describes the process of pausing to read the room. This requires, she says, that the therapist stop, listen, and observe. What is the energy of the people who are present? Is there receptivity to your visit right now? Is there activity occurring that suggests a need for privacy? If so, can you take a step back and wait until that activity is completed? Where is the patient situated, and what are the points of access for massage? The pause, says Smith, allows the therapist to get a feel for the dynamics already present in the space and to assess how they might enter "without a sense of intrusion" (Smith, 2017).

The speed with which we enter this space sets the gauge for the remainder of the session, including our movements around the room, our speech, and the speed of our strokes. Countless caregivers observing massage at the bedside have shared that even watching the work is very relaxing. As the patient's nervous system begins to settle, the caregiver's may follow suit. It is often said that one calm person in the room can change everything.

Touching story 4.1. Please slow down

I was new in this work when I arrived at the home of a patient whose elderly wife was the sole caretaker. The home was modest, and the patient's wife had a humble demeanor. The patient was comatose and frail, and the wife asked me if I could help reposition him in bed.

I had no hands-on experience with the use of a draw sheet at that time. I remember feeling nervous but attempting to project an air of competence. I grabbed two corners of the draw sheet on one side of the bed as I'd seen the aides do, pulling the sheet taut and waiting for the wife to do the same on the other side. And then the caregiver, whose name I don't remember but whose face I'll never forget, uttered these words to me: "You're moving too fast. You need to slow down." I felt my cheeks grow red as I muttered "sorry," and surrendered to a lesson

from someone whose wisdom and skill far surpassed my own.

Watching the woman and syncing my motions with hers, I lost my urge to hurry. I observed that repositioning the patient was not a precursor to care, but an essential part of care, in which respect and security are conveyed through calm, mindful movement. The experience changed forever how I move when I'm with a patient. From the moment I enter the space until I exit, my goal is to cause as little disturbance to the air molecules as possible. I endeavor, as my friend Susan Gee likes to say, to be the calm person in the room.

Introductions and consent

Informed consent, one of the cornerstones of ethical care, is straightforward when a patient can communicate with the therapist, or when a loved one can speak on behalf of a patient's known preferences. But this is not always the case at the end of life. The patient may be unable to speak and the family may be absent, or family may be present but have no idea how a patient would feel about massage. Even a patient who has enjoyed massage previously can experience a change in desire for touch. Consent is an ongoing inquiry *each time* massage is offered.

Good communication begins at eye level, sitting close to the patient, if possible. The patient is the center of the encounter and should be addressed directly, even if that person is nonverbal and others are present. This seems obvious but can take effort if others in the room are referring to the patient as "he," "she," or "they." When this occurs, I try to bring the patient into the conversation with comments such as, "You have a beautiful family," "I can tell that you are very loved," or "we are talking about what might feel good to you today." Whether the patient is able to speak or not, they are present and listening. I typically ask what name the patient likes to be called, and I use this preferred name when speaking to them.

Patients and caregivers may have questions or anxieties about how the session will work. I have learned that the word "massage" is not always helpful, as massage means different things to different people. What I offer instead is to apply some warm lotion to the skin. Most patients and caregivers are receptive to this offer, as the skin is nearly always dry at the end of life. I explain that the recipient does not need to undress or change position if they are comfortable. I clarify that the work is very gentle and so relaxing that many people fall asleep or remain sleeping through the session. I describe the areas of the body I might reach in the patient's current position, typically the neck, shoulders, arms, hands, legs, and feet, depending on what would feel good to them. The explanation is brief and to the point.

I use the same basic script, regardless of whether the patient can communicate verbally, and regardless of whether a caregiver is present. When patients are alone and unable to speak for themselves, I tell them where I plan to start by saying, "I'm going to caress your forehead very gently," or "I'm going to hold your hand and shoulder." I always hold the hand from underneath rather than covering the hand, which can feel confining. These noninvasive, respectful overtures are a form of requesting "tactile consent."

It may seem to therapists that we are relying on our intuition in this process. Intuition is a guide and a beginning, but it is not our road map. We must be willing to "trust but verify" our intuition with feedback from the patient. The list of common responses on pp. 68–9 can inform our conclusions regarding receptivity to our touch, or lack thereof. Family at the bedside can be invited to help us watch for these responses, as they know the patient best. Adverse responses should be honored as a message to lighten the pressure, move to a different area of the body, hold, or stop.

Personal note to the reader 4.1. Respecting touch preferences

There are some people who don't care for massage, even of the gentle variety. Touch preferences can be impacted by cultural or family norms, personality, sensory issues, or a history of trauma. Some humans enjoy being touched by people they love, but don't like being touched by strangers. A small percentage have an actual phobia of touch, and others simply prefer to be left alone. When a patient or caregiver declines massage, I try to clarify whether the preference is temporary (in which case they might want massage another day) or permanent (in which case I will document that the service was offered and declined).

At our inpatient unit, massage is offered to all our patients. This means that I am making "cold calls" where patients and families have not necessarily expressed interest in the service. Many have never had a massage before and have no idea what to expect. Others have had massage in the past and have expectations based on that experience. It's important to clarify what you're offering so that the patient knows what they are consenting to or turning down. This is the essence of informed consent.

Most patients and families at our IPU readily consent to massage when the service is described. A few are ambivalent but open to trying the service. I'll check in with them after a minute or two to see if they wish to stop or continue, assuring them that the choice is theirs. Many who are initially doubtful are pleasantly surprised and want to continue the session. A very small minority ask to stop the massage or display signs of increased agitation or pain. A small number decline the service without trying it, in which case I smile and say, "I understand. Is there anything else you need?"

A neutral response to massage, where the nonverbal patient demonstrates little to no observable reaction to being touched, is difficult to interpret and can be responded to in a variety of ways. At our unit, the massage therapists continue seeing patients who tolerate touch, for the benefit of caring presence and lubrication of dry skin. At other agencies, a documented benefit of the service is required for massage to become part of the care plan. Sometimes massage appears to have no impact on the patient but seems important to the family. So long as the patient does not have an adverse response, I am happy to honor the family's wishes.

Communication issues

Many conditions can impact communication, including amyotrophic lateral sclerosis (ALS), Parkinson's, dementia, brain injuries, hearing impairment, and cancers of the head and neck. Communication issues also occur when patients speak a language that is different from the language of the care providers. During the later stages of dying, nearly all patients become impaired in their ability to communicate their needs. They may become nonverbal, or they may remain verbal but unable to be understood. They may grow too weak to produce sound, even with great effort.

A person who cannot communicate their needs is extremely vulnerable. Care providers, including massage therapists, must watch for nonverbal signs that a patient is in pain or other distress. A grimace or frown, rapid respirations, increased heart rate, sweating, writhing, shifting in bed, guarding a body part, reluctance to move, moaning, groaning, and drawing the legs up are examples of possible distress. Sometimes signs are more subtle and require a deeper kind of listening. The therapist's job is to "hear" and discern the patient's needs, as best we can.

Touching story 4.2. The "unresponsive" patient

The RN didn't see much point in massage for the patient. "He's totally unresponsive," she said. Yet the family had requested massage for the man, so I entered his room. The patient was lying supine with his eyes closed. His

hands were curled. He was not moving. He did not respond to the sound of my voice. A visitor sat at the bedside. She did not speak English, so I pointed to my name tag which said, "Massage Therapist," pantomiming my intentions. She nodded her head to indicate consent on the patient's behalf.

I wish I had a video of what happened next.

After I warmed the lotion between my hands, I began to apply it to the patient's arm, moving slowly from his fingertips up the forearm, around the curve of his thin shoulder to the neck. The patient's eyebrows moved up and down, and he exhaled deeply. His curled fingers opened slightly, allowing me to place one of my hands inside his hand. I continued holding his hand, while my other hand gently massaged his upper extremity. The patient's eyebrows kept moving, at the same speed as my hand, it seemed.

The man's mouth fell gently open as I moved to his other arm. His breathing was very slow and relaxed by now. The visitor had moved closer to the bed, quietly observing. The patient occasionally sighed, with a soft sound of release. The massage was like a dance, each stroke inviting a small response, which then helped me know what to do next. When his breathing stopped for a moment, I stopped too, and simply rested my hands on the patient's body, feeling deeply connected with the rise and fall of his chest. Occasionally, I caressed his forehead.

Though it felt as if this choreography went on for a while, the session lasted all of 15 minutes. At the end of the visit, I rested one hand on the man's heart, and the other on the crown of his head. We breathed slowly together – the man, his visitor, and me. We all had our eyes closed by this time. As I slowly stepped away from the bed, the visitor stood and bowed to me. I bowed to her, and to the patient, in deep gratitude and quiet joy and with hardly any words at all.

Adapting the massage session

Communication with the dying and their companions should be guided by the dying person. If the dying person is quiet and others in the room are noisy, the therapist can support the patient by introducing quiet presence at the bedside. Not all patients are quiet or somber, however. Some are desperate for conversation, in which case the therapist can provide a listening ear. Some are humorous, engaging the therapist in playful banter that helps lighten a heavy situation. Part of caring presence is offering space for the dying person to be themselves. Other tips include the following suggestions.

- Slow down and keep it simple. Use brief, simple language to communicate who you are and what care you will be providing.

- Offer your settled nervous system, modeling a quiet, calm voice. If the patient or caregiver is hearing impaired, you may need to move closer or raise your volume.

- If a translation service is used, look at and talk to the patient and family, rather than the translator.

- If no translation is available, use other means to communicate. A friendly smile, pointing at your name badge, showing the patient or family the lotion container, or pantomiming massage to your own arm can convey your intention.

- If a shared language is available and the patient is verbal, offer neutral choices ("Would you like this or that?"). But be mindful of decision fatigue and the effort required for conversation.

- Use level 1 or 2 pressure for patients who are nonverbal, watching closely for nonverbal feedback.

- While eye contact can be a means of communication, it is not respectful in all cultures, or comfortable for all individuals (see Heads up 11.2, p. 203). Be aware of this possibility and follow the patient's or family's lead.

- There may be conversations happening in the room that don't involve you. Don't intrude unless invited.

- Don't be afraid to smile, laugh, or share tears, so long as your responses are consistent with the emotional tenor in the room. Our responses should be supportive rather than needful of attention or support.

- See pp. 168–9 for additional ideas for working with people who have impaired ability to communicate.

- Don't rush to fill a lull in the conversation. Use silence as a third hand.

The assessment

One of the most important tools utilized by clinical professionals is the physical assessment. This involves using the senses to access information about the patient for whom you are about to provide care. The assessment provides input to guide the session and to document the session for other team members. A touch therapist with well-developed assessment skills may be the person to notice something that others have missed.

Two assessment templates are provided in the Appendix of this book. The clinical assessment (on p. 215) is more detailed, intended to support therapists working in clinical environments. The simplified assessment (on p. 217) uses the letters A-B-C-D-E to focus on five key aspects of the patient's condition, an approach that may be helpful for new learners and those practicing in less clinical settings. Both templates are intended to organize the following information in a way that is easy for touch therapists to gather and record. The medical devices mentioned in this section are explained in Chapter 9.

Face, head, and neck

The patient's face provides an indication of their level of arousal and physical comfort. Are the eyes open, partially open, or closed? If the eyes are open, do they track movement or is the gaze fixed? The patient may be sleeping, awake and alert, or awake but groggy. They may be pleasantly confused or distressed with agitation.

If this is not your first visit, how does level of arousal compare to your previous visit? Decreased level of arousal may indicate decline, temporary fatigue, medication, or a change in emotional state (withdrawal or depression, for example). If this is a first visit, the nurse or caregiver might be able to indicate whether the level of arousal you're observing is the patient's baseline, or whether there has been a recent change.

Does the patient's facial expression indicate comfort or distress? Is there swelling of lips or other feature? Any signs of recent injury, including bruises, lacerations, or sutures? Is the patient wearing supplemental oxygen or breathing room air? Are there tubes in the nose, the mouth, or through the neck to support breathing, nutrition, or drainage? If the patient's head is covered, be aware that there may be a hidden injury or tumor. Patients sometimes wear caps to conceal these, though hats are also worn for warmth or modesty.

If the patient is verbal, are they able make their needs known? Is communication impacted by a slow thought process, difficulty finding words, or inability to put words together in a way that can be understood? Is speech slurred, mumbled, or whispered? Is the patient communicating symbolically, referring to travel, needing to "get out of here," "go home," or other common expressions of the dying experience? Communication can be impacted by disease, the dying process, medication, or a combination of factors.

Torso

Is breathing labored at rest, or with movement or conversation? Are the abdominal or accessory muscles being used to help the patient breathe? How fast are respirations? Normal is 12–20 respirations per minute. Is breathing even or erratic? Shallow or deep? Is breathing noisy with congestion or snoring? Are there periods of no breathing (apnea, see p. 98)? How long do the periods of apnea last?

Is the abdomen distended? Abdominal swelling may be due to constipation, tumors, or ascites from heart disease, kidney disease, liver disease, or cancer (see p. 98). The torso may be the site of implanted devices such as a port-a-cath or pacemaker. Are there visible tubes from the torso? These might include devices to empty urine from the kidneys, stool from the intestines, or fluid from the chest or abdomen. The abdomen is also a common site for needle systems to deliver medication.

Extremities

Are the extremities all present? Patients may be missing limbs, toes, or fingers from infection, diabetes, cancer, or congenital causes. Do the limbs appear to have normal tone, and is the patient able to move them? Is any tremor noted? Are there IVs in the arms, hands, or feet? Is there edema from heart disease, kidney disease, liver disease, or cancer? Is there a bracelet indicating a "restricted extremity"?

Are the fingertips clubbed, indicating chronic oxygen deprivation? Is there any discoloration to the extremities? Is toenail fungus present, indicating a need for gloves or avoidance of the area? A full assessment requires removing socks, a judgment call on the part of the therapist. If the patient is cold or actively dying, removal of socks may not be justified.

Are there pieces of jewelry, a hospital band, or elastic that seem too tight? If yes, can the item be removed, or do you need to report this to a caregiver or nursing staff? A bracelet that is meaningful to the patient might be moved to the opposite arm if edema is unilateral. A meaningful ring can be placed on a chain and worn as a necklace. In some cases, bracelets may need to be cut with scissors.

Skin

What is the color, temperature, and quality of the skin? The skin may be pale, flushed, or jaundiced (yellowing of the skin indicates liver involvement; the sclera, or whites of the eyes, can also be jaundiced, known as sclera icterus). Fingertips and lips may have a bluish or cyanotic tint,

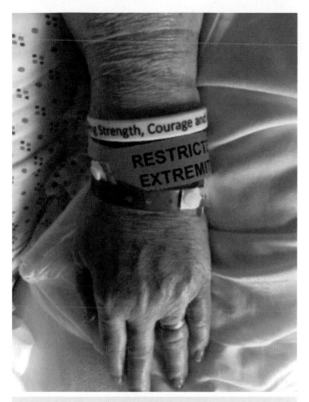

Figure 4.1
An example of edema causing jewelry to become too tight. Note the indentations on the skin above the bracelets. Two bands were removed with scissors, but it was too late to remove the ring.

(Photo by author.)

whitish, or "ashy." Look for rashes, abrasions, or scratch marks which might indicate pruritus, or itching. Lips are included in the skin assessment. Are they dry or cracked?

Is there skin-to-skin contact that is causing a breakdown in skin integrity? A common place for this to occur is between the heels when they are touching. Can a rolled washcloth be placed between skin surfaces to protect them?

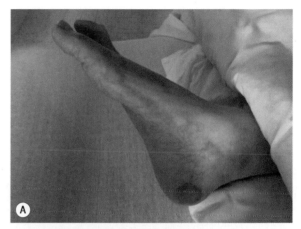

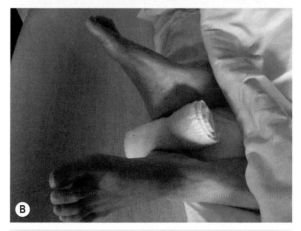

Figure 4.2
(A) Note the blister on the patient's heel where his heels had skin-to-skin contact. (B) The feet were gently separated, and a rolled washcloth placed between them to protect the skin from further breakdown.

(Photos by author.)

indicating low oxygen. A discolored (dark) band around the calves, with or without cool temperature, may indicate vascular disease. Reddened areas over bony prominences may foreshadow pressure injuries and should be reported to a nurse, along with rashes, blisters, or signs of infection not previously noted in the medical history.

Is there bruising or bleeding? Are there visible wounds such as skin tears, blisters, lacerations or pressures sores, or bandages that might be covering injuries? Are there surgical wounds, scars, or radiation burns? Is the skin dry? Is there surface peeling, flaking, or cracking? Dry skin in people with darker skin tones may appear dull, chalky, gray,

Assessing symptoms

Does the patient communicate the presence of symptoms? If verbal, ask "how is your pain right now?" Use the Edmonton scale to rate pain on a scale of 0–10 if the patient is willing and able, 0 indicating no pain and 10 indicating the most extreme pain imaginable. The Edmonton scale can also be used to rate shortness of breath, nausea, anxiety, or any other symptom.

If the patient is nonverbal, distress may be communicated by facial expression (furrowed brow, grimace, or frown). Grimace might be present at rest, or only when the patient moves. Other signs of distress include respirations faster than 20 per minute; restlessness, as if they can't get comfortable; sweating; and moaning, groaning, or crying out. Emotional symptoms are every bit as important as physical symptoms. The patient's demeanor, or affect, might be subdued, depressed, distraught, pleasant, or impossible to read. Severe symptoms are unlikely to respond to massage alone. Work with the patient or caregiver, if present, to determine whether the RN should be advised of symptoms. If in doubt, report your observations to clinical staff.

With practice, the assessment won't take more than a minute or two. Most observations can be accomplished while simultaneously entering the space and engaging with the people in it. Others may come to light as the session progresses. The assessment is a nonjudgmental form of perceiving which becomes second nature with practice.

Positioning and propping

Touch therapists will encounter people in a variety of positions based on comfort, activity level, and stage of decline. They may be seated on a chair, sofa, recliner, or wheelchair, or they may be lying in a hospital bed or a home bed of variable size. Massage can be provided in any of these locations, all of which can be made more comfortable, for both the patient and the therapist, with the use of pillows and other props.

The principles of good propping for the patient are akin to the precepts of restorative yoga, in which "the bones feel supported" so that the muscles can relax (Clark, 2015). This can be accomplished by filling empty space, such that

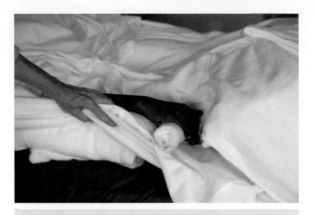

Figure 4.3
An example of filling space. A rolled washcloth provides support for the natural curve of the fingers, while folded towels placed under the fitted sheet are shaped to provide a supportive "nest" for the arms.

(Photo by Candice White.)

every part of the body has a surface to rest on. Another general principle of positioning is mindful smoothing and tucking. Patients on crumpled sheets can experience discomfort related to something as simple as a wrinkle or fold that causes skin irritation.

Positioning in the following pages will be divided into seated massage, reclining massage, and massage in bed, with a sidebar addressing the use of massage tables.

Heads up 4.1. What about massage tables for end-of-life massage?

Some massage tables are designed for portability by virtue of their slim design and light weight, such that they could be carried into a home environment. So why don't I use my portable table more often?

There are a number of drawbacks to the use of massage tables at the end of life. Many home hospice environments are crammed with equipment, making it difficult to find space for a table. A table that is carried from one patient setting to another must be thoroughly cleaned between uses. Careful handling of contaminated linen is also required, not to mention laundry at the end of the workday. But the biggest deterrents for me are concern about safe transfers and having to wake the patient at the end of a relaxing session. I prefer to provide massage wherever the patient is found or feels most comfortable sleeping, typically a recliner or bed. I use materials found in the home for propping, so there's nothing to carry in, remove, clean, or carry out.

There are patients who have a strong preference for a massage table as a way to normalize the massage experience. If you are willing to provide this experience, it can be nice during early decline so long as fall risk is managed. Stay near, or have a caregiver stay near, while the patient transfers on and off the table.

The principle of supporting the bones and filling space is just as applicable when using a massage table. A vinyl bolster under the knees will not suffice for comfort; use soft pillows instead. Many people with advanced disease are unable to lie flat, so you may need to create a means to elevate the head of the table. Prone (or face-down) positioning is rarely tolerated by people with advanced disease due to shortness of breath, abdominal swelling, nausea, or medical devices and tubes.

If you continue working with the patient over time, the patient will likely decline to the point that a table is no longer safe or appropriate. When this time comes, most patients are pleased to find that massage feels just as good in a recliner or bed as it does on a table.

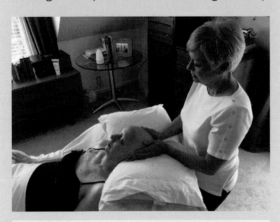

Figure 4.4
Adapted use of a massage table for this patient involved building up the head of the table to accommodate shortness of breath. Several pillows were squeezed under the fitted sheet to hold them in place, with a final pillow for the patient's head.

(Photo by author.)

Personal note to the reader 4.2. Propping ourselves

It was Irene Smith who enlightened me that propping is not just for the patient. Focusing on patient comfort to the exclusion of our own is not a sustainable way to work. I've also observed that empathic patients are keenly aware of whether *we* are comfortable. Their concern about us can keep them from fully relaxing.

Every therapist has preferred and habitual ways of working. Some of these preferences are ergonomically sound, others could likely be improved. As a precursor to specific positions for the patient, I invite you to consider the following questions:

- Do you prefer to work sitting or standing?

- If you prefer to stand, can the patient's body be raised to the right height for your comfort? If not, would sitting be better for this session?

- If you prefer to sit, what are the surfaces available to you? Is there a chair nearby, or one that can easily be moved to the bedside? Do you need to carry a portable stool? A stool carried from one patient setting to the next will need to be sanitized between uses but this may be worth the effort.

- If sitting, are you having to lean toward the patient? If you are leaning, can you move closer, or can you move the patient's body part closer to you?

- Would the use of a pillow under your arms allow your shoulders to relax?

- Would a pillow behind your back be helpful?

Attention to our own comfort at the bedside will increase the quality, longevity, and pleasure of our work.

Seated massage (chair, sofa, wheelchair, edge of bed)

Many people at the end of life are still *living*. Sitting on a chair or sofa allows them to be upright for eating, working, visiting with others, engaging in hobbies and legacy projects, watching television, reading, solving puzzles, and countless other activities. Sitting also provides a break from the confinement of bed, which lifts the spirits and protects the skin from pressure injuries (though it's important to know that pressure injuries can also result from prolonged sitting). In the case of a wheelchair, an additional benefit is mobility, allowing a physically impaired person to access more of the world. See p. 166 for more on wheelchairs.

Upright seated massage

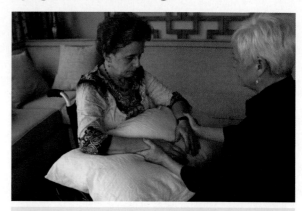

Figure 4.5
In this photo, the therapist is sitting on a stool to massage the hands and arms. A pillow in the patient's lap supports the upper extremities. When using a wheelchair, be sure to lock the wheels.

(Photo by Pamela Robison.)

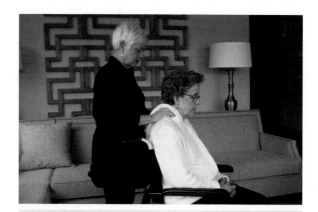

Figure 4.6
An advantage of seated massage is access to the back of the body. It is typically comfortable for the therapist to stand behind the chair or wheelchair to massage the head, neck, and shoulders. Patients who are able may lean forward slightly for massage to the lower back. Therapists must monitor seated patients at all times for signs of fatigue.

(Photo by Pamela Robison.)

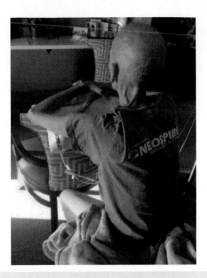

Figure 4.7

This variation on upright seated position provides excellent access to the back. The patient sat on the edge of her bed, supporting her arms on a chair. With the patient's permission, the therapist sat on the patient's bed behind her, using a disposable chux pad as a barrier. An empty pillowcase was used to protect the chair from lotion.

(Photo by author.)

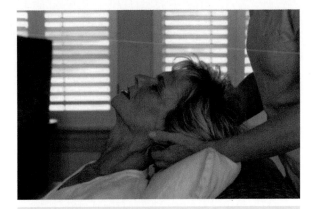

Figure 4.9

Standing behind the sofa is the easiest way to access the patient's head and neck. A small pillow or rolled towel can be used behind the neck for additional support if needed. If the sofa is pushed against the wall, the head and neck will be accessed from either side of the patient.

(Photo by Corrie Coleman.)

Massage in seated forward fold

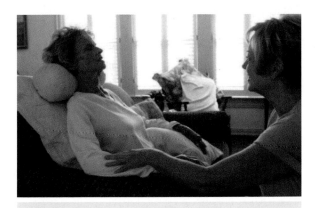

Figure 4.8

In this home session, the patient sat at one end of a sofa; a second armrest was created with a folded pillow. A pillow and neck roll provided good alignment and support for the patient's head and neck. The therapist sat on an ottoman that happened to be available.

(Photo by Corrie Coleman.)

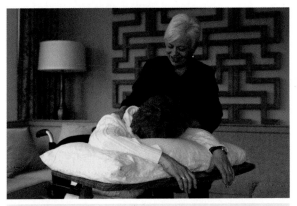

Figure 4.10

A forward-leaning position for accessing the entire back and upper hips can be created with an adjustable tray table and pillow. The patient can lean forward to rest, turning the head toward the left or right. One word of caution: consider the size of the patient and the stability of the tray to bear the patient's weight.

(Photo by Pamela Robison.)

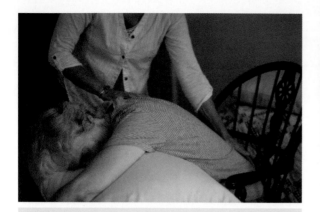

Figure 4.11
Another version of forward-leaning position in the home environment. The patient is seated in a chair, using a TV tray and pillow to support her upper body. As mentioned on the previous page (Figure 4.10), care must be taken not to exceed the weight-bearing capacity of the tray.

(Photo by Candice White.)

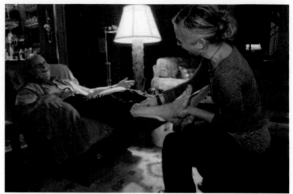

Figure 4.12
The recliner in this photo is covered with a large towel to protect upholstery from massage lotion.

(Photo by David Spence.)

Reclining massage (home recliner or geri chair)

A recliner is an excellent place to give and receive massage, providing superior patient comfort and ample access for the therapist. Many people find their recliners so comfortable that they sleep in them, especially if they have shortness of breath. A geri chair is a clinical version of a recliner, often found in inpatient environments and sometimes in homes.

Recliners and geri chairs provide excellent access to the feet and legs, with the therapist sitting on an ottoman or stool. The stool can be moved to either side of the chair to access upper extremities, shoulders, and neck. If the area behind the recliner or geri chair is accessible, the therapist may prefer to reach the patient's head, neck, and shoulders from behind as shown in Figure 4.6.

Massage in bed

Home beds

Most beds are pushed against a wall on one or more sides. The height of the bed is fixed. One side of the body will be

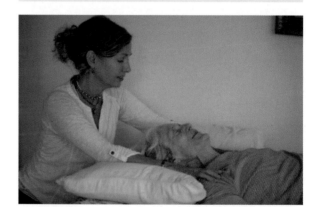

Figure 4.13
This twin bed was in a corner of the room, blocking access to one side and the head. The patient was able to lie with her head at the foot of the bed, providing access to the upper body. A portable stool and resting forearms on the patient's pillow made the experience comfortable for the therapist.

(Photo by Candice White.)

easy to reach, but the other side will be difficult unless the patient repositions midsession, which isn't always possible. Therapists must get creative and make the best of things. If the bed is tall, the therapist might work in a standing position; if the bed is low, sitting will be more comfortable. The patient will be either supine (face-up) or side-lying.

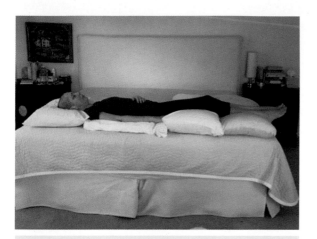

Figure 4.14
This patient was positioned crosswise at the end of a king-size bed to allow access to three sides of the body. The therapist used a portable stool to provide massage to the feet, right side of the body, head, and neck. With assistance, the client repositioned midsession with her head at the opposite side of the bed, providing access to the left side of the body. Note how propping was used to fill every contour.

(Photo by author.)

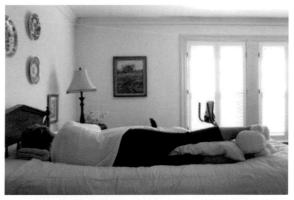

Figure 4.15
Side-lying alignment, using a folded towel under the patient's head, pillows under top arm and top leg, and a neck roll between the feet.

(Photo by Corrie Coleman.)

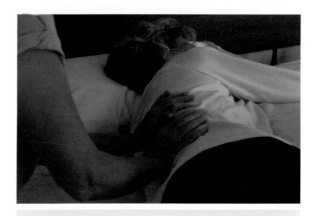

Figure 4.16
Back massage in side-lying position. The patient's top (or right) upper and lower extremities are also accessible. This bed was high enough that the therapist was comfortable in a standing position.

(Photo by Corrie Coleman.)

Side-lying position offers access to the back of the body and is very comfortable for some people. The general rule for propping is to support the spine in a straight line. This will generally require the bottom leg to be straight, the top leg to be bent at a comfortable angle, a pillow to be placed under the top leg, and another pillow under the top arm. If the legs are long and the top foot dangles, it will need an additional pillow for support. Patients who experience the difference a pillow or two can make in side-lying position tend to be amazed.

Hospital beds

Hospital beds, available in facilities and in many homes at the end of life, offer the same options for positioning as a regular bed with several advantages. The head of the bed (HOB) can be raised to facilitate respiration, while the foot can be raised to support the low back or to elevate lower extremities. For the therapist's comfort, bed height can be adjusted, and the narrow width of the bed allows better access to both sides of the patient's body. Despite these benefits, some patients resist the use of a hospital bed (see p. 167 for more on this topic). The heads of hospital beds are often pushed against a wall, and some have a headboard that cannot be removed. The solution is to work from the side of the patient.

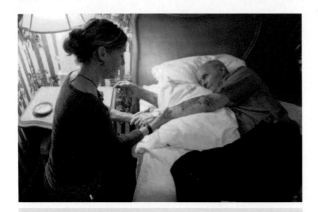

Figure 4.17
Side-lying massage can also be provided with the patient facing the therapist, which allows access to the top extremities from the front side of the body. The bottom arm can either be bent underneath the pillow or straight as shown above, depending on patient preference.

(Photo by David Spence.)

Most people in a hospital bed assume some variation of a semi-supine or Fowler's position, named for American surgeon George Fowler and known in nursing care as the "standard patient's position." In Fowler's position, the HOB is inclined at an angle of 30 to 45 degrees. In low Fowler's position, often preferred for sleeping, the HOB is barely elevated at a 15- to 30-degree angle. In high Fowler's, the HOB is more upright at 45 to 90 degrees, which is best for eating and drinking. People with cardiac or lung conditions often require high Fowler's position at all times.

A disadvantage of Fowler's position is pressure on the sacrum, making the patient more prone to pressure ulcers in this vulnerable area. Nurses often place a pillow under one of the hips to create a supported (or "off-loaded") leaning position. The sacrum can also be "floated" by placing pillows under both hips.

A smaller or shorter patient in high Fowler's might experience hanging elbows that don't reach the surface of the mattress. A pillow placed under each arm can improve comfort by giving the arms something to rest on.

Patients may also like pillows under their legs. A pillow may be used horizontally under the knees, with a second horizontal pillow under the calves and feet (Figure 4.18A). A variation is to place the pillows vertically, one pillow under one leg from knee to ankle, and a second pillow under the other leg from knee to ankle (Figure 4.18B). Anecdotally, most patients seem to prefer each leg on its own pillow, which allows the legs to splay more naturally.

A number of variations on side-lying position can be offered in the hospital setting. Patients who require high

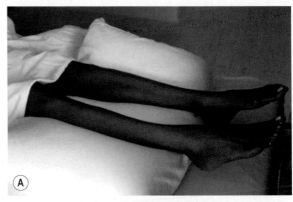

(A)

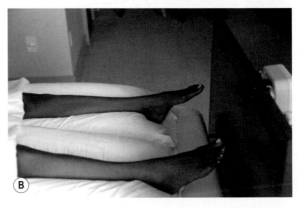

(B)

Figure 4.18
The heels can be floated whether pillows are horizontal (A) or vertical (B). The footboard of some hospital beds is easy to remove for better access to the feet, but foot massage can also be provided from the side of the bed.

(Photos by Candice White.)

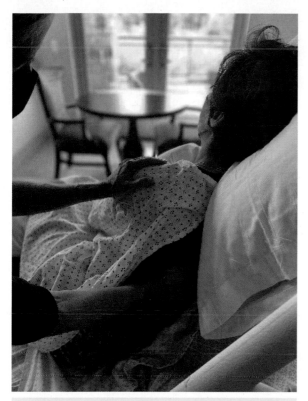

Figure 4.19
A patient who needs the head of the bed elevated can roll onto one hip, hugging a pillow for a modified side-lying position.

(Photo by Candice White.)

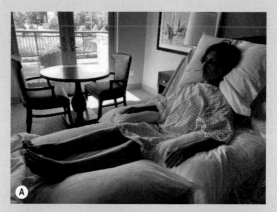

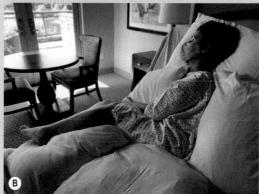

Figure 4.20
Five pillows in two different configurations. (A) A patient in high Fowler's position has one pillow under the head, one under each arm, and one under each leg. (B) A patient in side-lying high Fowler's has a pillow under the head, one under the top arm, one under the top leg, and the final two hugging the back of the body. The patient described these positions as "floating in a giant marshmallow."

(Photos by Candice White.)

Fowler's position to accommodate shortness of breath can sometimes roll onto one hip with a pillow to hug, providing access to the back.

Tip 4.1. How many pillows do we need?

It is ideal for every patient to have a minimum of five pillows. They may not always use all of them, but five are needed for many of the variations on positioning. Pillows in some institutional settings are scarce in number and poor in quality. Family can be encouraged to bring one or more favorite pillows from home but should be encouraged to use pillowcases with bright colors or prints to identify them easily.

To reposition or not to reposition

Depending on the area of the body that the patient desires to have massaged, the therapist will need to determine whether repositioning will enhance or compromise the patient's comfort. Things to consider include the patient's comfort in the current position, the patient's ability to tolerate a different position, the patient's energy level, and whether the process of repositioning will cause pain. It can be helpful to ask a verbal patient, "Are you comfortable in this position, or would you like to try something different?" I rarely reposition a nonverbal patient unless they appear to be uncomfortable.

The most common source of discomfort in Fowler's position is when the bend of the bed falls in the middle of the back, rather than at the bend of the hips. Patients may need help to be pulled up toward the head of the bed. A draw sheet is an indispensable tool for moving patients who can no longer move themselves. As the story on p. 52 indicates, caregivers and staff are experts who can educate therapists in the use of draw sheets for repositioning. Sometimes it is not repositioning that is required, but simple propping or padding to enhance the patient's comfort. A slim pillow under one hip or the other can create dramatic change, as can filling empty space between the patient's body and the surface below (see p. 58).

Tip 4.2. Princess Leia scroll

I learned this tip from massage therapists Nanci Newton and Erika Slocum, who teach oncology massage with Tracy Walton and Associates. The Princess Leia scroll is a fabulous way to provide lateral head support. It feels great to any client but may be especially helpful during active dying when the neck muscles may become too weak to support the head. The weight of the patient's head will anchor the roll in place.

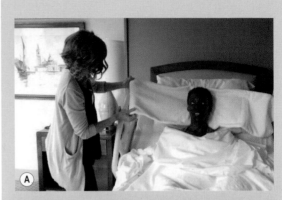

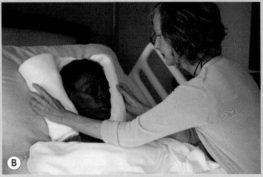

Figure 4.21

(A) Begin with a bath towel folded in thirds lengthwise. This is placed behind the patient's head with the ends extending on either side. Roll the edges of the towel down toward the bed, not up toward the ceiling. (B) Once the roll is complete on both sides, it can be adjusted as desired. Check to make sure the patient's ears are comfortably tucked.

(Photos by Candice White, first appeared in *Hands in health care*.)

The massage

Centering the hands

Many years ago, I had a brief and entirely unremarkable tenure as a potter. I loved the feel of a spinning lump of earth under my hands as I learned to center the clay.

The hands had to initiate contact with slow coordination, working as a unit. A firmness and a confidence were required, but also a willingness to hold steady and *wait* for the clay to warm and soften to the touch. The moment I felt my hand and the clay relax together in effortless contact, I could not help but smile.

It soon became clear that I was much better at centering clay than making a bowl. I have not thrown a pot in more than a decade, but I'll never forget that feeling which has stayed with me as a metaphor for massage. I introduce my hands to a patient in much the same way as I once centered clay, waiting for the skin and tissues to be receptive to a connection. I acclimate myself to the patient's breathing. I hold steady and wait for the moment when contact feels effortless. I still smile when this magic happens.

Centering, says acclaimed potter M. C. Richards, is the experience of saying "Yes, yes to what we behold. To what is holy and to what is unbearable" (Richards, 1989). I can't think of a better way to approach touch for a dying person.

The power of holding

It is difficult to convey the profound power of simply being held. I open and close every session by cradling the client's head, holding the hand and shoulder, or cupping the heart. I also use holds to signal a transition from one body part to another, punctuating transitions throughout the session with a moment of rest. The technique of holding will be mentioned repeatedly in this book.

That a simple hold is so noteworthy speaks to the fact that massage at the end of life is not really about technique. It is about deep, caring connection. It is about assuring another person's nervous system that you are safe to be with. We often say in this work that "less is more." But holding another human being is never less. In the end, it is everything.

Sequencing the massage

A full-body massage is typically a symmetrical experience, where everything done on one side of the body is done in the same order on the other side. At the end of life,

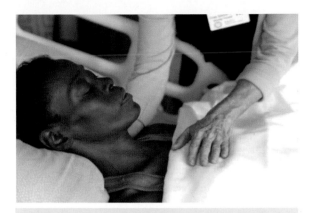

Figure 4.22
Holds are extremely calming and don't require access to skin. One hand on top of the body and the other hand underneath create the comforting sensation of being cradled. If you are ever in doubt during a session and need a minute, take a deep breath. Stop. And just hold.

(Photo by Candice White.)

symmetry becomes less important or entirely impossible. The therapist, with patient input, if possible, will select an area or areas of the body to be addressed. Factors impacting the sequence include the patient's symptoms, goals, and energy level. From a practical standpoint, sequence will also conform to the positions the patient can tolerate and what the therapist can comfortably reach.

There is no right place to begin or end. Some therapists prefer to work on the head prior to applying lotion to their hands and before touching the feet. There is also an argument to be made for completing work on one side of the bed (one shoulder, arm, hand, leg, and foot) before moving to the other side. If trust is still being established, it may be helpful to begin with a less vulnerable area of the body to assure the patient that a protected area will be treated with mindful tenderness.

As described in Chapter 3, the massage will consist of any combination of gliding strokes, compressions (using fingertips or a full gentle hand), light kneading, and holds. Applied slowly with a minimum of three repetitions or "passes," a sense of beginning, middle, and completion can be conveyed, even if the session is confined to a limited area. There is no end to the possible variations.

Working over cloth versus skin

People with advanced illness may be unable to dress and undress themselves, or they may be able to do these things but only with great effort. Even with assistance, dressing and undressing can require energy that may be in short supply. For this reason, most end-of-life massages are conducted with the patient "as is." Lotion can be applied to accessible skin. Areas covered by a gown or clothing are massaged over the cloth. Massage may need to be applied over a blanket if the patient is cold.

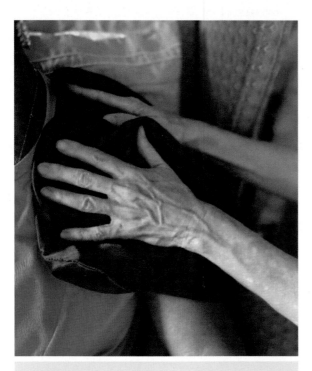

Figure 4.23
One option for working over cloth is to use a double-sided piece of silk which allows the hands to slide over fabric. If no such tool is available, a silk pillowcase can be adapted for this purpose.

(Photo by Candice White.)

Compression and petrissage work just as well over cloth as they do on skin. A gliding stroke may feel different over cloth but can be accomplished over most types of fabric. Skin may be accessed by slipping a hand under a loose sleeve or gown. If the patient is wearing socks, ask if they'd like you to remove them for foot massage and always put them back on when you're finished. I personally like to "get eyes" on as much skin as possible. As revealed in the description of the physical assessment, the touch therapist may be the one to first observe a problem with the skin that needs attention. Use a light touch (maximum of level 2) when working over cloth, due to the potential for unseen injuries.

Common responses to massage

Touch therapists should remain alert for feedback throughout the session. Responses can be subtle, profound, or anything in between. There may be tears, which are neither positive nor negative. The patient may be moved to share deeply personal information or reflections, or they may remain quiet. A verbal person can be asked an open-ended question, such as, "Any feedback on how this is feeling to you?" Whether the patient is verbal or nonverbal, observe carefully for changes in level of arousal, breathing patterns, facial expression, and mood. Below are some possible responses.

Positive responses

- Deep sighs or slower, deeper respirations.

- Eyes closing.

- Mouth falling open, with or without snoring.

- Eyebrows moving up or down.

- Face becoming more relaxed, softening of a frown or grimace.

- Softening of tense muscles or release of guarding behaviors.

- A soft, intermittent vocalization such as "ahhhh" or "hmmm."

- Squeezing the therapist's hand.

- Smiling.

Adverse responses

- Respirations that become faster or shallower.

- Clenching fingers or jaw, grinding teeth.

- Restless movement.

- Vigilant behaviors such as guarding or holding body parts rigid.

- Eyes that remain open and track the therapist's movements.

- Furrowed brow, grimace, or frown.

- More persistent vocalizations, moaning or crying out.

- Persistent startle reflex.

- Retracting from touch or moving a body part away from the therapist's hands.

Tip 4.3. Soliciting patient feedback

Patients often need assurance that they can decline, discontinue, or request changes to the session. Palliative massage therapist Ronna Moore shares a script she uses that empowers people to communicate feedback: "I have been a massage therapist for a long time, but I will never know what this will feel like to you. Only you can tell me that. So please let me know in whatever words feel right for you. You can say, 'Ronna, just stop.' If it feels good, tell me that too, so that we can do more of the same." Choices are presented in a neutral way, with no attachment on the part of the therapist.

Wrapping up: saying goodbye and other follow-up

When the session feels complete, I finish as I started, with a hold. I tune back into the patient's breathing and note any changes that I might want to record or need to share with the team. I offer a silent intention for the dying person's journey. And I thank the patient out loud for letting me spend time with them. I also thank the caregiver for trusting me with their loved one's care, or for any stories they shared with me. If the caregiver is occupied, I slip away quietly. I've learned not to offer the casual, "See you next week," but will respond in kind if the patient or caregiver are the ones to offer these words.

Many agencies consider the first visit to be an assessment or evaluation, in which the patient's response will indicate whether ongoing massage will be added to the care plan. My documentation after an initial encounter includes (1) a chart note for the visit and (2) a care plan indicating the frequency of ongoing visits and the interventions to be included. I make my care plan flexible to accommodate the patient's changing condition. My intervention often reads, "Light massage with emollient lotion to the upper and/or lower body as tolerated," so that my approach can vary from visit to visit. I include PRN (*pro re nata*, or "as necessary") visits so that frequency can increase to accommodate the patient's changing needs. The chart note is a record of the visit, including observations gleaned from the assessment, what was done during the visit, how the patient responded, and my plan for follow-up.

While the first visit presents an opportunity for an initial assessment, the dying process requires that assessment be an integral part of *every* session. Over time, whether dying is a short process or a long one, the therapist will observe changes in the patient's condition which warrant adjustments as described in Chapter 5. With experience, therapists develop comfort with this natural progression, along with an understanding of situations that should be reported to caregivers or healthcare providers. Concerns that merit reporting may include unmanaged symptoms, patient or caregiver distress, safety issues, and sudden changes in function or awareness. Staying within our scope of practice as a member of the care team sometimes means relaying new or sudden developments to a nurse or other expert.

What about caregivers?

Providing massage and other support for caregivers

Caring for someone at the end of life is physically, mentally, and emotionally grueling. While some carers report fulfillment in their roles, there is no doubt that many of their needs are sacrificed. Primary caretakers are often older with health problems of their own. Middle-aged caretakers may have demanding careers and multiple sets of parents in need at the same time. Younger ones may be coping with the demands of raising children in addition to work outside the home. Caregivers living at a distance endure the burden of travel and uprooted lives, often accompanied by guilt if they're unable to be present full-time.

Touch therapists are in a position to offer much-needed attention to these ordinary humans bearing extraordinary hardships. A brief shoulder massage or Reiki with lavender essential oil are examples of caregiver support that can be provided at the bedside. Even tiny gestures are appreciated. I once observed a daughter break into grateful tears over my offer of a pillow to support her arm as she held her dying mother's hand. Chapter 10 describes the profound potential of aroma and other therapies to support caregivers. Patients often benefit from knowing the carer is being cared for.

Some organizations provide massage for caregivers as an integral part of their services. In other agencies, caregiver massage flies under the radar, with tacit or assumed permission. Regardless of whether there is a formal protocol for intake and documentation, there are good arguments for limiting massage pressure to level 2 (level 1 if the caregiver is known to have any of the conditions listed in Table 3.1). At a minimum, I routinely ask if the caregiver has had lymph nodes removed or radiated. While the caregiver may generally be healthy, they are likely fatigued and grieving. Massage for them should not place additional demands on the body but should be an occasion for nurturing and tenderness.

Much of what the carer needs from us is the same as what the patient needs: calm, nonjudgmental presence that meets and supports them *where they are*. It may be privacy or silence that is needed, or it may be companionship in which to safely process what is happening. When carers seem to want to share, I try to ask open-ended questions such as, "Tell me about your dad," or "How did you two meet?" And then I try to stay quiet and listen. There may be laughter, tears, or deep emotion that makes speaking impossible. There may be a wall of self-control or distraction with electronics or phone calls that should not be breached. As always, we take our lead from patients and their families.

Other ideas for caring for the caregiver include the following:

- Notice whether the caregiver looks comfortable at the bedside and offer supportive propping as needed.

- Bring a blanket to a caregiver who is cold, even better if you can heat it in a dryer or warmer.

- Ask if the caregiver has remembered to eat and drink.

- Offer to bring the caregiver something to eat or drink if this is in your power.

- Make sure tissues are at hand.

- If the caregiver is distraught, ask if there's anyone you can call to come be with them.

- Validate and reassure. Tell the caregiver that they're doing a good job. Assure them there is no "right" or "wrong," only the best decisions we can make with the information available to us.

- Answer questions if you are able. Assist carers to access appropriate team members for questions outside your scope of practice.

Caregivers providing massage

Some of the most moving encounters I've experienced at the bedside have involved caregivers providing massage. Sometimes I enter a patient room to find that caregivers are already touching their loved one and there is nothing for me to improve on. In these cases, I offer them the

Touching story 4.3. Small things make a big difference

A cold January rain beat against the window of the hospice room where I sat at my mother's bedside. Mom was deep into the work of dying. She fussed and moaned and picked at her bedding, while I did what I could to soothe her. I felt so alone, just wanting us both to somehow get through the long night.

The hospice aide quietly entered the room in the early morning hours and asked if I would like anything. "Yes, please, a cup of tea." Shortly, he returned with a steaming Styrofoam cup. I would never choose to drink hot tea from Styrofoam! Momentarily disappointed, I took the cup in my hands. Immediately the familiar smell flooded me with good memories. The warmth and comfort of that small, imperfect gesture of kindness still touches and nourishes me all these years later.

LMT Glo Umphress, Mexico

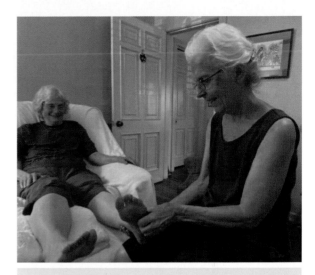

Figure 4.24
A caregiver provides foot massage.
(Photo by Candice White.)

ever had was a seven-year-old girl who helped provide massage for her aunt. She followed my every move with her tiny hands, repeatedly saying, "I wish she would wake up." I replied, "I know, I do, too. But you are helping her so much."

Suggestions for working in homes

- Most agencies require a risk assessment before services can be provided in a person's home, including such things as pedestrian and auto access, steps and stairs, the presence of guns, the presence of animals, hoarding behaviors, known drug use, and other issues which could impact staff safety. Smoke detectors and signage are required for homes where oxygen is provided. If safety is a concern at any time for any reason, discuss this with a supervisor or colleague. It's a good idea for others to be informed of your driving itinerary.

- Most pets are friendly and eager for extra attention from visitors, but they can also be protective and unpredictable. If you have concerns about a pet, it is reasonable to ask the owner to confine the animal while you are in the home.

warm lotion in my pocket and ask if there's anything I can do to support them. On other occasions, I sense that a family member would like to participate but needs encouragement, which I am happy to provide.

Caregivers sometimes ask if I need them to move out of the way. My answer is always, "Absolutely not! You are right where you should be." And then I ask if they'd like to help me. There isn't a right answer to this invitation. Some carers are grateful for the chance to *do something*, others are relieved to leave the bedside for a short break, or to simply observe. Any response is valid.

When carers do participate, it can be wonderful for them, and for the dying person. Some people appear to have a knack for massage. When this is the case, I share this observation with them. The youngest and best assistant I

- Families frequently express frustration when care staff show up unexpectedly or don't come as promised. When scheduling home visits, set a realistic time that you can commit to, then request a "grace period" of 15 minutes on either side of the appointment. Tell the client that you'll call to advise if your arrival will be outside this time range.

- Be sensitive to household preferences, such as not wearing shoes inside the home.

- Asking to use someone's bathroom can feel intrusive. Many field therapists feel more comfortable using public facilities between home visits, though this can be challenging in rural areas.

- Wear a name tag. If you don't work for an agency that provides this, order one online with your name and role. This is helpful to patients and families who likely have multiple providers visiting the home.

Suggestions for working in group homes

- Seeing more than one patient at a single facility is an excellent way to increase efficiency.

- In addition to facility staff, the therapist might need to communicate with family members or hospice team members who wish to be advised of visits.

- Every facility has a protocol for guests entering and departing. Protocols change during outbreaks of flu, C. diff, and other infections.

- A name tag is helpful and may even be required.

- If you're working in a memory care center, there will be codes for entering and exiting the elevator and the building. Take care not to allow a resident to follow you in or out.

- Scheduling for massage will revolve around meals, group activities, and patient care. Sometimes it makes sense to provide the touch session in a public area of the facility. An example is a shoulder massage for a patient listening to live music.

- Take time, as you are able, to develop rapport with care staff, roommates, and other residents.

- If the session is provided in a patient's room, be sure to knock before entering, even if the door is open.

Suggestions for working in the hospital or IPU

- Store your things in a designated area and enter the patient room with as few items as possible.

- Sanitize hands on the way into the room and on the way out, known as "foam in, foam out" or "gel in, gel out." This does not take the place of handwashing, which should occur immediately prior to and following each visit.

- Knock on a patient's door before entering, even if the door is open. This room is their home for the present.

- If the medical team, social worker, or chaplain is present, tell the patient you'll return later.

- If there are visitors present, ask if it's a good time or if the patient would prefer that you return later.

- Generally, refrain from sitting on the patient's bed, unless doing so is the only way to reach them for massage. If this is the case, ask the patient's permission and put down a fresh chux pad as a barrier, then dispose of the chux before leaving the patient's room.

- Don't use the patient's private bathroom.

- Eat and drink only in designated areas.

- Beware of medical wipes in the hospital environment. Some are for sanitizing surfaces and are not safe for hands!

- A name tag will likely be required.

Conclusion

In Chapter 4, we crossed the threshold of the dying person's space with an expanded focus in which we create room for the unknown. Whether verbal or nonverbal, the patient and the patient's companions become our guides for the session, an experience that is "never the same twice," according to palliative massage therapist Lee Ball. "Never the same tools needed, and nothing that can be planned for. Even seeing the same patient will be different each time" (Ball, 2021).

Tools for the session include the physical assessment, positioning and propping, centering the hands, and sequencing the massage. These tools must be used with humility, flexibility, and deference to patients and their loved ones. Permission is sought each time we offer touch, and listening becomes more nuanced as the dying process unfolds. Chapter 5 will illuminate the stages of dying, what to expect, and how to respond.

References

Ball, L., 2021. Comment regarding massage for people at the end of life. [email] (Personal communication, 18 January).

Clark, B., 2015. *The why, what & how behind using yoga props*. [online] Available at: <https://www.elephantjournal.com/2015/01/the-why-what-how-behind-yoga-props>.

Richards, M.C., 1989. *Centering: in pottery, poetry, and the person*. Middletown, CT: Wesleyan University Press.

Smith, I., 2017. *How to be receptive to physical & emotional challenges of hospice*. [online] Available at: <massagemag.com/receptive-physical-emotional-challenges-hospice-44346>.

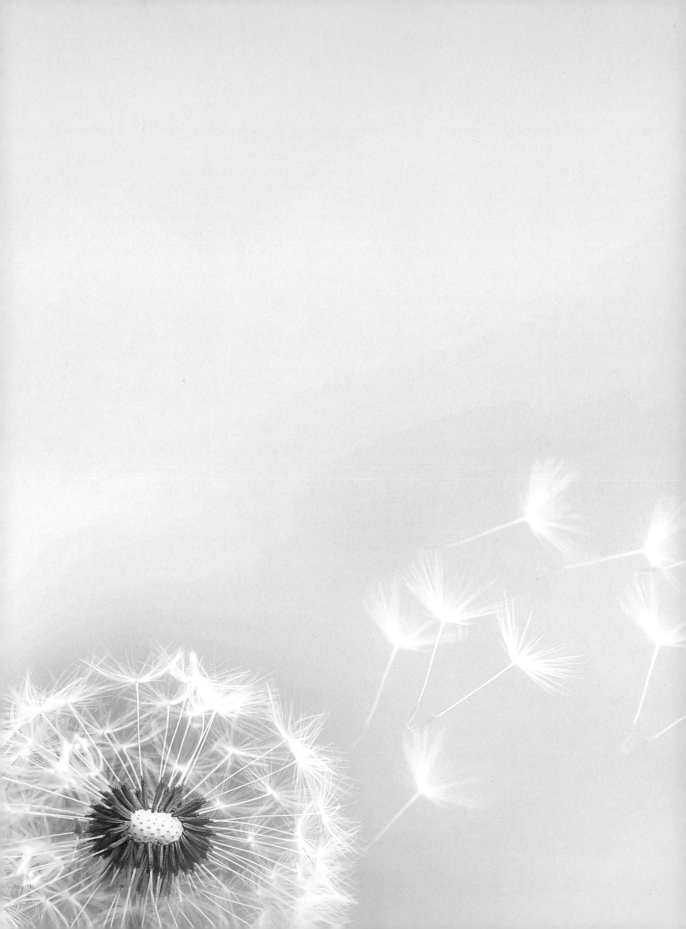

Stages of dying

I never thought dying would be so easy.
                    –Actual patient

I never thought dying would be so hard.
                    –Actual patient

Dying is often compared to birth, both natural processes for which the body is genetically designed. Like birth, the dying process has common patterns that can be described in stages, each marked by predictable changes that are less frightening when understood. In the case of dying, symptoms are largely due to the body's efforts to conserve a waning supply of energy. Energy is shifted away from functions that are less urgent for short-term survival, such as digestion, elimination, and circulation to the extremities. The most vital functions are preserved for as long as possible, including the heartbeat, breathing, and brain function to keep them both going. In the later stages of dying, the vital organs begin to shut down in a relatively systematic order. But this does not mean that dying *looks* or *feels* orderly, or easy. Leaving the body often requires great effort and usually some discomfort.

For both the dying person and their loved ones, dying represents an extraordinary physical, emotional, spiritual, *and* psychosocial process that can feel quite chaotic. As one caregiver puts it, "Dying is not a journey, it's a roller coaster" (Powers, 2020). For many people, concerns about relationships, regrets, and unfinished business are more distressing than the physical aspects of dying. Touch therapists must care for both the physical body *and* the spirit, discerning common themes while allowing for individual differences. There is likely no richer or more complex human experience than the natural end of life.

Chapter 5 will address common changes during the last six months of life, beginning with early decline and ending with the aftermath of the last breath. Physical changes will be described, along with some common emotional responses of patients and their loved ones. The goal is not to reduce the dying process to a tidy checklist, but to prepare touch therapists for a range of sights, sounds, smells, and feelings they might witness, and to normalize these experiences in a way that reduces fear. With familiarity, we can move beyond fear to a more grounded place from which to support others who might be hurting or fearful.

Specific suggestions for the therapist are offered in this chapter for each stage of dying. Most of these pertain to massage, but some will seem outside the scope of a typical massage practice. In the words of Merrill Collett, author of *Stay Close and Do Nothing*, work with the dying sometimes means "doing the next thing to be done" (Collett, 1997). If a need is pressing and requires no special skill, a touch therapist at the bedside can help with simple things that contribute to patient comfort, such as moistening the mouth or brushing the hair. Because the stages are fluid, it is recommended to read this chapter in its entirety in case suggestions in one stage are helpful for another.

It is unlikely that any one person will experience all the changes listed in this chapter. *Most* people will experience *some* of them, but progress through the stages is rarely linear, nor is the timetable predictable. There can be movement back and forth between stages, or a person can seem to get stuck in a stage. Just as some births are more difficult than others, death seems to come harder and take longer for certain people. Any discussion of the stages of dying must be accompanied by a great deal of humility and tolerance for the unknown.

Early decline (3–6 months before death)

For some patients, the beginning of the dying process is defined by the decision to stop active treatment. For others, the "beginning of the end" is only clear in hindsight. There might be a precipitating event such as a fall, a new infection that does not respond to treatment, or an unseen threshold that is breached in the body by advancing disease. Treatment, if continued, has diminishing returns. If the disease trajectory has been long, patients and their loved ones are likely exhausted. If diagnosis is recent, there may be shock and devastation at the news of disease that is already widespread and untreatable. How people arrive at the threshold of the dying experience will impact their responses and needs.

Physical changes

The patient in early decline is likely to be experiencing one or several symptoms, possibly including fatigue, pain, anxiety, and/or insomnia. If hospice or palliative care is involved, opioids and other medications will likely be introduced to address these symptoms. New side effects may result, including constipation and sedation.

Patients who stop curative treatment during this period may feel relief, though some treatment side effects are long-term or permanent. Examples of lasting side effects include ongoing pain from surgery, neuropathy, and lymphedema. The degree to which people function in early decline is quite variable, depending on diagnosis, age, and overall health. Some are still active and living independently, though they are likely to be coping with new limitations as disease becomes more advanced. Reduced appetite is common, as the body shifts energy away from the work of digestion.

Emotional and psychosocial adjustments

The emotional adjustments to early decline can be extreme, as patients come to terms with a diagnosis that is likely to be fatal. There may be denial, disbelief, or anger. Grief related to losses already endured may surface, along with fear of losses to come and anxiety about an uncertain future. The patient may express any or all of these emotions, or none of them. Loved ones will also be experiencing a wide range of feelings, which may or may not correspond at any given time to what the patient is experiencing. There may be conflicts between family members regarding whether to stop or continue active treatment. If hospice is started, the day of admission can be difficult for all concerned. Understanding and compassion are needed as patients and their families adjust to a changing care plan that offers comfort rather than a coveted cure.

on, especially if I find the content to be banal or disturbing. I must remind myself at these times that it is I who must conform to the dying person's preferences, rather than the patient who must conform to mine.

Collett reports that some of the hardest hospice work he ever did was to care for a man who spent his last days watching TV soap operas. Yet Collett says of this experience, "Wanting to change ourselves is good, wanting to change our patients is not" (Collett, 1997). Another of my favorite authors, Sallie Tisdale, writes that we must notice our urges to "put our own veneer on someone else's experience" (Tisdale, 2018). It is the dying person who decides, says Tisdale, whether to spend the current moment listening to music or watching "The Walking Dead."

This concept of total acceptance applies to every aspect of another person's dying experience. We must be willing to let go of our personal opinions regarding the ideal location of death, the interventions chosen or not chosen, religious or cultural observances, habits, and beliefs that differ from our own. Read more about this in Chapter 11.

Adapting the massage session for early decline

It is a gift for a touch therapist to be involved at the early stage of decline, allowing time to build rapport and to discover the patient's preferences. Find out who the important people are in the patient's world and get to know them. They are part of the unit of care for hospice and palliative services and will eventually become the patient's appointed gatekeepers. Follow the patient's lead in validating what this time means for them and what they need to get through it. Early decline can be a busy stage, with decisions and arrangements to make, visitors, final projects, and meaningful experiences such as travel. "Dying," says Joan Halifax, "is a full-time job" (Halifax, 2008). There may be days when massage takes a back seat to other activity and days when massage provides a desperately needed break in the action.

Given the demands of early decline alongside growing fatigue, it is likely that the therapist will arrive to find the patient sleeping at some point. It can be helpful early in the patient–therapist relationship to ask if the patient would prefer to remain sleeping or to receive massage even if they're not awake. This exchange creates a dynamic in which the patient's choices are honored at each step of the dying process.

Other adjustments during early decline include the following:

- Evaluate the location of massage to ensure safety and comfort.

- Session length may be 30–60 minutes, depending on energy level and symptoms.

- Level 2 pressure is safe for most people and most parts of the body.

- Level 1 pressure should be used for severe symptoms (see Table 3.1).

- Limited use of level 3 pressure may be appropriate for some people during early decline, as indicated on p. 34.

- Patients may tolerate a variety of positions, including seated, supine, reclining, or side-lying.

- Explore patient preferences regarding aromatherapy, music, positioning, and massage.

- Allow patients to do what they can for themselves. Ask before providing assistance.

- Focus on symptom support; see Chapter 6 for ideas.

- Call ahead to confirm each appointment, and don't take it personally if the patient cancels.

- Intense emotion warrants a shorter, gentler session. Quiet holds can be very effective.

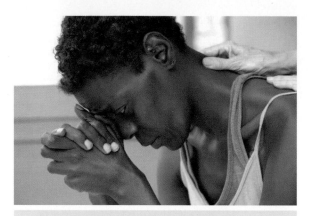

Figure 5.1

Each stage of dying involves loss and grief, as the patient and loved ones adapt to new realities of the disease progression. Denial, anxiety, fear, anger, and sadness are all normal reactions. Acceptance of whatever arises during the massage session will help the patient feel heard and supported.

(Photo by Candice White, first appeared in *Hands in health care*.)

Touching story 5.1. Daniel in early decline

I met Daniel soon after he was admitted to hospice for advanced liver cancer. He was referred for massage by his nurse to address anxiety and right shoulder pain. When I called to make the first appointment, Daniel told me that he had never had a massage before. But he knew that a table was involved, and he stated unequivocally that he wanted "the whole nine yards." I packed my table and drove to the working-class suburb where Daniel lived with his wife, Cici.

Daniel's truck, parked in the driveway, had multiple bumper stickers. One of them said "Not as mean, not as lean, but still a marine." The others were too indecent for me to share. Daniel answered the door, a wiry

pistol of a man who sized me up with a bit of wariness. Cici, in contrast, threw her arms around me as if we were long-lost friends.

Daniel went out to his garage to have a cigarette while I set up my table. I soon learned that he was a chain smoker and would need to sandwich his massage sessions between smokes. I felt a little nervous watching him get onto my table. Despite his energy, he was very thin and a bit unsteady on his feet. I stood nearby while he managed to position himself supine. Cici assisted me to place pillows under his head and knees.

I slowly began to work, providing level 2 pressure to Daniel's head, neck, shoulders, arms, hands, legs, and feet. The only area I avoided was a bandage on his right forearm. Daniel engaged in a bit of banter, which included multiple attempts to get me to use deeper pressure on his right shoulder.

In response to Daniel's request, I brought focused attention to the shoulder with some level 2 fingertip pressure. I covered every inch of the scapula, using a combination of small circles and static compressions. I ended the session with a two-handed hold to the shoulder, one hand on top, and the other slipped underneath, between the fitted sheet and the surface of the table. Daniel lay quietly while my hands cupped his shoulder. He seemed to sink into a trance-like state, and Cici thanked me profusely, saying it was the most relaxed she'd seen him in their 20 years of marriage. The session lasted 40 minutes.

I wasn't sure that Daniel would want another massage, given his disappointment over the lighter pressure. But Cici called me the next day and asked when I could come again. We set up a weekly schedule and my affection for this couple quickly grew. One day when I arrived, Cici was furious with Daniel. He had apparently found his truck keys and driven himself to the store for cigarettes and soda while she was mowing the backyard. Daniel grinned when Cici told me the story, clearly pleased with himself.

But for all the teasing and bravado, it was clear that Daniel was becoming weaker. I gently suggested that we try a massage in his recliner, and he didn't resist. He still needed a cigarette prior to every massage, so I began to tag along with him for this ritual. Cici wouldn't let Daniel smoke in the house, so we sat out in the garage, shivering in our coats and hats, while Daniel smoked and told me stories about his life.

Late decline (1–3 months before death)

In late decline, every organ is working harder and losing efficiency. The heart is not pumping as effectively, which leads to slowed circulation and reduced oxygen to the extremities and other organs. The dying person has less energy, further loss of appetite, and reduced fluid intake. The body attempts to hold onto fluids and to store them in the arms and legs, where they cause the least harm. Symptoms experienced previously may increase in severity, and *new* symptoms are likely to emerge. The medical team will respond by adding or changing medications. Patients in late decline are often on opioids and other medications to control pain, anxiety, and other symptoms. Bowel management becomes an ongoing issue. A growing supply of supportive medical equipment may be needed, causing the home environment to change. An example is supplemental oxygen, which may be introduced to reduce the sensation of air hunger.

Physical changes

Patients in late decline may experience any of the following symptoms:

- Increased sleep, up to 16–20 hours per day.
- Sore muscles and joints from prolonged inactivity.
- Disease-related pain.
- Poor appetite with accelerated weight loss, unless fluids are retained from cardiac problems or use of steroid medication.
- Growing weakness with increased fall risk. Patient may need assistance to walk or become unable to walk.
- Dehydration with electrolyte disturbances (drowsiness and confusion).
- Dry skin, possibly with itching.
- Jaundice, or yellowing skin, with liver conditions.
- Edema, often in one or both lower extremities or the abdomen.
- Incontinence.
- Constipation.

Emotional and psychosocial adjustments

Pride and personal dignity may suffer as the patient becomes dependent on others for care. The patient might need assistance to use a bedside commode, urinal, or bedpan. If the dying person has been living alone, they will begin to need more help to manage activities of daily living. If the patient remains at home, the demands on the caregiver are increasing. Additional help or a change in location may be necessary, adding to stress and frustration. Many people experience financial hardship with increased expenses of care. For those who must give up their homes, the sense of loss can be profound. This anguish may be compounded if beloved pets are involved.

Due to the realities of late decline, the patient's anxiety may be increasing, adding to the intensity of other symptoms such as pain or shortness of breath. Loved ones who remain in denial may blame decline on "too much medication" or other perceived problems with the care plan. Grief and fear may be high for both patients and families. As mobility becomes challenging, the patient's world grows smaller. The dying person begins to withdraw from others during this stage, which may represent a need for solitude to complete inner work. Another notable phenomenon is that the dying person's relationship to material things begins to change. While the bedside or tray table might have held books, toiletries, and electronic devices, those items begin to disappear. The exceptions seem to be cell phones and religious objects for those who find them meaningful.

Heads up 5.1. Near death awareness

With increasing periods of sleep, the patient's reality begins to shift in a way that others may dismiss as confusion. Patients may see deceased loved ones. They may use symbolic language to describe their experiences. This language often reflects the patient's interests or how they spent their time. An architect, for example, might talk about needing to "climb the stairs," while an accountant might speak of getting his "numbers in line."

Near death awareness (NDA) is a term to describe a broad range of experiences unique to the dying process, including visions and end-of-life dreams. NDA differs from delirium or hallucinations, in that NDA occurrences are reported with detail and clarity and are usually comforting rather than disturbing. Common themes include the presence of deceased loved ones, preparing for travel, and visions of another realm. Another recurring feature of NDA is that some patients know with accuracy when death will occur.

People who share NDA with others should be supported rather than dismissed. Helpful responses include listening with openness and curiosity, accepting what the patient is sharing, and validating whatever meaning the patient assigns to the experience.

Adapting the massage session for late decline

- Length of the session might be 20–40 minutes.

- Maximum of level 2 pressure, level 1 pressure for conditions indicated in Table 3.1.

- Reevaluate the location of massage for safety.

- Limit or seek assistance with transfers due to fall risk.

- Reevaluate patient positioning, adding pillows and other soft props for comfort.

- Apply emollient cream liberally to dry skin.

- Refer to Chapter 6 for specific symptoms and Chapter 7 for specific diseases.

- Offer gentle range of motion for patients who request it (see p. 193).

- Model calm presence in everything you say and do.

- Listen with open curiosity. "Tell me more: what do you see?"

- Acknowledge the efforts of the caregiver. "You're doing a great job."

- Communicate concerns and changes to the medical team.

Touching story 5.2. Daniel in late decline

I arrived at Daniel's one morning to learn that he had fallen during the weekend. His injuries included a broken right arm, multiple skin tears, and scattered bruises. He was in a lot of pain and hadn't gotten out of bed that morning. I told Cici that it was no problem, he could receive massage in his bed. She seemed relieved and took me into the bedroom.

The room was dark, but even so, I could see that Daniel was a mess. His right arm was in a sling, and he had numerous bandages and several nicotine patches. I ascertained that Daniel wanted a back massage that day. He was able to turn onto his left side, with several pillows to cushion his injured arm. He was cold, so I worked over his shirt and the blanket. I noticed when I moved my hand to his low back that he was wearing a disposable brief.

Daniel recounted visits from three of his grown children with whom he had recently reconciled, reunions that brought him great joy. He also told me his dead mother had been visiting him, and that he found comfort in these meetings. I sat on a stool at the edge of the bed, providing gentle caress to Daniel's head and neck, and holds to his posterior shoulders, lumbar, and hips. Even working over Daniel's clothing and covers, I could feel every bone in his small body. The session lasted 20 minutes, and Daniel was sleeping when I finished.

I exited the bedroom to find Cici on all fours, peering under the sofa. She explained that Daniel's fingers had grown so thin that he'd lost his wedding ring. We talked about Daniel's pain, which he had described to me as being 8 on a scale of 1–10. Cici had already phoned his nurse, who was on her way to see Daniel. I was very relieved to hear this. I was eager for another member of the team to assess and attend to his discomfort.

Pre-active dying (1–2 weeks before death)

During pre-active dying, the patient's level of consciousness and arousal begin to change. There may still be moments of lucidity, but the patient primarily becomes semi-responsive. They may wake for brief periods when their name is spoken or when they experience pain. The patient has little appetite or thirst and will not be eating or drinking much. The body still produces fecal matter, and the care team will want the patient to have a bowel movement every third day or so to prevent stool from hardening in the colon, a condition known as impaction. Urine decreases in quantity and becomes darker in color (tea-colored). Both urinary and bowel incontinence are the norm at this point, requiring disposable underwear or a urinary catheter.

The body's oxygen and carbon dioxide receptors are no longer functioning well, and the patient may begin to experience changes in breathing. Cheyne–Stokes refers to a pattern of shallow breathing with short periods of apnea, or no breathing. It is as if the body is practicing for letting go of respiration. Edema may occur or worsen in the upper or lower extremities and sometimes throughout the body. Unless the patient has a vascular disease, the extremities are still warm during pre-active dying.

Physical changes

- Decreasing level of arousal.

- Patient may sleep with eyes open, half open, or closed.

- When eyes are open, the dying person may stare past people and objects in the room.

- Blood pressure decreases.

- Heart rate may be faster or slower, or alternate between the two.

- Body temperature changes. Skin may feel hot or cool, or alternate between the two.

- Respiration becomes irregular. It may be faster or slower, or alternate between the two.

- Fatigue grows extreme. The patient may be too tired to speak or chew.

- Swallowing becomes difficult, with risk of aspiration and pneumonia. The clinical team may suggest thickened water or juice.

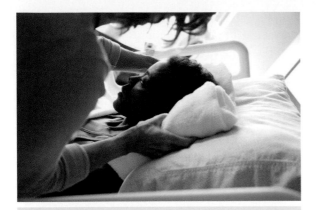

Figure 5.2

In pre-active and active dying, the patient's eyes may be open or half open, though the patient otherwise seems to be sleeping or unconscious. Here, the therapist uses a rolled towel to provide bilateral support to the head.

(Photo by Candice White, first appeared in *Hands in health care.*)

- Delivery system for medicines may change from oral to sublingual. In hospital and inpatient settings, IVs may be used.

- Dehydration increases, causing dry mouth and skin.

- Patient likely becomes bedbound, with growing risk of skin breakdown.

Emotional and psychosocial adjustments

Less is known about the emotions as dying progresses due to decreasing communication from the dying person. The patient appears to be withdrawing from the world, spending increasing amounts of time in a place that the living do not comprehend. The following are common observations that may speak to emotional or psychosocial dynamics, though these behaviors are frequently attributed to physical changes in the body.

- There may be agitation, picking at clothes or bed linen, or restless movement.

- There may be repetitive movements, such as bringing the hand to the mouth.

- The patient may reach for something unseen.

- They may seem to see or hear people who are not present to others.

Adapting the massage session for pre-active dying

- Length of the session might be 15–30 minutes.

- Maximum of level 2 pressure, level 1 pressure for conditions listed in Table 3.1.

- Speak quietly to the patient, telling them who you are and what you are doing before you touch them.

- Prop as needed to provide support and prevent skin breakdown.

- Continue application of lubrication to dry skin, including the face and lips. Avoid open skin.

- The patient may indicate thirst. If water, thickened liquids, or ice chips are on the patient's tray table, it may be presumed that the therapist can assist the patient to access these. The head of the bed may need to be raised to facilitate swallowing.

- Be on the alert for tight jewelry or wrist bands if edema is present. These may need to be removed for safety (see Figure 4.1).

- A damp, folded washcloth can be placed over open eyes if they appear red and dry.

- Provide a calm, supportive environment to accept whatever arises.

- Do not interfere with random movements the patient might be making (Peralta, 2017).

- Offer gentle and unconditional support to the family as their grief intensifies.

Tip 5.1. Offering massage during pre-active or active dying

The space around an imminently dying person is hallowed ground. The massage therapist who enters this space must be especially sensitive, particularly if it is a first encounter with the patient. Once a patient is no longer speaking, a surrogate decision maker will consent to or decline the massage session. Loved ones are understandably protective and may be resistant to massage for a number of reasons. They may feel it is too late for the patient to benefit. They may have preconceived notions regarding massage, which make them assume it would be painful or "too much." Or they may feel that their few remaining hours are too precious to share with anyone outside the patient's inner circle.

One tip for entering this delicate situation is to entirely avoid use of the word "massage," as described in Chapter 4. Loved ones are generally more open to the idea of light lotioning to honor and care for dry skin. The therapist should assure the family that the session will be brief and gentle, with no need to undress or move the patient. The family can be invited to assist the therapist in observing any responses that might indicate the patient does not wish to be touched (see p. 69). Loved ones sitting or standing close to the patient should be assured that they are not in the way. The session should be fashioned in a way that accommodates their rightful presence at the bedside, either by confining massage to an area of the body that the therapist can reach without displacing family or by inviting the family members to participate in the massage. In the event of an unfavorable response, the session should be dialed back or discontinued. An attitude of

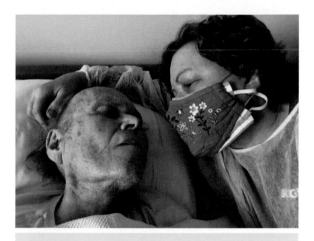

Figure 5.3
Loved ones are understandably protective as people become more vulnerable during the dying process.

(Photo courtesy of Merilynne Rush.)

quiet humility can go a long way in assuring loved ones that the dying person is safe in your hands (Spence, 2021, first appeared in *Hands in health care*).

Touching story 5.3. Daniel in pre-active dying

Cici called the following week to let me know that Daniel had been taken by ambulance to the hospice inpatient unit (IPU) to address his pain. He'd also developed nausea and vomiting. She told me that he was complaining bitterly that the nicotine patches didn't help, and he was too sick to smoke. The unit would not have allowed it anyway. When I arrived at the IPU to visit Daniel, Cici was swabbing his mouth with a sponge dipped in Dr Pepper. Daniel managed to smile, but I could see that his body was failing. His abdomen was swollen with ascites, and his skin and eyes were very yellow. I wasn't sure if the jaundice was new, or if his bedroom had simply been too dark for me to see it.

Daniel closed his eyes and appeared to drift off. Cici left to get lunch. I provided light caress to Daniel's head and forehead, gently combing his long hair with my fingers. I applied warm lotion to his dry face, and salve to his lips. He sighed deeply and his breathing slowed. His skin felt very warm to the touch. I dampened a washcloth and laid it over one arm and then the other, providing level 1 massage on top of the washcloth. I folded the washcloth and placed it across Daniel's forehead. I finished the massage at Daniel's feet.

Cici returned to the room and let me know that the medical team was working to get Daniel's pain under control so that she could take him home. She'd promised him that he could die in his own bed. It was important to him, and therefore important to her. She told me that the only good thing that had happened that week was that she had found Daniel's wedding ring.

What happened next is one of the highlights of my massage therapy career. Cici said, "I wish it weren't too late for us to renew our vows." I was quiet for a minute, and then I looked at Cici, and she looked at me. Truthfully, I was thinking we could call a chaplain. But Cici would have none of that. We approached the bed, and she spoke Daniel's name until he opened his eyes. I recited what I could remember from countless weddings I've attended, something along the lines of "Do you, Daniel, take Cici to

be your lawfully wedded wife? To have and to hold from this day forward?" Daniel said yes. Cici began to cry and then she said yes, too. They kissed. And I thought to myself, as I often do, that nothing in massage school could ever have prepared me enough for this job.

Active dying (1–3 days before death)

Active dying is a term that is often misused to describe the lengthy process of dying in general. In truth, active dying refers to a short period, typically one to three days, that immediately precedes death. A person who is actively dying is referred to as imminent. While the difference between pre-active and active dying may seem subtle when described on paper, there is no mistaking this last phase. Family or staff will often say, "There's been a change."

One of the hallmarks of active dying is that the dying person may appear to be sleeping deeply, as if they are in a coma. They may not respond to their name, but might still respond to pain by grimacing, moaning, or crying out when being repositioned. Clinical practice is to reposition every two hours to prevent skin breakdown, though many families request that the dying person be undisturbed. Comfort care will include sponge baths, cleaning and moistening the mouth, and keeping the perineal area clean and dry.

It must be remembered that the dying person may be acutely present, even if they don't seem to be. It is agreed that hearing remains until the end, and that experiences may be magnified in a body that is becoming more porous. Joan Halifax reports that her father, when asked, "How are you feeling?" replied without hesitation, "*Everything*" (Halifax, 2008). Care staff will often suggest a quiet environment with low light to reduce stimulation.

Heads up 5.2. The last surge

The imminent patient has likely not taken food or fluids for one or more days. An occasional exception occurs when a patient has a last surge of energy. They may suddenly wake up and request a favorite meal, a visit with a certain person, or other desires seemingly out of nowhere. This surge may last minutes, hours, or even a day, startling loved ones and creating the illusion of a miraculous recovery. When this last surge of energy is complete, however, the end is often very near.

Personal note to the reader 5.2. When people linger and who "should" be there

The timing of death is a variable that creates disquiet for many people. Loved ones frequently ask "how long it will be" so that they can arrange their lives to be present at the end. The problem is that we are not very good at predicting when the end will be.

Some people linger beyond reasonable expectation, while others die suddenly from an "exit event" that catches everyone off guard. A person who is expected to live for months can die abruptly, while an imminent patient in the next room may still be alive a week later. The dying often wait for people to arrive, but they are just as likely to wait for people to leave.

Our team has observed that there is often a developmental component to a prolonged death. Younger people often take longer to die, as do some elderly people with dementia who perceive themselves to be young. People may hold on to reach a certain milestone, and then die quickly afterward. Care providers may urge the family to assure the dying person that it is "okay to go." The team also supports reaching out to estranged family members, leaving the dying person alone from time to time, and arranging for last rites and other observances. Sometimes these measures seem to help. But ultimately, death comes when it comes.

My suggestion to every touch therapist is to be open but not attached to the possibility that the dying person has chosen you to be present. You may have never met the patient before, but they could be waiting for someone with calm energy to be at the bedside. It could

Changes in skin color and temperature are another indication of active dying. Mottling is common (see Figure 5.4), typically beginning in the lower extremities. The lips, tips of the ears, fingers, or nail beds may be tinged with blue, indicating cyanosis from lack of oxygen. The skin may appear waxy or pale. Mottling and cyanosis are often accompanied by cool skin temperature unless the patient is running a fever. The body's internal thermostat is not well regulated during active dying and may change from hour to hour. Fever will be treated with acetaminophen (paracetamol), either by suppository or placed under the armpit where it dissolves through the skin.

The timing of death remains mysterious but can be predicted with more certainty as it draws closer. Clinical staff observe signs such as falling blood pressure, weak or absent pulses, and pupil reactivity to estimate a range of hours when death is likely. Family will be informed of these observations so that they can prepare. Many people have strong feelings about being there for the moment of death, or *not* being there. Some families gather at the bedside for the final hours, referred to as the vigil. Families may share stories, music, or prayer according to their customs. Loved ones may say their goodbyes in person or via phone, FaceTime, Skype, or other technology if the internet is available. There may be laughter or tears, sometimes both. For others, the vigil is a very quiet time.

be that they do not want their surviving loved one to be alone at the moment of their death. Or it could be that the dying person is alone and does not wish to be. If the patient's breathing pattern changes suddenly while you are in the room, I urge you to stay. Something might be happening that you are meant to be part of.

Physical changes

The electrolyte disturbances that occur with dehydration produce a natural anesthetic in the body. These endorphins, combined with reduced brain function, allow most people to die peacefully. It is almost as if the body is already detaching from the process, though experts agree that the dying person can still hear and sense the presence of others. Pain medications are continued to ensure comfort. Once urination ceases, there is a slight risk of involuntary twitching called myoclonus. These movements may be due to opioid metabolites and are managed by changing or rotating medication. If terminal restlessness occurs, medications will be given to reduce anxiety.

The sounds of dying can be unusual and disturbing when misunderstood. One of these sounds is the proverbial "death rattle," a gurgling that can be heard as air passes over secretions in the throat. These secretions accumulate when the dying person is no longer able to swallow or cough. The family may worry that the patient is drowning or struggling to breathe, but end-of-life experts agree that this is generally not the case. The airway is kept open by the sternocleidomastoid muscles in the neck, which cause the head to extend and the mouth to stay open. Some patients snore loudly, and others make rhythmic sounds that may resemble moaning, humming, or the sound "ah." Care staff educate families to watch for signs of true discomfort, such as facial grimace or restlessness. When the dying person's face is lax and smooth, it can be assumed that they are comfortable. My personal observation is that some patients seem to be soothed by the vibrations of their own sounds. The combination of sound, breath, and rhythm is in fact used in many traditions as a way to center and calm the mind.

Dying can also involve strange smells. A particular odor sometimes emanates from the dying person in the last hours of life. It is a sweet-but-sour smell, likely due to chemical processes in the dying body. There may be other smells that are less pleasant, especially in the case of intestinal cancers or severe wounds. Some traditions keep the doors and windows closed so the soul does not escape too soon. Others call for an open window to allow the soul to leave the body. This practice, when possible and endorsed by the family, has the benefit of bringing fresh air into the room.

A summary of these and other changes during active dying appears below.

- Extremities may become mottled and cold to the touch. Mottling is typically progressive, though it can also come and go (see Figure 5.4).

- There may be terminal fever.

- The face may begin to change as the tissues relax, with temporal wasting, bossing (or smoothing) of the forehead, drooping or disappearance of the nasolabial fold, and pinning of the ears such that they flatten against the head (Peralta, 2017).

- Eyes are glassy and may be half open.

- Some people experience terminal restlessness, attempting to climb out of bed. There may be a sense of "needing to get out of here."

- There is scant urine of a dark brown color, or no urine output.

- Breathing is irregular, with lengthening periods of apnea.

- The head is typically extended with the mouth open.

- The accessory muscles of the chest and abdomen may be working hard to assist the failing lungs.

- Mouth and skin may be very dry.

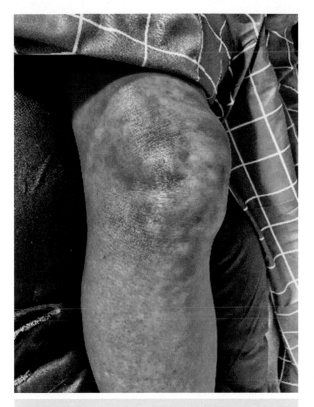

Figure 5.4
Mottling is a red, purple, or dark discoloration that often appears during active dying. The most common places for mottling to begin are the feet or knees. In people with darker skin tones, temperature changes can be a more reliable indicator of mottling. Skin that is mottled will feel cool or cold to the touch.

(Photo by the author.)

Adapting the massage session for active dying

- Massage of short duration (10–15 minutes) with focus on the upper body.

- Level 1 pressure, light caress, or holds.

- Speak quietly to the patient, tell them who you are and what you are doing.

- For congestion, try raising the head of the bed. Otherwise, don't reposition the patient for massage unless the family requests it.

- Add blankets as needed for warmth but avoid electric blankets due to risk of burns.

- If fever is present, remove heavy covers. Apply cool, wet washcloths to the forehead, gently sponge the limbs, or wrap the hands and feet.

- Continue to moisturize dry skin and lips.

- A dry mouth can also be soothed with a moistened swab or washcloth.

- Essential oils can be incorporated into the massage if the family desires.

- Be sensitive to any change in desire to be touched, indicated by facial grimace or acceleration in breathing.

- Care and attention shifts to the family.

Touching story 5.4. Daniel in active dying

Daniel did make it home, and I did get to see him one more time. He was lying supine in the bed he shared with Cici. His eyes were partly open, but he did not look at me or respond to me when I spoke his name. His breathing was shallow and irregular. I uncovered his lower body to see that his feet were splotched with purple. I covered him back up and pulled my stool close to his ear.

I placed one hand on the top of Daniel's head and the other over his heart. I thanked Daniel for letting me spend time getting to know him. I told him that he and Cici had inspired me. I wished him peace and ease. And then I sat quietly, as his breaths came sporadically. His face was soft, and he appeared to be comfortable. He didn't seem to need much.

The session was very short, about 10 minutes long.

Cici was crying at the kitchen table. I approached her and asked if I could do something for her. I stood behind her and placed my hands on her shoulders. She leaned back in the chair and closed her eyes, inhaling and exhaling deeply for a few minutes while tears rolled down her cheeks. I moved to the side of the chair, placing one hand on the back of her neck and the other hand over her heart. We breathed together quietly for another minute, and then I kissed the top of her head before hugging her goodbye.

The last breath and beyond

The last breath is typically peaceful, with respirations growing farther apart until they stop. Robert Chodo Campbell refers to the ensuing stillness as the "silence of the leaving" (Campbell, 2016). If family is present, the moment can understandably be extremely emotional. A touch therapist who happens to be at the bedside when death occurs can provide comfort to the family along with an offer to assist with whatever they might need. This could include calling hospice, who will send a nurse to pronounce the death after confirming there is no heartbeat. Hospice typically encourages families to spend time alone with the body if the family wishes to. It is appropriate to ask, "Would you like me to stay with you, or would you prefer to have some privacy?"

What happens next will likely be informed by cultural, religious, or individual preferences. Immediate post-mortem care may be provided by nursing staff, by the family, or by the family's appointed representatives. This may include washing the body and putting on a fresh gown or sheets. This last stage of care for a person's body is imbued with the same respect and reverence which hopefully defined their care while dying.

Touching story 5.5. Care for the dying does not end with death

On a handful of occasions, I have had the honor of assisting with postmortem care at our inpatient unit. This is the story of my first time. I entered the room with one of our aides, Marta. She filled a basin with warm water, adding a few drops of soap. Marta mentioned that she also added toothpaste to the water to give the body a fresh smell. I watched as Marta donned gloves and dipped a washcloth into the basin, wringing it out so that it was barely damp. She gently washed the patient's face, ears, and neck. She washed the arms and legs, uncovering and recovering each limb with utmost care. Marta hummed an African hymn as she worked. The patient looked peaceful, as if he were sleeping.

Marta had me help her roll the patient gently onto his side so that she could check his brief. The patient was clean and dry, so there was no need to change his clothing. The back side of his body was dark purple from blood pooling, which Marta said was normal. We replaced the top sheet with a fresh one. We neatly folded the top of the sheet, leaving the patient's arms exposed in case family wanted to hold his hand. I said a silent blessing as I combed the patient's hair. With that, our care of the body was complete.

Before we exited the room, we bundled up the dirty linen and trash. We moved flowers and boxes of tissue to surfaces where they could be seen and accessed. We straightened the chairs and opened the balcony door, as it happened to be a sunny day. I thanked Marta for allowing me to participate. We hugged briefly, and I walked toward the family to let them know that everything was ready for them.

Post-mortem care varies from place to place. In some settings, a "chin strap" (a scarf, a tie, or rolled piece of bed linen) is tied under the chin to hold the mouth closed. Marta did not do this, as it's not standard practice on our unit. She turned off the patient's oxygen and removed the nasal cannula but did not remove his IV. She explained that the latter is done only when the family requests it.

The purpose of post-mortem care is to prepare the patient for viewing by the family. The intentions are to honor the patient's body and to provide comfort for loved ones in their grief. What I learned from the experience is that the care we provide to the dying does not end at the last breath. I have a newfound appreciation for the work of undertakers and others who support the various rituals of preparing our earthly bodies to reach their final destinations, a job that is still carried out by family members in many parts of the world. It is yet another sacred opportunity on the continuum of care that we are honored to be part of, and for me, it was a perfect way to bid farewell.

Conclusion

I was not there when Daniel died the day after my last visit. Cici called to tell me about it. She had climbed into bed with him and was holding him as his breathing slowed, then stopped. It was clear that she was pleased with how the end happened for him. Not because it was easy, but because Daniel's irascible, "splendidly maddening" spirit was honored at each step of the way (Saunders, 1965).

Daniel was one of the most singular people I've ever met. His story will never be repeated. And yet he shared with every other person on the planet some remarkable similarities in his stages of dying. Through early decline, late decline, pre-active dying, active dying, and his last breath, Daniel experienced physical changes that are universal to the human experience. But the way he lived out his last months, days, and hours was uniquely his own. Cici still talks about the comfort he found in being touched at each stage of dying.

Death can be a "gentle unraveling" (Gershten, 2013) or an arduous struggle. It is typically a combination of both. Chapter 6 will address the struggle, specifically some of the most common symptoms at the end of life and how massage can help.

References

Campbell, R., 2016. *Awake at the bedside: contemplative teachings on palliative and end-of-life care.* Somerville, MA: Wisdom Publications.

Collett, M., 1997. *Stay close and do nothing: a spiritual and practical guide to caring for the dying at home.* Kansas City, MO: Andrews McMeel Publishing.

Gershten, M., 2013. The five psychological stages of dying and medical issues around death. In: Holecek, A. *Preparing to die: practical advice and spiritual wisdom from the Tibetan Buddhist tradition.* Boston and London: Snow Lion. Ch. 8.

Halifax, J., 2008. *Being with dying: cultivating compassion and fearlessness in the presence of death.* Boston, MA: Shambala.

Peralta, A., 2017. *The process of dying.* [patient handout] Duncanville, TX: Palliative Medicine Consulting Services.

Powers, E., 2020. Discussion of her father's death. [conversation in person] (Personal communication, 20 March 2020).

Saunders, C., 1965. *Watch with me: the founding of St. Christopher's hospice.* [pdf] Available at: <http://endoflifestudies.academicblogs.co.uk/wp-content/uploads/sites/22/2014/04/Watch-with-Me-full-text-2005.pdf>.

Spence, C., 2021. Sacred time: touch at the end of life. In: MacDonald, G. and Tague, C. *Hands in health care:*

massage therapy for the adult hospital patient. 2nd ed. Edinburgh: Handspring. Ch. 14.

Tisdale, S., 2018. *Advice for future corpses (and those who love them): a practical perspective on death and dying.* New York: Simon & Schuster, Inc.

Wilner, L.S. and Arnold, R., 2015. *The palliative performance scale (PPS).* Fast Fact #125. [online] Available at: <https://www.mypcnow.org/fast-fact/the-palliative-performance-scale-pps>.

Additional resources

Callanan, M., 2012. *Final gifts.* New York Simon & Schuster.

Hartman, V., 2012, 2009. Circle of life: hospice and palliative massage workshops. Dallas training notes, Concord training notes.

Karnes, B., 2019. *Gone from my sight: the dying experience.* Vancouver: Barbara Karnes Books, Inc.

Marks, A. and Marchand, L., 2015. *Near death awareness.* Fast Fact #118. [online] Available at: <https://www.mypcnow.org/fast-fact/near-death-awareness>.

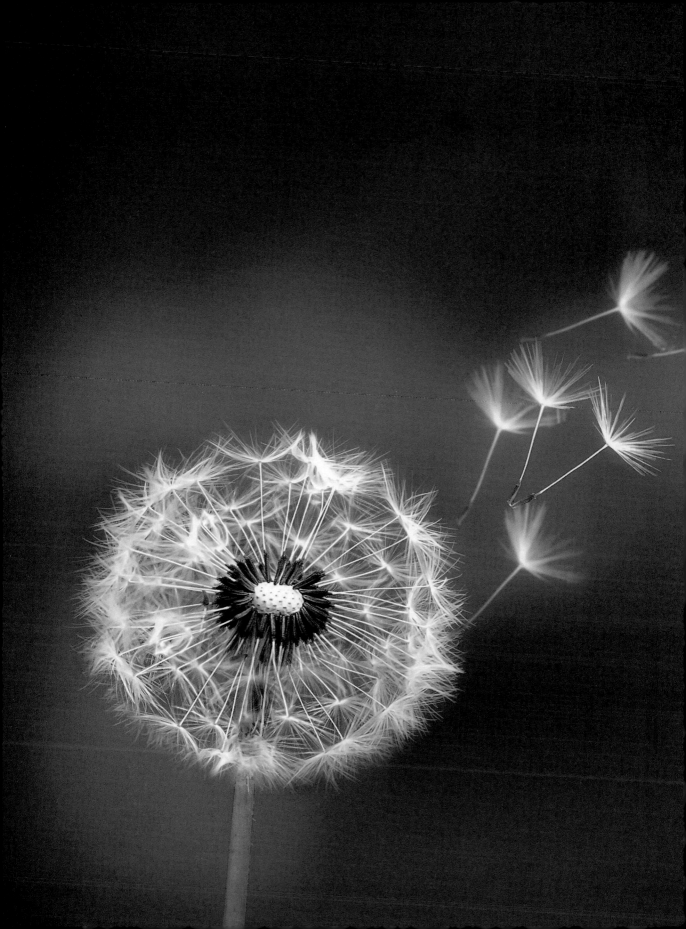

Diving deeper 2

Common symptoms at the end of life   95

Common conditions   117

Medications in end-of-life care   145

Equipment, devices, and procedures   165

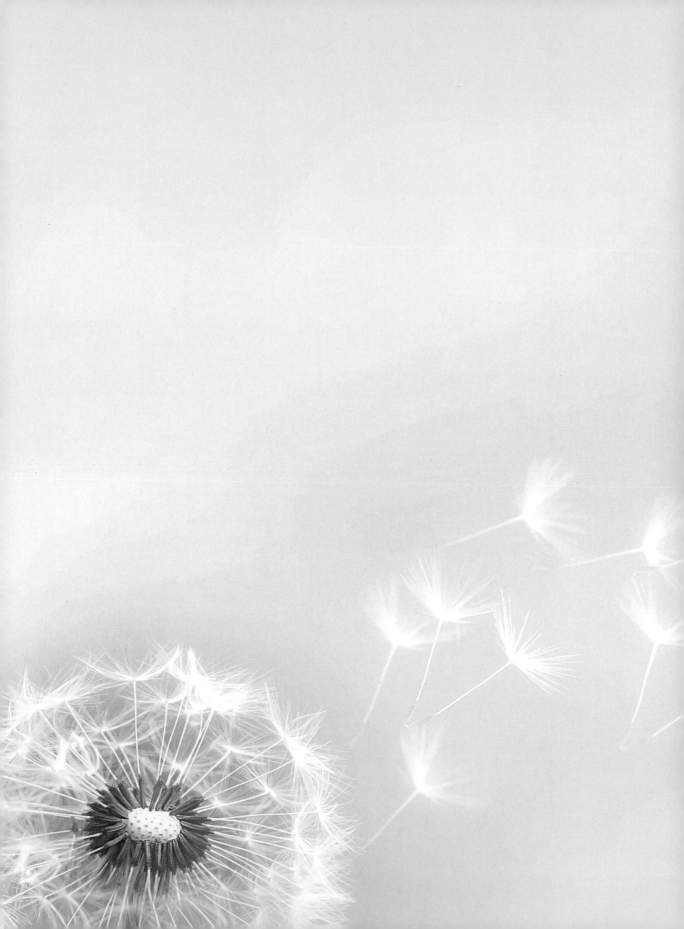

Suffering is only intolerable when nobody cares.

–Cicely Saunders

My favorite definition of the word symptom, read long ago in a source I cannot remember, is that a symptom is an "unwanted experience." What I like about this perspective is that the emphasis is not on the pathology of disease, but on the experience of that disease for the person who is impacted. By the time a person reaches the end-stage of any disease, they have likely endured countless unwanted experiences. Yet the meaning, importance, and response to any symptom is highly individual. Some people seem to become inured to suffering, denying or minimizing what looks to be intolerable. Others experience significant distress from a source that is not obvious to anyone else. Symptoms are perceived by the person experiencing them, while signs are physical evidence that can be observed by others. Both symptoms and signs contribute to the clinical assessment, but it is the patient's experience that drives the care plan.

The concept of "total suffering" was first identified by Cicely Saunders to describe the holistic experience of dying which includes physical, psychological, social, and spiritual dimensions. It is the role of the interdisciplinary care team to help patients find relief for their unwanted experiences across these dimensions, as defined and prioritized by each patient and their appointed decision-makers. Touch therapists can be an excellent addition to this team approach, providing skilled care that can relieve multiple components of suffering.

Chapter 6 will address 25 of the most common symptoms at the end of life, focusing on adjustments to the massage session that may be needed and comfort measures that may help. Many symptoms can be managed effectively by an integrated palliative approach. But it must be acknowledged that it is not always possible to eliminate every discomfort of dying. Anguish, grief, and other distress can be normal responses to death, and piecemeal efforts to excise this suffering may unintentionally diminish and sterilize the dying experience. Caring does not always mean the elimination of suffering; sometimes it means acknowledging and *sharing* it (Taboada, 2021). Portions of this chapter first appeared in *Hands in health care* (Spence, 2021).

Anorexia and cachexia

One of the first signs of decline in a terminal patient is loss of appetite, or anorexia. Anorexia is a natural result of the body's inability to make use of food. The digestive process (chewing, swallowing, breaking down and moving food through the digestive tract, and eliminating waste) all require energy. As the energy available for these processes becomes scarce, several factors can contribute to impaired food intake, including fatigue, early satiety, nausea with or without vomiting, and difficulty swallowing. End-of-life nutrition can be further complicated for some patients by poor oral health, ill-fitting dentures, pain, and shortness of breath.

Cachexia refers to the extreme wasting of muscle that results from anorexia. Cachexia can accompany almost any terminal diagnosis, including cancer, acquired immunodeficiency syndrome (AIDS), kidney disease, liver disease, congestive heart failure (CHF), chronic obstructive pulmonary disease (COPD), dementia, and aging. Anorexia and cachexia involve systemic inflammation and the release of cytokines, chemicals that interfere with the absorption and synthesis of nutrients. Even if the dying person could consume enough calories to sustain life, the body would be unable to break down and use them. In short, people don't die because they aren't eating. Rather, they don't eat because they are dying (Bahti, 2012). For this reason, artificial nutrition and hydration are rarely beneficial at the very end of life and can cause problems including congestion, edema, infection, aspiration of food into the lungs, and subsequent pneumonia (see p. 177). Corticosteroids may be used on a short-term basis to temporarily increase appetite, but side effects, including insomnia, can outweigh benefits.

Anorexia and cachexia can be extremely hard for loved ones, as they are undeniable signs of advancing disease. Eating is associated with the will to live and rituals that bind people together. Families often say, "If he would just eat something," indicating grief, frustration, and misunderstanding about the role of anorexia in the dying process. It is not uncommon for there to be conflicts about food between patients and their loved ones, who may have difficulty understanding why the medical team is not taking a more aggressive approach toward nutrition and hydration.

Hospice philosophy is to allow the patient to control eating and drinking, while providing support to manage the risk of choking or aspiration. For people who are able to swallow, small amounts of favorite foods may be offered. This is known as "pleasure feeding," which can be assisted by care staff or family as needed. Ideal foods are soft and bland. Bites must be small, and time allowed for swallowing. Thickened liquids are often easier to swallow because they flow more slowly down the throat. The team also supports families with education and compassionate support, including encouragement to explore meaningful connections that don't involve food. Spouses, partners, parents, siblings, and friends, even very young children, can be taught to provide gentle touch as a means to nourish the dying person.

Adapting the massage session

- Length of massage session should be shortened to reduce demands on the body.

- Level 2 pressure is usually well tolerated by people with mild to moderate cachexia.

- Level 1 pressure should be used for severe cachexia, indicated by temporal wasting (see p. 33 for photo).

- Bony prominences are at risk of skin breakdown. "Floating" the heels with pillows and frequent position changes to protect the sacrum are strategies to protect fragile areas.

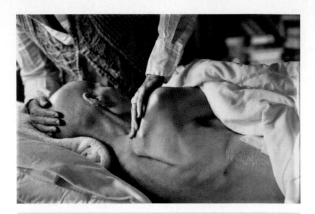

Figure 6.1
A rolled washcloth fills space between the patient's neck and the pillow below. Therapists should avoid massage directly over bony prominences that may be very sensitive.

(Photo by Candice White, first appeared in *Hands in health care*.)

- Pillows or rolled towels can be used to fill hollow spaces, providing a sense of cushioning and support as shown in Figure 6.1.

Anxiety

Most people experience at least *some* degree of anxiety at the end of life, and for many, this symptom can be extreme. Loss of control, fear of the unknown, separation from loved ones, unresolved regrets, worry about family or finances, and preexisting anxiety or trauma can be contributing factors. Pain and other symptoms can cause or worsen anxiety, and anxiety in turn can magnify pain, shortness of breath, nausea, diarrhea, and insomnia. Common signs of anxiety include restlessness, heightened vigilance, wishing to remain awake or keep the lights on, irritability, or a persistent need to control the environment. An anxious person often presents as a demanding patient for caregivers and staff.

While antianxiety medication is often needed, massage can be a helpful part of the care plan. Anxiety responds most favorably to slow engagement, both on and off the body. A therapist who is mindful of the speed with which they move, speak, initiate contact, conduct the touch session, and exit the room creates a very different energy than a therapist who is not mindful of these things. Calm, caring presence in the face of anxiety and fear may, in fact, be the biggest gift we have to offer others. Anxious patients and families may be comforted by our composure in the same way that passengers on an airplane experiencing turbulence are reassured by the calm demeanor of their flight attendants.

Of note, anxiety in patients with dementia or nonverbal patients may present as extreme restlessness, including inability to be still, attempting to get out of bed for no known reason, or insistence on looking for "lost" items. The reactions of these patients must be closely monitored to assess whether massage is making things better or worse. Even patients who have previously enjoyed massage may reach a point, temporarily or permanently, when they do not wish to be touched. Assessment for changes in response to massage should therefore be ongoing, providing patients with choice and control.

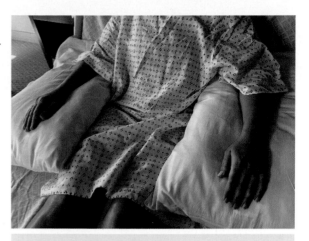

Figure 6.2
Pillows under the arms give the upper extremities something to rest on, conveying a sense of security and support. Good propping can communicate to the nervous system that it is safe to let go.

(Photo by Candice White.)

Adapting the massage session

- Promote a sense of control by asking the patient or family whether there is any area the patient protects and might wish not to be touched.

Tip 6.1. Propping to reduce anxiety

Anxious patients, both those who do not tolerate touch and those who do, will benefit from attentive propping. Pillows and other soft materials (rolled towels, washcloths, blankets, and pieces of foam) can be used to create contours that conform to, cradle, and hold the patient's body. One example of this is placing pillows beneath each arm when the patient is in high Fowler's or seated as shown in Figure 6.2, a common vigilant position for anxious patients.

- Support patient preferences for positioning, offering extra propping for security.

- Full-handed level 2 or level 1 pressure should be employed, depending on the patient's condition, including holds, gentle compression, or slow gliding. Monitor the patient's response to massage and adjust the treatment accordingly.

- Soothing music or calming essential oil can help some people, but take care not to overstimulate with too many interventions at once.

- A favorite blanket or pillow, stuffed animal, or religious article, such as a rosary or other prayer beads, is often seen at the bedside. Therapists can place these items on or near the patient as a way to connect them to something familiar and soothing.

- Sometimes it is a family member who expresses anxiety through irritability or excessive demands on the care team. Slowing and deepening your own breath will help you to remain grounded in compassion and may soothe the anxiety of others.

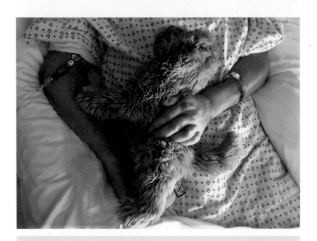

Figure 6.3
Comfort or "transitional objects" can include personally meaningful items that convey love and security. These can be very helpful for a person with anxiety.

(Photo by author.)

Apnea

Apnea is defined as the temporary cessation of breathing. End-of-life apnea is a natural and progressive process, which takes place as the respiratory system begins to shut down. Respirations during this transition may be fast, slow, shallow, deep, or any combination of these features, punctuated by periods of no breathing at all. This variable breathing pattern is a hallmark of active dying referred to as Cheyne–Stokes breathing, though it may occur intermittently during an earlier stage. As active dying progresses, periods of apnea may increase to up to a minute or longer, with lots of waiting in between. Apnea may be accompanied by silence and stillness, or by noisy breath sounds if secretions are present (see p. 111 on secretions).

One example of matching the massage session to the patient's energy level can be for the therapist to stop moving during an episode of apnea, simply resting the hands on the patient's body. This also provides the opportunity for the therapist to monitor the duration of apnea for charting or reporting to the medical team. It is not unusual, as the patient relaxes, for periods of apnea to grow longer during massage.

Adapting the massage session

- Apnea signals that the patient is in the active stage of dying. Level 1 pressure or holds are indicated.

- The session may be brief, as short as 10–15 minutes in length.

- Though apnea is not distressing to patients, it can be difficult for loved ones to witness. Clinical staff will ideally provide education that touch therapists can endorse with active listening and calm support.

Ascites

Ascites is the accumulation of abdominal fluid that can occur in advanced liver disease, kidney disease, CHF, and many cancers, including cancers of the ovary, breast, colon, stomach, pancreas, or lung (Kinzbrunner and McKinnis, 2011). The volume of fluid can be quite large, resembling late pregnancy and causing shortness of breath, loss of appetite, nausea, vomiting, edema in the lower extremities, and reduced mobility. Medical management will depend on the cause. For nonmalignant ascites, diuretics and reduced salt and fluids may be recommended, though this approach is generally not effective when cancer is the cause. Paracentesis, a bedside procedure in which fluid is removed through a needle, can provide immediate relief (see p. 176), but the fluid generally returns and may increase in volume following efforts to remove it. A permanent catheter system may be placed in the body to drain ascites on an ongoing basis. Risks include fatal hypotension (low blood pressure), bleeding, dislodgment, tube blockage, and infection.

Adapting the massage session

- People with ascites often prefer a seated position or the head of the bed elevated for ease of breathing.

- Some patients will not want their abdomen to be touched; others will be comforted by level 1 holds or light effleurage to the abdomen.

- Use level 1 or level 2 pressure for all other areas of the body, including lower extremities with edema.

- Avoid drains and catheters, if present, due to risk of infection.

Confusion, delirium, and terminal restlessness

Confusion is sometimes described as altered mental status, or AMS. AMS may be part of a disease process, such as dementia, renal failure, liver failure, brain cancer, or cancers that metastasize to the brain. Other causes include pain; medications (especially steroids, opioids, and benzodiazepines); infection (particularly urinary tract infections); dehydration; electrolyte disturbance; fever; a full bladder; constipation; hip fracture; hypoxia (lack of oxygen to the brain); and acidosis (build-up of acid in the blood from kidney disease, lung disease, or diabetic ketoacidosis). An accumulation of opioid metabolites in the body, once urination ceases, is another possible cause.

Confusion can range from mild and benign to severe and disturbing. There may be forgetfulness, rambling speech, picking at bedclothes, or random hand motions. A common and more severe form of confusion in the final days of life is known as terminal agitation or terminal restlessness, characterized by tossing and turning, repeated attempts to get out of bed, or pulling off clothing. Less common but more extreme is terminal delirium, which may cause the patient to hallucinate, cry out, or become combative. These behaviors are distressing for patients, families, and professional caregivers. When the source seems clear, the care team will attempt to treat delirium, but if death is imminent, it may be necessary to palliate this symptom without determining or reversing the cause.

Confusion, delirium, and terminal restlessness should not be conflated with near death awareness (NDA), in which people experience the presence of deceased relatives and other premonitions of death. NDA, described in Chapter 5, tends to be characterized by predictable experiences, which are often described with clarity and are comforting to the patient. Confusion, delirium, and terminal restlessness have a more random quality and the potential to be disturbing when severe. Delirium and terminal restlessness may require around-the-clock observation or sedation to keep the patient safe. Sometimes confusion is relieved by the presence of familiar loved ones. At other times, visitors seem to be a complicating factor. Reducing stimuli, such as lighting, noise, and activity, is generally helpful. For some patients, slow, grounding touch by a therapist or family member may be soothing. For others, touch is a source of stimulation that causes arousal rather than comfort. Therapists working in the inpatient environment should check with nursing staff prior to visiting patients with agitation. If staff members have worked hard to get a restless patient settled, they may not want that patient touched.

Chart talk 6.1. A+O X 1–4

Medical charts often describe patients as alert and oriented on a numeric scale, based on level of awareness and responsiveness to their environment. This is also referred to as A+O, or AAO, or AO, followed by an "X" and a number as follows:

AO X 1 – the person is "oriented to self or person." They know their own name, and the names of significant others.

AO X 2 – the person is "oriented to person and place." They know where they are.

AO X 3 – the person is "oriented to person, place, and time." They know the date and day.

AO X 4 – the person is "oriented to person, place, time, and situation." They know what has happened to them, where they are, and why. For example, they know they are at the hospital because they had a fall.

Adapting the massage session

- Create a calm, quiet environment.

- Speak softly and clearly, identifying yourself by name. Briefly explain what you are about to do and that your intention is to help them feel better.

- Reorient without contradiction, assuring the patient that you are with them, and they are safe.

- A slight change in position or gentle range of motion can sometimes help with agitation.

- Visual and hearing aids, if worn, can help.

- Level 2 holds may provide a sense of grounding.

- Do not attempt to restrain restless or repetitive movements, but do alert family or staff immediately of any situation that seems unsafe or distressing to the patient.

- Monitor reactions to massage to ensure that touch is helping rather than making the problem worse.

- If the patient is fearful, stay calm and present.

Constipation

The body continues to produce stool up until the very end of life, even after eating has stopped. But numerous factors can interfere with the ability to produce bowel movements. Narcotics are the number one cause of constipation at the end of life. Decreased consumption of food and fluids, reduced activity level, decreased efficiency of the digestive system, and lack of privacy all interfere with normal habits of elimination. Certain conditions, such as Parkinson's, cerebral infarction, multiple sclerosis, and abdominal malignancies, to name a few, are associated with higher risk of constipation (Kinzbrunner and McKinnis, 2011).

Suffering related to constipation can be substantial. Abdominal distention, nausea, vomiting, pain, fever, and intermittent diarrhea can occur. Unabated, constipation can lead to fecal impaction and bowel obstruction, which are extremely painful and potentially fatal. The care team will likely initiate a bowel regimen of stool softeners and laxatives when opioids are used, with more aggressive interventions if necessary. Though not a replacement for these measures, massage can be very effective for some patients, either to promote digestion through general relaxation, or to provide direct stimulation for peristalsis through abdominal massage. Several studies endorse abdominal massage to reduce symptoms, decrease time between bowel movements, and improve quality of life (Turan and Atabek Aşt, 2016; Lämås et al., 2011).

Tip 6.2. Abdominal massage

Food moves up the ascending colon on the right side of the abdomen, across the transverse colon, then down the descending colon on the left side of the abdomen before entering the sigmoid colon and exiting the body through the rectum and anus. Abdominal massage using two-handed light effleurage or a gentle wavelike motion similar to that used in manual lymphatic drainage (MLD) should be applied in a clockwise direction, with level 1 or 2 pressure adjusted to ensure the patient's comfort (see Figure 6.4).

Abdominal massage can be performed over clothing or directly on skin and can be taught to patients so that they can perform it on themselves. This is a gentle, noninvasive technique, but should not be used if indwelling abdominal catheters are present (feeding tubes or peritoneal catheters), or when obstruction is present or suspected. Because patient feedback is essential, massage to the abdomen should not be performed on a nonverbal person.

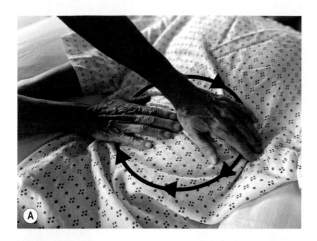

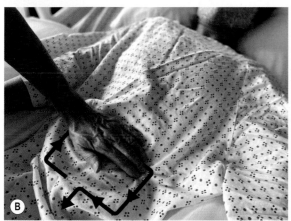

Figure 6.4

Two different methods for abdominal massage. (A) Two hands can be used to provide gentle effleurage in a clockwise circular pattern; the movement is fluid and continuous. Alternately, one hand is used (B), pressing down lightly with the palm, then rocking the hand in a wavelike motion; the hand is then picked up and placed down again to repeat the motion, gently encouraging movement of bowel contents through the intestines, as indicated by the black arrows. Gas and stool can often be felt as hard areas or lumps. Patients who experience positive results are often motivated to perform these techniques on themselves. Studies suggest that best results are achieved with a minimum of daily practice.

(Photos by Candice White.)

Adapting the massage session

- Most patients with constipation prefer a supine or semi-reclining position.
- Check with medical staff to rule out partial or total obstruction before providing abdominal massage. The presence of catheters in the abdomen should also be assessed.
- Use level 1 or level 2 pressure when providing abdominal massage, always in a clockwise direction with patient feedback to guide comfort. Abdominal massage should be relaxing for the recipient.
- Patients who are willing can be taught abdominal massage.
- Foot reflexology can be used as an alternative to abdominal massage, using thumb walking to trace digestion on the soles of the feet; see Figure 6.5.

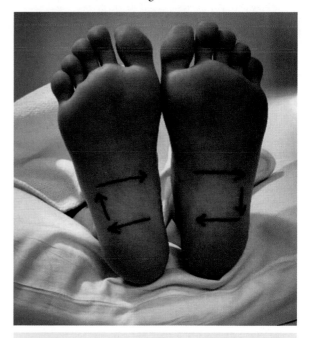

Figure 6.5

The therapist's thumb will inch along the path indicated by the arrows, using pressure that is comfortable for the patient.

(Photo by author.)

- An acupressure point in the hand may also be effective for constipation. See Figure 6.10(B) on p. 108 to locate Large Intestine 4 in the fleshy muscle between the index finger and the thumb.

Depression

Research suggests that *most* patients with advanced illness do not experience clinical depression, but rather normal grief in response to the dying process. Grief is an "adaptive, universal, and highly personalized response to the multiple losses that occur at the end of life" (Widera and Block, 2012). While grief can cause tremendous suffering, it does not require medical intervention. Depression, on the other hand, may warrant medication, and studies indicate that it is undertreated. Risk factors for depression include poor symptom control, family or personal history of depression, substance abuse, poor social support, and financial distress (DiBello, 2015). While diagnosis and treatment are outside the scope of practice for touch therapists, we can participate as members of the care team to help identify patients who might benefit from more support.

Adapting the massage session

- When a dying person or caregiver expresses sadness or other distressing emotion, helpful responses include active listening and validation of feelings as a legitimate response to a challenging situation.

- People who are grieving may experience occasional feelings of hopelessness, but these are typically interspersed with an ability to experience pleasurable activities, which may include massage.

- Other members of the care team, including social workers and chaplains, are trained to provide grief support.

- The following signs may indicate depression and should be evaluated by a clinical professional: excessive feelings of guilt, shame, or hopelessness; persistent withdrawal from family, friends, and activities; persistent loss of interest and pleasure; thoughts of suicide (Widera and Block, 2012).

- If you are concerned that a patient may be depressed, it is important to share this with the care team so that it can be addressed.

Diarrhea

Diarrhea can be a distressing problem for people at the end of life, leading to abdominal pain, dehydration, electrolyte imbalance, fatigue, and skin breakdown. There may be odor or a frequent need for clothing or linen changes that causes embarrassment or social isolation. Common causes of diarrhea include the overuse of laxatives to combat constipation; other medications, including antibiotics; malignancies of the pancreas and gastrointestinal tract; AIDS; bowel disease; and infections such as C. diff (Kinzbrunner and McKinnis, 2011). "Overflow diarrhea" can occur with severe constipation, fecal impaction, or partial obstruction, as liquified stool may be all that the patient can pass (Alderman, 2015). A palliative approach will depend on the cause but may include medication.

Adapting the massage session

- The massage session may be delayed or interrupted by diarrhea.

- Patient dignity must be prioritized. If diarrhea is known to be an issue, the therapist might address this at the beginning of the session by assuring the patient that they can request to stop the massage at any time.

- If C. diff infection is known or suspected, the therapist should wear gloves and a gown in accordance with agency protocols. Hand sanitizer is not effective against C. diff. Hands will need to be washed thoroughly with soap and water.

Dyspnea (shortness of breath)

Dyspnea is a common and extremely distressing symptom that can accompany primary lung cancer, cancers that metastasize to the lungs from elsewhere in the body, COPD, pulmonary fibrosis, CHF, or amytrophic lateral sclerosis (ALS). Dyspnea can also occur in advanced diseases that cause fluid to collect in the abdomen, such as heart, renal, or liver failure. The dying process itself can cause shortness of breath, as the body's O_2 and CO_2 receptors begin to fail. Respiratory distress is a very frightening symptom for patients and their loved ones. Shortness of breath leads to anxiety, and anxiety in turn increases the sensation of air hunger.

Dyspnea is addressed by the medical team with supplemental oxygen, medications to open the airway, and small doses of morphine to reduce the patient's perception of breathlessness. Diuretics may be used to manage congestion in the lungs. While massage does not address the root causes of dyspnea, it does reduce anxiety and can therefore have a positive impact on this symptom. Massage can provide relief to accessory muscles which are working overtime in the dyspneic patient, including pectoralis major and minor, latissimus dorsi, serratus anterior and posterior, scalenes, sternocleidomastoid (SCM), and intercostals (muscles of the chest, neck, shoulders, back, and between the ribs).

Adapting the massage session

- Patients with respiratory distress will be unable to lie flat. Seated, high Fowler's position, or forward leaning will likely be most comfortable.

- Level 2 pressure is usually well tolerated, level 1 if widespread bruising is present.

- Cooler temperature and circulating air may be helpful.

- Some patients are helped by gentle tapotement (light taps with the fingertips, no greater than level 2 pressure) applied over the posterior lungs (see Tip 7.1 for more information).

- Be sensitive to any pressure over the chest, even resting hands, which may feel like constriction.

- Reflex points for the lungs are located in the ball of the foot. Static or circular pressure to this area can be comforting for the patient.

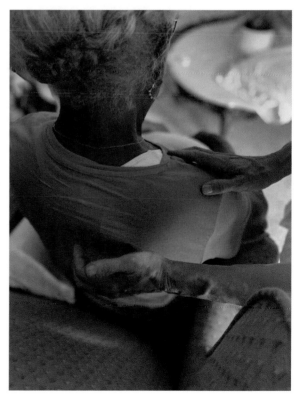

Figure 6.7
Gentle tapotement is applied with relaxed fingers and should feel calming to the patient.

(Photo by Candice White.)

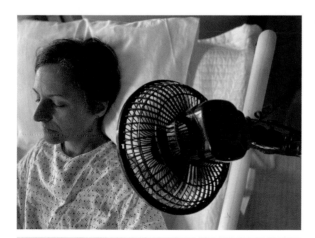

Figure 6.6
A small fan that clips to the bedrail can provide cool, direct airflow that relieves the sensation of dyspnea.

(Photo by author.)

Edema and lymphedema

Fluid overload, or swelling, often occurs at the end of life as the body loses its ability to process, absorb, and eliminate fluids. Edema is a general term to describe this fluid overload, which may happen anywhere in the body. The extremities are a common place for edema to occur, often in the feet or legs, but also in the hands or arms. Edema in the extremities is called peripheral edema and may occur on one side (unilateral) or both sides (bilateral).

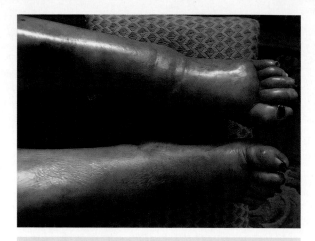

Chart talk 6.2. Pitting edema

The medical chart may describe pitting edema rated by a score of 1–4. These numbers describe the response of the tissue when gently pressed by the examiner's finger as indicated below.

Pitting edema +1 – a depression is barely visible (2 mm) and disappears immediately.

Pitting edema +2 – slight indentation (3–4 mm) that disappears in 15 seconds or less.

Pitting edema +3 – 5–6 mm depression that disappears in 10–30 seconds.

Pitting edema +4 – deep indentation (8 mm) that remains visible for more than 20 seconds.

Figure 6.8
The tissues of a person with edema can feel water-logged from fluid overload, or tight and hard with shiny skin. Gentle strokes toward the heart often feel good to the patient.

(Photo by author.)

Edema that occurs in the abdomen is called ascites, described on p. 98. Edema can also be generalized all over the body, a condition called anasarca. Lymphedema is a specific type of edema that may occur as a complication of cancer, explained in greater detail on p. 37 and p. 122. All types of fluid retention can cause discomfort or pain. When severe, both edema and lymphedema can cause weeping of fluids through the skin pores, creating a risk of infection. The medical team may treat edema with diuretics. Diuretics are not effective for treating lymphedema. The approach for touch therapists to fluid overload is the same, regardless of cause. Goals include patient comfort and the maintenance of skin quality.

Adapting the massage session

- Elevate edematous extremities to provide comfort.

- Level 1 pressure or holds if swelling is severe, level 2 if mild to moderate.

- Be cautious with areas of skin that may have thinned due to swelling.

- No massage should be given to a weeping area of the body. Very gentle holds may be provided *over* a waterproof pad, if desired by the patient.

- Strokes should be directed toward the heart.

- See p. 125 for specific information regarding MLD for lymphedema.

Falls

Falls are unfortunately very common at the end of life. Aging and disease both impact strength, gait, visual-spatial perception, and balance. Other risk factors include hearing impairment (Lin and Ferrucci, 2012), cognitive impairment, peripheral neuropathy, and muscle atrophy from limited physical activity. Certain conditions increase fall risk, including heart disease and neuromotor diseases such as Parkinson's. Numerous medications impact the central nervous system, causing dizziness, drowsiness, confusion, and sedation, all associated with falls. Environmental factors include objects on the floor, poor lighting, and rugs. Falls may happen when people are reaching for items, or when they become disoriented in a new environment. Improper footwear and incontinence may contribute. Injuries may result in bruises, swelling, broken bones, wounds requiring bandaging or stitches, and/or life-threatening hemorrhage.

Adapting the massage session

- Take care to ensure that patient transfers are safe. If the patient is not able to transfer independently and help is not available, provide massage wherever the patient is found.

- Remember to lower the hospital bed, if raised for massage.

- Return bedrails to upright position if they were lowered for massage.

- Return anything that was moved for massage to its original location, including furniture, overbed tables, mobility devices, and personal items.

- Be aware that bed alarms and cameras are used in some settings to monitor patient safety. One type of bed alarm is a thin pad placed under a fitted sheet that senses changes in motion or pressure. Another involves a pull cord that attaches the patient's gown or clothing to the bedsheet or pillow. The alarms will sound *very loudly* if the patient attempts to leave bed.

- Report safety concerns to staff or family and document accordingly.

Fatigue

Given the significant demands that end-stage diseases place on the body, fatigue is a normal part of the dying process. At the end of life, people experience incremental loss of energy for activities they once took for granted: the ability to walk across a room, take a shower, dress by themselves, sit in a chair, have a conversation, or finish a meal. Some of the causes can be addressed – anemia, insomnia, and infections, for example. But the reality is that there is no medication to treat end-of-life fatigue. A major focus of the care team is to help patients and loved ones adjust their expectations to new realities. Dying people sleep more as they decline. Moments of wakefulness become a gift to be enjoyed to the fullest. The role of the massage therapist is to provide a session that is supportive and nurturing, never demanding. The pressure and duration of the massage, conversation during the session, undressing, and repositioning all require energy that is in short supply for the patient. Therapists must also be mindful of socializing with staff in areas where patients could be impacted by noise. A restful environment helps patients get the sleep they need, so that they can conserve energy for experiences that are meaningful to them.

Adapting the massage session

- Maximize the potential for rest by avoiding massage around mealtimes, expected visitors, and other activities which might interrupt the restful aftermath of gentle touch.

- The patient's preferred sleeping position can be a nice option for massage. But reposition sparingly, as movement and transfers require energy.

- Level 2 pressure is used for mild or moderate fatigue. Level 1 or holds are preferred if fatigue is extreme.

- Minimize conversation. Some patients need "permission" to close their eyes and rest.

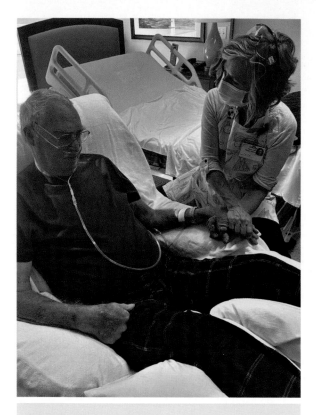

Figure 6.9
Patients with severe fatigue often experience a "bed-to-chair existence." Working on the patient where found is one way to conserve a waning supply of energy.

(Photo by Beth Giniewicz.)

- Shorten session length to match the patient's energy level.

- Place needed objects such as drinks, snacks, remote controls, eyeglasses, tissues, and trash cans within easy reach.

Fever

Fever is another common symptom at the end of life, potentially caused by infection, inflammation, and certain cancers, including lymphoma. Fever may accompany some brain injuries, perhaps due to trauma of the hypothalmus. Deep vein thrombosis and pulmonary embolism

have also been cited in the literature as possible causes of fever (Strickland and Stovsky, 2015). During active dying, fever may be intermittent with periods of chill. There may be excessive sweating, called diaphoresis, in which the dying person's clothing and bed linen become soaked. Regulation of body temperature may become chaotic, with parts of the body feeling hot to the touch and others feeling cold.

Fever is often cited in massage school as a contraindication to massage. At the end of life, however, light touch can be very comforting to someone with fever. The medical team may or may not treat a fever with medication, depending on whether the patient appears to be uncomfortable. The drug of choice at our inpatient unit is acetaminophen (paracetamol), given orally if the patient can swallow. For patients unable to swallow, acetaminophen can be placed under the armpit for absorption through the skin, a much less invasive alternative to rectal suppository.

Adapting the massage session

- Level 1 pressure is used for active fever.

- Warm blankets should be removed. The top sheet can remain for modesty or light cover as needed, folded if desired to expose the feet.

- A cool or tepid damp washcloth can be used to sponge the body, placed across the forehead, or wrapped loosely around the feet. A waterproof pad under these wet compresses will keep the bed dry. As the cloths absorb heat from the body, they should be refreshed under cool or tepid water.

- A small fan may be helpful.

- Monitor closely for signs of chill.

- Report fever to clinical staff for observation and treatment as needed.

Fractures

Fractures can occur in terminal patients due to falls and diseases that compromise bone health. A decision must be made by the clinical team regarding repair. Surgery on hips and other long bones of the body has inherent risks and involves a long and difficult recovery. When a patient is dying, a more compassionate approach can be to stabilize the joint and to provide pain control while the body does whatever healing it can on its own. Factors to consider are anticipated life expectancy, overall bone health, and goals and wishes of the patient and family.

Adapting the massage session

- Do not reposition patients with untreated fractures without assistance from medical staff.

- The injured area may need to be supported for protection or avoided altogether.

- A level 1 hold might be tolerated as the fracture heals.

- Level 1 or 2 pressure may be appropriate elsewhere on the body.

Hiccups

Hiccups at the end of life have numerous possible causes. Most are related to issues in the gastrointestinal system or metabolic changes. Some medications can cause hiccups, including corticosteroids, benzodiazepines, chemotherapy, and opioids. Diaphragmatic irritation can also occur from tumors, infection, or inflammation (Phillips, 2005). When the cause is known, the clinical team will treat accordingly. In many cases, however, the cause will be unknown.

Chronic or intractable hiccups, defined as hiccups lasting longer than one month, can be quite distressing, inhibiting the ability to eat, drink, converse, and sleep. The affected person may suffer weight loss, dehydration, fatigue, anxiety, and social embarrassment. When a patient's quality of life is affected, the team may attempt relief with medications, described on p. 155. There is also evidence that acupuncture can help some people (Zhang and Gong, 2020). Remedies such as holding the breath or breathing into a paper bag may have merit, in that they increase carbon dioxide which can inhibit hiccups.

Adapting the massage session

- There is not much for the touch therapist to do, other than support the affected patient with comfortable positioning and massage that feels good.

- The abdominal and intercostal muscles may be tender. Holds or light massage to these areas may be helpful.

Nausea and vomiting

Nausea with or without vomiting may occur at the end of life from numerous causes, including constipation, gastrointestinal obstructions, renal or liver failure, elevated calcium levels, side effects of medications, brain tumors, or anxiety (Wood, 2010). The medical team will manage nausea and vomiting according to cause if known, using antiemetic drugs (see p. 155). Touch therapists can provide nonmedical support that may help some patients. If severe, the affected individual may prefer to delay massage until nausea and vomiting are controlled.

Adapting the massage session

- A person with nausea will likely prefer high Fowler's or upright position.

- Avoid wearing perfume or using scented massage products, as smells can trigger nausea and vomiting.

- Essential oils, including ginger and peppermint, may be helpful (see p. 187). One to three drops can be placed on a cool, wet washcloth around the back of the neck or front of the throat, or on a tissue that the patient can hold or lay on the chest.

- Increase air flow by opening a window or placing a small fan in the room.

- Two acupressure points may relieve nausea for some people: Pericardium 6, or P6 (MSKCC, 2019), and Large Intestine 4, or LI4 (WebMD, 2019). These can be accessed by the touch therapist and taught to the patient and caregivers. The pressure should be firm but not painful, applied for two to three minutes in a circular motion, then repeated on the other wrist or hand (see Figure 6.10).

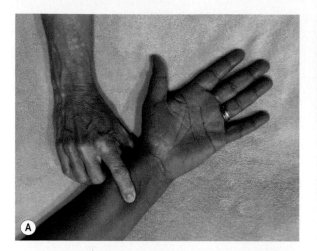

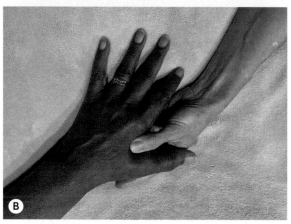

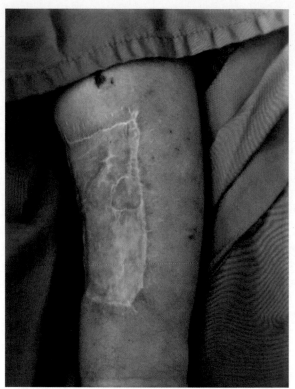

Figure 6.10
Figure (A) demonstrates P6 for nausea, located three finger-widths from the crease of the wrist. Figure (B) demonstrates LI4 in the fleshy muscle between the thumb and first finger. Pressure applied to LI4 may help with nausea or constipation.

(Photos by David Spence.)

Figure 6.11
This patient reported pain at the site of a skin harvest to rebuild his esophagus. Though his head and neck wounds appeared to be more significant, it was the pain in his arm that bothered him most.

(Photo by author.)

Pain

Pain can be very complex at the end of life. Dying doesn't in and of itself cause pain. There are terminal patients who have little to no pain. But most have *some* degree of pain, and most need medication to cope with pain during the dying process. Pain can be caused by terminal disease; a concurring disease; treatments such as surgery, radiation, or chemotherapy; inactivity; inadequate propping; wounds; infection; amputations; old injuries; or arthritis. Pain can occur with any diagnosis, though some diagnoses are more closely associated with pain than others. An example of this is bone cancer or cancer that has metastasized to bones. As stated in the introduction to this chapter, pain is rarely confined to a physical phenomenon, but most often complicated by mental, emotional, social, or spiritual suffering.

Patients are often asked to rank their pain using the Edmonton scale of 0–10. Pain is treated according to the patient's perception of severity, using a stepladder approach developed by the World Health Organization. Mild pain is treated with aspirin, acetaminophen (paracetamol), ibuprofen, or other mild pain reliever. Moderate pain, or pain that does not respond to mild pain relievers, is treated with a "light" opioid such as codeine. Severe or persistent pain warrants the use of a stronger opioid such as morphine. One important aspect of pain management is the concept of dosing on a routine schedule rather than waiting for pain to occur, as it can take longer to control pain once it manifests. Sudden spikes of "breakthrough pain" may occur with activity, or intermittently for unknown reasons. Breakthrough pain is treated with additional doses of medication as needed. The goal is to provide a level of pain management that is consistent with an acceptable level of comfort for the patient.

Pain is also treated according to type. Pain caused by tissue damage or inflammation in the skin, muscle, tendons, or internal organs is referred to as nociceptive pain. Pain from nerve damage, such peripheral neuropathy from diabetes or some chemotherapies, is referred to as neuropathic pain. Chapter 8 describes the medications used to address various types of pain. Of note, bone pain, though considered to be nociceptive, is often treated with some of the same strategies and medications as neuropathic pain.

It is important for every member of the care team, including touch therapists, to understand the patient's beliefs, goals, and concerns related to pain control. There are patients, family members, and some medical professionals who are resistant to the use of opioids, even at the end of life. Morphine, considered to be the gold standard in pain control, has come to be associated with death in the minds of many people. Fears about addiction are common, as are concerns about drug tolerance, or the need for increasing doses of medication that may eventually become ineffective. Chapter 8 addresses these misunderstandings, just as the clinical team will address them with patients and their families.

Another possible obstacle to pain control is that some patients and loved ones wish for the patient to remain awake and alert. This rationale may have validity since pain medications can cause drowsiness that may interfere with meaningful interactions, especially during the first days of use. After a period of adjustment, however, medication can actually help people to be *more* alert (Dear, 2019). As patients decline, it is typically not medication but fatigue and changes in brain function that cause them to sleep more and interact less. One strategy the care team may use is to offer time-limited trials of medication so that patients and families can see for themselves the cost versus benefit of better pain control. In the end, patients and their surrogate decision makers have the final say. There are patients with belief systems that find meaning and value in suffering. Professional caregivers must work closely with patients and their loved ones to achieve an approach to pain control that best supports the patient's wishes, which may change over time.

Touch therapists can provide nonmedical interventions for all types of pain, approaches that are most likely to be helpful when pain is mild to moderate in severity. Patients with extreme pain (a pain score of 7 out of 10 or greater) may be unable to tolerate or enjoy touch until their pain is managed with medication. That said, there really is no downside to a trial of massage, topical analgesics, or hot and cold compresses, if the patient is open to these strategies.

Adapting the massage session

- Ask about pain if the patient is awake and responsive. It can be helpful to have the patient rate their pain from 0 to 10 if they are willing and able.

- Allow the patient to determine comfortable positioning. Additional propping may be helpful for pain, using the principles outlined in Chapter 4.

- Adapt pressure with patient input. Patients with pain might tolerate level 2 pressure, level 1 pressure, gentle holds, or no touch at all.

- If the patient is receptive to gentle touch, begin with an area of the body that does not have pain, proceeding to the painful area after trust is established.

- Pain may be helped by a warm or cool compress (see p. 188). If the area is too sensitive, wrapping the *opposing* extremity can provide sensory distraction (Rice, 2020).

- Certain types of pain may respond to pain patches or topical analgesics (see peripheral neuropathy below).

- Even patients who appear to be sleeping or unconscious can feel pain. Touch therapists should observe potential signs of pain including facial expression, muscle tension, shifting as if to get more comfortable, moaning, crying out, and rapid breathing (respirations faster than 20 per minute).

- If the patient is awake at the conclusion of the massage, a post-session pain score can be solicited. A comparison to the pre-session score can be a way to assess the benefit of massage.

- A patient in severe pain should not be left alone. Report severe pain to the clinical team and remain with the patient if possible. Holding the patient's hand, empathic presence, and providing reassurance that help is on the way may give some comfort until an intervention can be accessed.

Peripheral neuropathy

Peripheral neuropathy (PN) occurs when nerves become damaged or destroyed, interfering with messages from the brain and spinal cord to muscles, skin, and other parts of the body. PN may be described as numbness; tingling; prickling; electric-like pain; a feeling of burning or freezing; sharp, stabbing, jabbing, or shooting pain; or a combination of these sensations, which may be constant or episodic. Symptoms often occur in the feet or hands. Some patients describe a sensation of wearing an invisible sock or glove. There may be associated cramping or twitching, difficulty with balance or walking, muscle weakness or loss of function, and trouble sleeping due to discomfort.

The most common causes of PN at the end of life are diabetes and kidney disease, but PN can also be a long-term side effect of surgery, radiation, and certain chemotherapies used to treat cancer. HIV/AIDS can cause PN. Sometimes, however, the cause is unknown, or idiopathic.

Evidence for treatment of PN is inconsistent, largely because responses are highly individual. Massage and topical analgesics are helpful in some cases. A doctor's order may be required for analgesics to be applied to the skin in some settings.

Adapting the massage session

- Responses to massage on areas of the body with PN vary widely. The affected areas may be too sensitive for touch, but many patients are surprised at the benefit they receive from gentle massage.

- The therapist will need to explore with the patient whether touch is tolerable and what kind of touch feels best: level 2 or level 1 pressure, gliding versus static compressions, over socks or directly on the skin, or avoidance of the affected area.

- Topical capsaicin has been shown in several studies to benefit some patients with PN. An over-the-counter strength of 0.075% is recommended (Mason et al., 2004).

- Emla is an over-the-counter cream, sometimes used to numb the skin prior to an injection or procedure. It contains lidocaine and prilocaine and may help some people with PN (Coyle et al., 2008).

- Application of 5% prescription-strength lidocaine gel or cream has also shown promise for some patients (Mason et al., 2004).

- Keep in mind that the patient with PN may be at increased risk of falls.

Pruritus (itching)

Itching is a common and distressing symptom at the end of life, which can interfere with sleep, exacerbate anxiety, and lead to skin tears and infection from scratching. Pruritus may be a feature of end-stage liver or kidney disease, leukemia, lymphoma (especially Hodgkin's), multiple myeloma, pancreatic cancer, biliary (bile duct) disease, HIV, multiple sclerosis (MS), aging, or fungal infection, or may be a reaction to opioids or other medications, which may be temporary or ongoing. Itching may also be an allergic reaction to laundry detergents, soaps, or some other environmental exposure. Treatment of pruritus involves eliminating the cause when possible. A combination of topical and systemic approaches will likely be needed. Some of the topical analgesics recommended below may require a doctor's order or approval for use in clinical settings. Therapists should clarify such policies with their supervisors.

Adapting the massage session

- Treating dry skin is an important aspect of management. Use a highly emollient product.

- Encourage frequent reapplication of lotion. Consider leaving sample product with the family to reapply.

- Avoid scented products (Perdue, 2016) as these may exacerbate itching.

- Cooling agents such calamine or 0.5–2% menthol cream may counteract itching. Lidocaine or Emla cream may be helpful (Von Gunten et al., 2020).

- A cooler room may be helpful, as overheating increases itching.

- Cold compresses may be helpful (Perdue, 2016).

- Triamcinolone acetonide cream, a prescription cortisone, may be added to massage cream and applied to the skin under clinical supervision.

- Consult the clinical team prior to massage for any rash that has not been diagnosed.

Secretions

Some diseases reduce the ability to clear the airway, resulting in excess saliva and respiratory secretions that gather at the back of the throat. This may occur with brain injuries or neurological diseases such as Parkinson's and ALS. People with tracheostomies may also have difficulty with secretions. Mechanical suctioning may be used to clear a trach tube or to keep a patient's airway open, or

patent. Family caregivers often learn to provide suctioning and become quite proficient.

Terminal secretions are sometimes a feature of active dying when patients have lost the ability to swallow and cough. These secretions may sound like congestion, crackling, or gurgling (see p. 86). They are not thought by end-of-life experts to cause discomfort to the patient, but the sounds can be very distressing for loved ones. The medical team may therefore attempt to treat secretions with medications (see p. 155). Suctioning can be distressing for the patient and may not be helpful since secretions often occur too far down the respiratory tract to reach.

Adapting the massage session

- Repositioning can sometimes ease terminal secretions. The patient may be placed in side-lying or side-leaning position, with the head turned to the side to support drainage (Bickel and Arnold, 2015).

Seizures

Seizures may occur at the end of life from brain tumors, strokes, epilepsy, infection, substance abuse, metabolic imbalances, and electrolyte disturbances. Symptoms that may or may not be visible include jerking, twitching, or tremors; stiffening of the body; drooling; repeated blinking, blank staring, or other unusual eye movements; sudden difficulty speaking, confusion, or memory loss; or recurring movements such as chewing, lip smacking, or clapping (HPNA, 2015). There may be a loss of consciousness. If seizures are recurring, the medical team will attempt to identify their cause and treat accordingly with medication (see p. 155).

Adapting the massage session

- Seizures may be triggered by stimuli that are particular to the individual. Therapists should inquire about any known triggers.

- Touch of any kind, even gentle touch, can be a seizure trigger, making massage inappropriate for some.

- Adjustments may include dim lighting, turning off ceiling fans, using unscented products, and reducing noise.

- Should a seizure occur during the session, the patient should not be restrained or left alone, and nothing should be placed in the mouth. Cushion the bedrails with pillows if the patient is in bed and turn the patient's head to the side if possible. After the seizure is over (it may last several minutes), reorient the patient to the environment. Reposition the patient, if possible, in side-lying position with the head turned to the side.

- Seizure activity should be reported to the caregiver or staff.

Skin changes

Touch therapists working in end-of-life care are likely to encounter a range of skin changes unlike anything they've ever seen before. Advanced illness can cause extreme variations in skin color, including jaundice (yellow or orange tones suggesting liver or bile disease) or cyanosis (blue or purple tones suggesting lack of oxygen). The skin may appear dark or red in areas of the body that have poor circulation, a DVT, infection, or subcutaneous bleeding. Over time, skin texture may be become hard, wrinkled, or leathery due to these issues. Chronic edema and lymphedema can also cause changes in skin texture.

Many of the skin changes observed at the end of life do not require special adjustments to a gentle massage session. They often represent signs of disease that can be observed rather than symptoms that are felt by the patient. As noted elsewhere in this book, dry skin, also known as xerosis, will benefit from lubrication during massage.

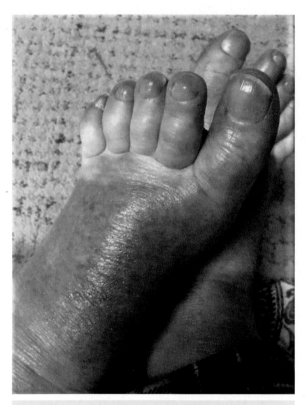

Figure 6.12
Edema and erythema in this patient's feet were normal for him during the last six months of life, causing no distress on his part. The color always became lighter following a level 1 massage, a response that lasted a day or two and which the patient found "interesting." Clubbed toenails as shown in the photo are a common indication of advanced lung disease.

(Photo by author.)

Chart talk 6.3. Terms for skin changes

The terms below describe skin changes often found in advanced disease. Touch therapists should be aware that bruises may be less apparent on skin with more melanin. When providing massage for people of color, be alert for swelling and areas that are darker than the surrounding skin.

Contusion – synonymous with a bruise. Bleeding under intact skin from an external trauma. Usually tender and resolves within two weeks, with color changes during the healing process.

Erythema – red skin which blanches (or lightens) with pressure. May or may not cause pain or itching.

Purpura – bleeding under the skin, which may appear red or purple, or dark brown or black in darker skin. Caused by underlying disease or a vascular problem, not trauma. Usually not painful. May be chronic due to the ongoing nature of the cause.

Petechiae – very small or pinpoint purpura that are red, purple, brown, or black.

Ecchymoses – larger area of purpura.

Tremors and myoclonus

Involuntary muscle movements, or tremors, can occur with many terminal diagnoses, including stroke, traumatic brain injury, neurodegenerative diseases such as Parkinson's, substance use, substance withdrawal, and liver or kidney failure (NINDS, 2021). Shaking can also be caused by certain medications, especially corticosteroids and bronchodilators used for shortness of breath. Tremors may be intermittent or constant, but typically have a rhythmic or repetitive quality that is sometimes described as shaking.

Myoclonus is a different type of involuntary movement sometimes seen at the end of life, described as twitching or jerking that is sudden, brief, and potentially startling (DeMonaco and Arnold, 2015). Myoclonus may be caused by metabolic abnormalities from liver or kidney failure, low sodium, or low blood sugar; electrolyte disturbances; central nervous system damage from tumors, stroke, seizures, and encephalitis; or medications including opioids, anticonvulsants such as gabapentin, antidepressants, and some antibiotics. Previously tolerated medications may become problematic as urination slows during the dying process, causing a build-up of metabolites that would normally be excreted from the body.

Whereas mild tremors may be tolerated by the affected person who becomes accustomed to them, severe tremors and myoclonus can be distressing for patients and families, disrupting sleep and making coordinated movements difficult. If a cause can be identified and addressed, the clinical team will make changes accordingly. Massage *may* be helpful for certain types of tremors that are triggered or worsened by anxiety (Riou, 2013). Otherwise, there is not much for a touch therapist to do, other than be aware that shaking or sudden jerking may occur. If the symptom is new or disturbing for the patient, it should be reported to clinical staff.

Wounds (skin tears, fungating tumors, fistulas, and pressure injuries)

Like all other organs, skin has the potential to fail at the end of life. Risk factors for skin failure include aging, immobility, poor nutritional status, impaired immunity, long-term use of certain medications including corticosteroids, edema, lymphedema, and poor circulation. Distress from wounds can range from mild discomfort to intense and unremitting pain. Healing is often compromised, resulting in chronic wounds that may remain open until the patient dies. Any disruption of skin integrity creates a risk of infection that can become systemic and hasten death.

Common wounds at the end of life include skin tears, lower-extremity ulcers, fungating tumors, fistulas, and pressure ulcers. Skin tears typically occur from a preventable accident, such as a fall, friction, or minor impact with a fingernail, jewelry, or equipment. Lower-extremity ulcers, fungating wounds, and fistulas, in contrast, are typically caused by disease processes and are *not* preventable. Fungating wounds occur when cancer breaks the surface of the skin, most commonly in breast cancer or head and neck cancer. These malignancies can create hollow craters in the body that can be quite deep, or large growths with either a smooth surface or wrinkled appearance resembling a cauliflower. Pain and itching can be extreme with a fungating wound, but many patients are more bothered by the embarrassment and social isolation caused by continuous bleeding, fluid discharge, and odor. Fistulas can cause these same problems internally, namely: leaking of stool, urine, or blood from one body cavity into another through abnormal passages or holes that develop between organs.

Pressure injuries are another common wound at the end of life, previously known as pressure ulcers, decubitus ulcers, or bedsores (see p. 36). These tend to occur at bony prominences such as the heels, sacrum, and shoulders, but may also be seen on the ears of people who favor sleeping on one side. The injury begins underneath the surface of the skin, first presenting as a red area that often progresses to an open ulcer. Standard protocol in many settings for at-risk patients is to reposition the patient every two hours to prevent these ulcers. But even with conscientious care, skin breakdown can occur. One variety of pressure ulcer that is particularly hard to avoid is a Kennedy ulcer that sometimes occurs in the final weeks or days of life. These wounds can develop very suddenly. They may be red, yellow, or black and are often in the shape of a pear or butterfly. Kennedy ulcers usually occur on the sacrum or tailbone, but may also happen on the heels, arms, elbows, or calf of the leg.

Since wound healing may not be possible at the end of life, the care team's efforts will focus on the patient's comfort and dignity. The skin will be kept clean and dry, and pain medication (oral or topical) will be provided in anticipation of repositioning, wound care, and dressing changes. Special mattresses and medicated dressings may be used. Odor management may involve the placement of charcoal or coffee grounds under the patient's bed.

Adapting the massage session

- Skin that is not intact should not be touched, with or without gloves.

- Therapists should keep nails short and avoid wearing jewelry on fingers or wrists.

- Healing skin (with intact scabbing, no redness) may be incorporated into the session by working over the sheet or wearing gloves (Werner, 2019).

- "Float" the heels of people confined to bed by placing a pillow under the lower leg (see p. 64).

- Side-lying position for extended periods at the end of life should be avoided, to prevent pressure on the greater trochanter of the hip. Floating one hip or the other to create a side-leaning position may be safer and more comfortable for the patient.

- Red areas over bony prominences must be treated with great care (maximum of level 1 pressure if tolerated by the patient) and reported to caregivers or staff. Precautions can be taken to shift the patient's weight away from these areas.

Xerostomia (dry mouth)

More than 75% of hospice patients experience dry mouth, or xerostomia, which can lead to pain and infection (Reisfield et al., 2009). Dry mouth can cause nutritional impairment due to chewing and swallowing difficulties and loss of taste. Speech can become unintelligible, resulting in frustration for patients and loved ones. Causes of xerostomia include medications such as opioids and antihistamines, history of radiation to the head and neck, dehydration, and diseases such as HIV, diabetes, and kidney failure. The clinical team will likely omit unnecessary drugs, substitute less-drying ones, or reduce dosages. Sugarless gum and candies may help, along with saliva substitutes. Touch therapists can support affected patients by encouraging the use of lip balm and assisting patients to drink sips of water as desired from a cup, sponge, spoon, or straw. It can be assumed that these items are safe if they are present at the bedside. If not, the therapist should check with carers or staff before introducing fluids into the environment. Some patients are NPO (*nil per os*, Latin for "nothing by mouth") to prevent choking.

Conclusion

Dying people face significant challenges that can interfere with quality of life during their final months. Managing these symptoms is the essence of hospice and palliative care. An interdisciplinary team is ideal for addressing "total suffering," which may involve physical, mental, emotional, social, and spiritual components. Skilled touch, adapted for safety and comfort, can be an invaluable contribution to this care. While dying will likely present a range of unwanted experiences, good palliative care offers the best possible odds of a dignified and peaceful death. It is the dying person who defines what this means to them. It is our job to listen and respond.

References

Alderman, J., 2015. *Diarrhea in palliative care.* Fast Fact #96. [online] Available at: <https://www.mypcnow.org/fast-fact/diarrhea-in-palliative-care>.

Bahti, T., 2012. Myths about the dying process. *CURE,* [e-journal] (11)2. Available at: <https://www.curetoday.com/view/myths-about-the-dying-process>.

Bickel, K. and Arnold, R., 2015. *Death rattle and oral secretions.* Fast Fact #109. [online] Available at: <https://www.mypcnow.org/fast-fact/death-rattle-and-oral-secretions>.

Coyle, N. et al., 2008. *Understanding peripheral neuropathy.* [e-book] New York: Cancer Care, Inc. Available at: <https://media.cancercare.org/publications/original/10-ccc_neuropathy.pdf>.

Dear, J., 2019. *What does it feel like to die? Inspiring new insights into the experience of dying.* New York: Kensington Publishing Corp.

DeMonaco, N. and Arnold, R., 2015. *Myoclonus.* Fast Fact #114. [online] Available at: <https://www.mypcnow.org/fast-fact/myoclonus>.

DiBello, K., 2015. Grief and depression at the end of life. *The Nurse Practitioner,* [e-journal] (40)5, pp. 23–28. Available at: <http://dx.doi.org/10.1097/01.NPR.0000463781.50345.95>.

HPNA Nursing Resource Guide, 2015. *Seizures.* [online] Available at: <www.goHPNA.org>.

Kinzbrunner, B. and McKinnis, E., 2011. Gastrointestinal symptoms near the end of life. In: Kinzbrunner B. and Policzer J. *End-of-life care: a practical guide.* 2nd ed. New York: McGraw-Hill. Ch. 8.

Lämås, K. et al., 2011. Experiences of abdominal massage for constipation. *J Clin Nurs.,* [e-journal] 21(5–6), pp. 757–765. Available at: Wiley Online Library <https://onlinelibrary.wiley.com>.

Mason, L. et al., 2004. Systemic review of topical capsaicin for the treatment of chronic pain. *BMJ,* [e-journal] 328(7446), p. 991. Available at: <http://doi:10.1136/bmj.38042.506748.EE>.

Lin, F. R. and Ferrucci, L., 2012. Hearing loss and falls among older adults in the United States. *Archives of Internal Medicine,* [e-journal] 172(4), pp. 369–371. Available at: <http://dx.doi.org/10.1001/archinternmed.2011.728>.

Memorial Sloan Kettering Cancer Center (MSKCC), 2019. *Acupressure for nausea and vomiting.* [pdf] Available at: <https://www.mskcc.org/pdf/cancer-care/patient-education/acupressure-nausea-and-vomiting>.

National Institute of Neurological Disorders and Stroke (NINDS), 2021. *Tremor Fact Sheet.* [online] Available at: <https://www.ninds.nih.gov/Disorders/Patient-Caregiver-Education/Fact-Sheets/Tremor-Fact-Sheet>.

Perdue, C., 2016. Management of pruritus in palliative care. *Nursing Times,* [e-journal] 112(24), pp. 20–23. Available at: <https://www.nursingtimes.net/clinical-archive/end-of-life-and-palliative-care/management-of-pruritus-in-palliative-care-13-06-2016>.

Phillips A., 2005. *The management of hiccups in terminally ill patients.* [pdf] Available at: <cdn.ps.emap.com/wp-content/uploads/sites/3/2005/08/050802The-management-of-hiccups-in-terminally-ill-patients.pdf>.

Reisfield et al., 2009. Xerostomia. 2nd ed #182. *Journal of Palliative Medicine,* [e-journal] 12(2), pp. 189–190. Available at: <http://dx.doi.org/10.1089/jpm.2009.9670>.

Rice, D., 2020. Discussions of common conditions, symptoms, and medications. [conversations in person, via Zoom and telephone] (Personal communication, 12 August 2020, 23 September 2020, 25 September 2020, 7 October 2020, 22 October 2020).

Riou, N., 2013. Massage therapy for essential tremor: quieting the mind. *Journal of Bodywork and Movement Therapy,* [e-journal] 17(4), pp. 488–494. Available at: <http://dx.doi.org/10.1016/j.jbmt.2013.03.007>.

Spence, C., 2021. Sacred time: touch at the end of life. In: MacDonald, G. and Tague, C. *Hands in health care: massage therapy for the adult hospital patient.* 2nd ed. Edinburgh: Handspring. Ch. 14.

Strickland, M. and Stovsky, E., 2015. *Fever near the end of life.* Fast Fact #256. [online] Available at: <https://www.mypcnow.org/fast-fact/fever-near-the-end-of-life>.

Taboada, P., 2021. *Caregivers' ability to deal with suffering.* [online] Available at: <https://hospicecare.com/policy-and-ethics/ethical-issues/essays-and-articles-on-ethics-in-palliative-care/caregivers-ability-to-deal-with-suffering>.

Turan, N. and Atabek Aşt, T., 2016. The effect of abdominal massage on constipation and quality of life. *Gastroenterology Nursing,* [e-journal] 39(1), pp. 48–59. Available at: <http://dx.doi.org/10.1097/SGA.0000000000000202>.

Von Gunten, C. F. et al., 2020. *Pruritus.* Fast Fact #37. [online] Available at: <https://www.mypcnow.org/fast-fact/pruritus>.

WebMD, 2019. *What to know about acupressure points for nausea.* [online] Available at: <https://www.webmd.com/balance/what-to-know-about-acupressure-points-for-nausea>.

Werner, R., 2019. *A massage therapist's guide to pathology: critical thinking and practical application.* 7th ed. Boulder, CO: Books of Discovery.

Widera, E. W. and Block, S. D., 2012. Managing grief and depression at the end of life. *American Family Physician,* [e-journal] (86)3, pp. 259–264. Available at: <https://www.aafp.org/afp/2012/0801/p259.html>.

Wood, G. J. et al., 2010. Management of intractable nausea and vomiting in patients at the end of life. In: McPhee, S. et al. *Care at the close of life.* San Francisco: McGraw-Hill. Ch. 7.

Zhang, Z. and Gong, C., 2020. Intractable or persistent hiccups treated with extracranial acupuncture. *Medicine,* [e-journal] 99(20), e20131. Available at: <https://doi.org/10.1097/MD.0000000000020131>.

Here's the most important thing: I want you to see me as a whole person, not as a disease.
  –Christine Longaker

Extensive knowledge of diseases is not a prerequisite to providing safe, comforting touch for people at the end of life. "It is far more important to know [the] person a disease has," said Hippocrates, "than what disease the person has." But a working knowledge of common terminal diagnoses will help us to be more aware, empathic, and able to anticipate and accommodate issues that might impact the touch session.

Those who work in healthcare settings will benefit from a basic level of clinical literacy in order to interpret the medical chart and to interact with the medical team, even if it is only to know what questions to ask. Members of the care team are constantly learning from one another. At the same time, we learn from patients and their care providers, who often become experts in their conditions. Patients become our teachers, as they help us determine what works for them.

It is important to remember that many people at the end of life are coping with more than one disease. It's common, for example, for a person to have both heart disease and kidney disease, which tend to occur together. Other people have two or more diseases that appear to be unrelated. For some patients, the list of concurring conditions can be quite long. Conditions can interact with and complicate one another, as can the treatments to address each. Treatment can, in fact, take a greater toll on both patient and family than the disease itself. By the time a person gets to the end-stage of a terminal diagnosis, their quality of life may have been negatively impacted for some time.

This chapter will address common causes of non-sudden death, including heart disease, cancer, dementia, lung disease, kidney and liver disease, brain injuries, neurodegenerative diseases, and HIV/AIDS. Common complications are described for each disease and complications that can occur with multiple conditions appear at the end of the chapter.

Two key points warrant consideration. The first is that end-stage disease is often a product of healthcare received or not received over the span of a person's lifetime. Access to quality care, barriers to services, and related factors are highly variable across the globe, between countries, and within communities. Vulnerable people and populations suffer differently, even when they suffer from the same disease. This book endeavors to address a range of experiences in developed countries, while acknowledging that disparities abound. The end of life and the conditions that lead to it are universally challenging. The goal of hospice and palliative care is to address those challenges with compassion for all people.

The second point is that massage, *with appropriate modifications*, can be a welcome part of the palliative care plan for any terminal condition at any stage of disease. The conditions described in this chapter make huge demands on the affected person, impacting body, mind, and spirit. The disease history, including treatment, often results in trauma that is stored in the body that we are now touching. Some patients and loved ones share parts of their stories with us, but it is not necessary for us to know the details of these narratives. It is only necessary to keep our hearts and hands tender, knowing that the bodies we touch have been through a lot.

Personal note to the reader 7.1. About the photos in this chapter

Unlike many of the images in this book featuring close-ups of pathologies for learning purposes, the photographs in Chapter 7 capture an essence of wholeness that speaks to the human spirit and a range of lived experiences. The people we touch are so much more than their diseases. They are multidimensional in their personalities, their talents, and their quirks. The captions in this chapter are my love letters to them, and convey my deep affection and abiding gratitude.

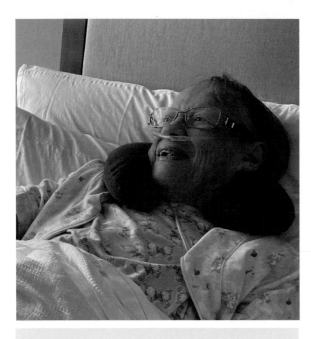

Figure 7.1

At the age of 91 with a terminal illness, Corinne remained engaged in life. She loved visiting with family, friends, and hospice staff, especially her massage therapist, whom she coached on how to make a perfect pot roast. When the therapist returned to work the following week, Corinne greeted her with raised eyebrows. The pot roast was indeed perfect.

(Story provided by Lisa Castillo, photo by author.)

Heart disease

Also known as cardiovascular disease, or CVD, heart disease is the leading cause of death worldwide and often occurs alongside kidney disease and diabetes (WHO, 2017). It is a frequent comorbidity for unrelated diseases of aging, such as dementia.

People with advanced heart disease are likely to experience extreme fatigue, fluid overload, and shortness of breath. Constricted arteries can block blood flow and oxygen, causing tissue damage, or ischemia, which can happen anywhere in the body. CVD is considered end-stage when symptoms are significant even when the patient is at rest, or when it is no longer possible to engage in minimal physical activity without pain or dyspnea.

By the time a person reaches the end of life with heart disease, they have likely survived numerous crises, hospitalizations, and treatments. Patients may have endured grueling interventions such as a heart transplant or coronary artery bypass grafting (CABG), which is the most common surgery for cardiac patients. Touch therapists may encounter large surgical scars on the chest, along with scars on the lower extremities where arteries or veins have been harvested to repair blocked vessels elsewhere. There may be residual tenderness or altered sensation at these sites.

Some cardiac patients have implanted devices that can be seen or felt under the skin. These include pacemakers and implanted defibrillators, described in Chapter 9. A more complicated implanted device is the left ventricular assist device (LVAD), which involves a permanent "driveline" or cable connecting the patient to a machine worn outside the body. Surgery, implanted devices, and medications improve and extend life for people with heart disease, but they are not a cure. As end-stage disease progresses, patients typically need help with decisions regarding the burdens and benefits of interventions that may interfere with a peaceful death (see p. 178). Palliative and hospice professionals can help with these decisions, along with providing support for symptom management.

Chart talk 7.1. Cardiovascular terms

The medical chart may use different terms and abbreviations related to heart disease. Cardiac conditions often present in clusters, or combinations of the following.

Atherosclerotic cardiovascular disease (ASCVD) – occurs from plaque build-up in the arteries that blocks blood flow.

Cardiomyopathy – a general term for disease that causes the heart muscle to become enlarged or stiff.

Congestive heart failure (CHF) – occurs when the heart muscle becomes too weak or damaged to circulate blood through the body.

Coronary artery disease (CAD) – refers to heart disease occurring in the arteries.

Coronary heart disease (CHD) – broad term synonymous with cardiovascular disease, or CVD.

Ischemic heart disease – another term for heart disease caused by narrowed arteries.

Myocardial infarction (MI) – also known as a heart attack, an acute disruption of blood flow that results in damage or death to part of the heart muscle.

Peripheral artery disease (PAD) – disease from plaque build-up in the arteries of the extremities, typically the legs.

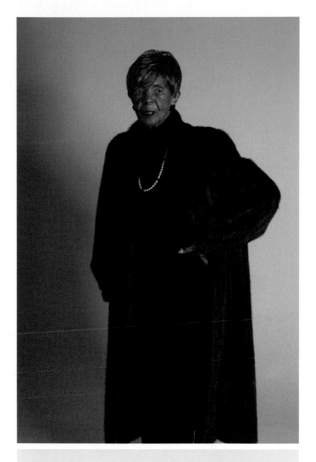

Figure 7.2

Nana, pictured at her 101st birthday party. Her family reports that she was the first African–American to have an office position with the US government. She worked as a freight rate analyst, purchasing her own home in the 1960s. Nana's granddaughters describe her as a "tiny person with a big personality." Her health began to fail following a heart attack which occurred two weeks after this photo was taken.

(Photo courtesy of patient's family.)

Common symptoms

End-stage cardiac patients are often middle-aged or older and medically complex, presenting with at least several of the following symptoms:

- Shortness of breath (dyspnea).
- Decline in endurance with minimal activity.
- Extreme fatigue.
- Edema in the lower or upper extremities.
- Ascites.
- Pain or cramping in the lower extremities, due to edema or constricted blood flow.

- Chest pain.

- Pain from chest tubes or previous surgeries.

- Changes in appetite.

- Weight loss, known as cardiac cachexia.

- Dry or discolored skin.

- Cold feet or toes, or wounds on the lower extremities that won't heal due to poor circulation.

- Depression.

- Anxiety.

Touching story 7.1. Get along home, Cindy

I will always remember with great affection a patient named Andy, an 86-year-old Navy veteran with congestive heart failure. Despite his decline, Andy enjoyed flirting with his female healthcare providers. When he learned my name, he broke into the old Bob Wills song "Get Along Home, Cindy," which became the soundtrack for our sessions. Due to shortness of breath, it took Andy a long time to get through the song. But he sang it to me every time I visited, until he reached a point in his decline where he began sleeping through his massage. When that day came, I began singing "our song" to him.

Adapting the massage session

A vigorous massage is inappropriate at any stage of cardiovascular disease, but particularly at the end of life. These patients are at high risk of deep vein thrombosis (DVT) and bleeding. Short, gentle sessions are indicated, with the focus on an area of the body of the patient's choosing. Neck and shoulders, or hands and feet can be good options. Management of excess fluid in the body from

cardiovascular disease is an issue for the medical team, not a goal for the touch therapist.

Below is a summary of suggestions for modifying the massage session:

- Short session (20–30 minutes) addressing one or two areas of the body.

- Level 1 or 2 pressure, depending on patient energy and skin integrity.

- Positioning with the head elevated, due to dyspnea.

- Patients who have both dyspnea and ascites will need to adjust the head of bed (HOB) for comfort. Too low will restrict breathing; too high will crowd a distended abdomen.

- Positioning for comfort if patient is wearing an LVAD device.

- Elevation of edematous extremities.

- Slow, grounding strokes or light compressions interspersed with static holds to ease anxiety.

- Avoid expenditures of the client's energy (transfers, conversation, even turning in bed can be exhausting).

- Avoid wounds and implanted devices.

- Strokes toward the heart if extremities have edema. The intent is to provide comfort, *not* to move fluid.

- CHF is an absolute contraindication to manual lymphatic drainage.

- Follow oxygen precautions if O_2 is present (see p. 41).

Cancer

Cancer is the second leading cause of death worldwide (WHO, 2018), but the most common diagnosis in hospice and palliative care (NHPCO, 2020). Like heart disease, cancer may present as the terminal diagnosis, or as a secondary diagnosis alongside another terminal disease. There are a growing number of cancer survivors worldwide, which means that many people have a history of cancer, either recent or remote. Given the prevalence of this disease and the adjustments required for massage, touch therapists who wish to work with people at the end of life would do well to pursue oncology massage training. In fact, many of us who specialize in palliative or hospice massage began our careers in cancer care.

Oncology massage training focuses on the effects of surgery, chemotherapy, and radiation, and how to adapt massage to safely accommodate these treatments and their aftermath. In end-stage cancer, patients are likely suffering from long-term effects of treatment *in addition to* the burdens of advanced disease. Solid tumors grow large enough to wreak havoc in the body, causing obstruction, nerve compression, broken bones, bleeding, open wounds, and disfigurement. By the end of life, cancer can be so widespread that it impacts nearly every function of the body, including eating, breathing, elimination, mobility, and cognition.

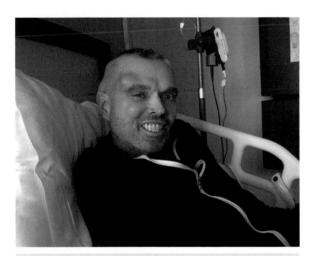

Figure 7.3
Michael's spirit and personality were unaffected by tumors on his head and face, caused by multiple myeloma. Each time care staff entered the room, he routinely asked, "How are *you*?" He liked to surprise us by frequently changing hats from a large collection which he kept at his bedside, including ball caps from favorite sports teams, fedoras, berets, and a pith helmet that he liked to wear on Fridays. Told by a doctor in 2015 that he had 21 days to live, Michael announced he would prove the doctor wrong. He lived another five years.

(Photo by author.)

There are more than 100 types of cancer, each presenting differently. It is not necessary or practical for touch therapists to develop expertise in each type of cancer, though such learning is likely to occur from experience over time. More important is an understanding of the lasting impact of cancer treatment, common end-stage symptoms, and complications that require adjustments to massage for safety and comfort. Several of these complications are described below.

Common complications

Bleeding and clotting issues are both common with end-stage cancer. Cancer patients are up to seven times more likely to develop a DVT, while simultaneously at greater risk of bleeding when anticoagulants are used to treat the clot (Komatsubara and Diuguid, 2016). Bleeding may occur as a side effect of cancer treatment; an example is low platelets, known as thrombocytopenia, from radiation or some chemotherapies. Bleeding may also be caused by the cancer itself, such as:

- Blood in the urine (hematuria) from bladder, kidney, or prostate cancer.
- Bloody cough (hemoptysis) from lung cancer.
- Vaginal bleeding from gynecological cancers.
- Rectal bleeding from gastrointestinal (GI) cancers.
- Nosebleeds, bleeding from the gums, or easy bruising from leukemia, lymphoma, or cancer that spreads to bone marrow.

Bleeding may come from wounds or from any orifice of the body, such as the mouth, nose, rectum, or vagina. It can also be internal, which may or may not result in visible bruising. If cancer invades a vascular area of the body or if it erodes major arteries, the quantity of blood can be significant and quite distressing for patients and caregivers. When the risk of catastrophic bleeding is high, the medical team sometimes attempts to prepare the patient and family. Dark sheets and towels may be kept at the bedside along with gloves and clinical waste bags. The potential for clotting and bleeding problems is a pressure precaution for massage, as indicated in the guidelines on p. 36.

Lymphedema typically occurs when lymphatic vessels or lymph nodes have been removed or damaged during cancer treatment, but can also be caused by advanced cancer if tumor growth crowds lymph nodes so that they can't function properly. Lymphedema is typically unilateral, on the side of the body where lymph nodes have been removed, radiated, or obstructed by disease. A person with cancer of the left breast, for example, is at risk of developing lymphedema in the left arm. Someone with an intestinal or reproductive cancer may develop lymphedema in the lower extremities, pelvic region, or genitals. An oral or neck cancer may result in swelling of the tongue, lips, or face.

Lymphedema can be a chronic, progressive, and distressing problem without intensive intervention. Patients with access to specialized care may benefit from combined decongestive therapy, or CDT, involving compression bandaging and MLD. Many people have never had their lymphedema managed, and others discontinue the demands of CDT at the end of life. When MLD is offered in the hospice setting, it must be adapted by a skilled practitioner to numerous contraindications. The intent to move fluid from one area of the body to another must be accompanied by an understanding of the bigger changes taking place in the body as it declines.

Pathological fractures are broken bones that occur from disease. Bones can be vulnerable to fracture due to primary cancers in the bone such as sarcoma, lymphoma, or multiple myeloma. Pathological fracture may also occur from cancers that metastasize to the bones, especially breast, prostate, and lung (Damron et al., 2020). As stated in Chapter 3, bones can be so compromised by disease or radiation used to treat disease that they fracture spontaneously. Common sites of pathological fracture include the ribs, spine, and long bones of the extremities. Cancer in bones is typically very painful, as are fractures. Massage will need to be used with extreme caution or avoided altogether in affected areas.

Hypercalcemia is a high level of calcium in the blood, a common complication of advanced cancers of the lung,

head and neck, esophagus, breast, kidneys, lymphoma, and multiple myeloma (Siddiqui and Weissman, 2015). Calcium is an essential mineral that works in balance with magnesium to regulate bone health, muscle function, and the transmission of nerve impulses to and from the brain. Cancer can disrupt this balance, potentially causing cognitive symptoms (sedation, delirium, coma); GI symptoms (anorexia, nausea, vomiting); and renal symptoms (dehydration, thirst, excessive urination). People with hypercalcemia may also have musculoskeletal problems, such as twitches, cramps, bone pain, and fractures. In advanced untreatable cancer, a palliative approach would be to manage symptoms with the goal of optimizing the patient's comfort.

Obstructions can be caused by malignancies that compress or block normal passages in the body. One common type of obstruction is bowel obstruction, also referred to as an ileus, which can prevent food, fluids, and gas from moving through the intestines. Obstruction can be due to a tumor, hardened stool that cannot pass, or scar tissue that forms in the intestines following surgery or radiation. The obstruction may be partial or complete. Cancers commonly associated with bowel obstruction are GI and gynecological cancers. Symptoms include abdominal pain, swelling (or distention) of the abdomen, nausea, vomiting, and inability to have a bowel movement. It is also possible for liquid stool to seep around the obstruction, causing diarrhea. A palliative approach to bowel obstruction may include resting the bowel with IV or tube feeding for a few days, or placement of a nasogastric (NG) tube that can be used with mechanical suction to remove stomach contents (CCS, 2020). NG tubes are described in Chapter 9.

Another common obstruction is superior vena cava syndrome (SVCS). SVCS occurs from blockage of a major vein in the mediastinum, which carries blood from the head, neck, upper chest, and arms. SVCS is most often caused by lung cancer but can also result from other cancers including breast, colon, esophageal, or non-Hodgkin lymphoma, when tumors press on the superior vena cava or invade surrounding lymph nodes. A blood clot in the vein can also cause this syndrome. Symptoms include shortness of breath, cough, and swelling of the face, neck, upper body, and arms. Jugular vein distention (JVD) may be visible as a bulge on the right side of the neck. The medical team may use medications including steroids, diuretics, or anticoagulants, depending on the cause (ASCO, 2020).

Spinal cord compression occurs when the spinal nerves become constricted or damaged by tumors on the vertebrae. Spinal cord compression can occur anywhere from the top of the cervical spine to the bottom of the lumbar spine. Symptoms may include new or worsening back pain; weakness and loss of sensation in the arms, hands, or legs; and loss of bowel and bladder control (Robson, 2014). Symptoms at the end of life will likely be managed with pain medication and steroids to reduce inflammation.

Common symptoms

In addition to the complications described above, people with end-stage cancer may experience any of the following:

- Pain (from tissue damage, tumor compression, fractures, or treatment).

- Peripheral neuropathy (see p. 110).

- Changes in body appearance and function.

- Loss of function in the affected organs.

- Dysphagia (difficulty swallowing) in cancers of the head and neck.

- Dysphasia (slurred or unintelligible speech) or aphasia (no speech) in cancers of the head and neck.

- Nausea, vomiting.

- Weight loss, anorexia, cachexia.

- Constipation.

- Jaundice in liver or biliary cancers, or cancers that spread to the liver or bile duct.

- Xerostomia (dry mouth).

- Weakness, fatigue.

- Loss of mobility.

- Fluid overload, including lymphedema, edema, and ascites (see p. 104).

- Dyspnea, pleural effusions (see p. 141).

- Wounds, including fistulas and fungating tumors (see p. 113).

- Depression.

- Anxiety.

Touching story 7.2. Shorter, slower, softer

Jamal's chart described a 31-year-old man with a terminal diagnosis of malignant neoplasm of the long bones in his left lower extremity. He lived with his parents, worked as a sound engineer, and was a single father to an eight-year-old son.

On a routine visit for outpatient care, Jamal walked to the clinic, pushed the door open, and suffered a pathological fracture to his right humerus. The next day, he experienced tingling in his lower extremities and became unable to walk. An MRI revealed pathological fractures at T4 and T8 along with spinal cord compression. He was also found to have metastatic disease to the lung with malignant pleural effusions.

Jamal was admitted to hospice and transferred to our IPU to address symptoms of pain, anxiety, and shortness of breath. He was bedbound with paralysis in his legs and severe pain in his back and arm. He was described in the chart as alert and oriented with periods of forgetfulness. The nurse described him as sullen and withdrawn.

I entered Jamal's room to encounter him sitting in bed watching cartoons with his son, who was wearing Spider Man pajamas. Jamal did not make eye contact with me but asked me to come back later. I returned in the afternoon to find him alone with the lights off and shades drawn. His eyes were open, but he did not say a word or acknowledge me, just nodded his head to indicate consent for the massage.

I started with his left tattooed arm, gently spreading warm lotion across his skin. I worked slowly up the left shoulder and lingered there with some gentle petrissage. He closed his eyes and sighed. Moving to the other side of the bed, I avoided his right arm but let my hands rest without pressure on his right shoulder, one hand cupping the front of his shoulder and the other hand cupping the back. After holding this area for a few minutes, I moved my hands to the posterior neck, making small circles with my fingertips at the base of his skull. I finished the massage with light caress to his temples and brow.

The session lasted 20 minutes and addressed only the upper body. I used level 1 pressure while holding the right shoulder, and level 2 pressure elsewhere. I expected to leave the room without any exchange of words. But Jamal opened his eyes while I was lowering his hospital bed. "Thank you," he said, looking at me for the first time, "that helped a lot."

Adapting the massage session

Adaptations for oncology massage fall into the categories of site (areas to avoid or approach with caution), positioning, and pressure (MacDonald, 2014). For end-stage cancer patients, lighter pressure is likely the most important accommodation to be made. Among the reasons are increased risk of DVT or bleeding, risk of fractures, and risk of lymphedema. Most cancer patients will be at life-long risk for lymphedema in the treated area.

Depending on the location of disease, people with end-stage cancer may rely on devices to assist failing organs. Examples include colostomies, pleural tubes, nephrostomies, tracheostomies, and feeding tubes, which the touch therapist should be aware and mindful of during the session (see Chapter 9). Remember that the session must be adapted regardless of whether cancer is the terminal diagnosis or a concurring diagnosis. Even if cancer is in the distant past, a history of cancer and cancer treatment will have a bearing on massage.

The list below includes additional recommendations.

- Shorter session, based on energy level and general condition.

- Level 1 or 2 pressure.

- Positioning per patient preference, with supportive propping to accommodate comfort throughout the session.

- Ask if there are areas of the body that the patient protects. It may be necessary to avoid or simply hold areas of extreme sensitivity.

- Massage may be provided over clothing or to exposed skin.

- Begin with massage to an unaffected part of the body to develop a sense of comfort and trust.

- Avoid indwelling tubes, devices, and open wounds.

- Avoid massage directly over a tumor, though the warmth of resting hands or Reiki may be comforting.

- Massage is contraindicated in an area with partial or complete obstruction (bowel, superior vena cava, or elsewhere). Resting hands or Reiki are safe if tolerated by the patient.

- The direction of strokes should be toward the heart. However, avoid strokes toward areas with compromised lymph nodes: the groin in cancers of the lower body and torso, the armpit in breast cancer, or the neck in head and oral cancers.

Heads up 7.1. MLD precautions at the end of life

There are numerous potential contraindications for manual lymphatic drainage (MLD) at the end of life. Therapists who practice this therapy must be informed about concurring conditions that would prohibit or restrict the use of MLD. Caution must be used not to increase fluid return to the heart and kidneys if they are compromised, which is often the case with end-stage disease. Any patient who cannot lie flat due to shortness of breath is likely not a good candidate for MLD.

If MLD is determined to be safe, the length of the session should be adjusted to the patient's energy level, generally shorter than a conventional MLD treatment. MLD might also be confined to one area of the body rather than the full protocol. The therapist may need to work around medical devices and limited access to bare skin. The goal of the session is comfort and relaxation rather than an aggressive attempt to treat.

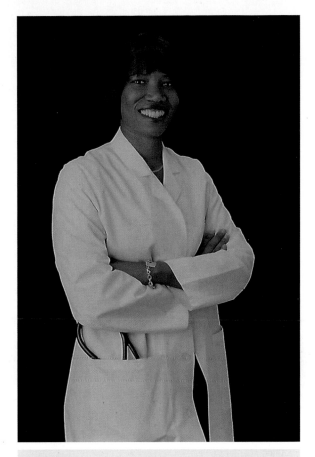

Figure 7.4

Dr. Felicia was a physician with more than 500 online patient reviews, consistently describing her as calm, compassionate, and "lovingly direct." She was known by family and friends for her droll sense of humor and was nicknamed "Warrior Queen," as she continued providing excellent medical care to others through radiation, chemotherapy, and a double mastectomy. It is clear from comments posted on social media after her death that her patients had no idea she was ill.

(Photo courtesy of the patient's family.)

Dementia

People affected by dementia, both patients and their loved ones, endure a long disease trajectory with profound losses on multiple fronts – physical, mental, emotional, financial, and social. It has been described as "loss in slow motion," eventually impacting every facet of the affected person's identity. There are many different types of dementia, including Alzheimer's disease, vascular dementia, Lewy body dementia, and frontotemporal dementia. Dementia is often a concurring diagnosis and is a feature of numerous conditions, including brain cancer, brain injuries, Huntington's disease, some types of Parkinson's, and substance abuse. Dementia is common worldwide and likely to increase as our global population ages (WHO, 2019).

Symptoms vary but typically involve changes in memory and personality. The toll on caregivers is extraordinary, given the extended prognosis, difficult behaviors to manage, and eventual need for around-the-clock supervision. Due to the intensity of these demands, facility placement is common.

125

One issue in addressing dementia is the difficulty of defining "end of life" for people affected by this condition. Indicators used to establish hospice eligibility include swallowing difficulties leading to weight loss, aspiration pneumonia, recurring infection, and skin breakdown (Ross and Sanchez-Reilly, 2018). Urinary tract infections (UTIs) are common, often causing a sudden increase in confusion and agitation. UTIs and pneumonia may be treated with antibiotics to alleviate symptoms, though antibiotics typically become less effective as the end of life approaches.

Chart talk 7.2. The FAST scale

The Functional Assessment Staging scale (FAST), developed by Dr. Barry Reisberg in 1984, is a seven-point ranking system used to describe decline in individuals with dementia. Scores are based on cognitive function and ability to perform activities of daily living. A score of seven typically indicates hospice eligibility (Reisberg, 1984).

Common symptoms

- Pain.
- Loss of mobility.
- Loss of language.
- Difficulty swallowing, "pocketing" food, risk of aspiration.
- Loss of interest in food, weight loss.
- Constipation.
- Incontinence.
- Anxiety.
- Depression.
- Withdrawal. May sleep much of the time.
- Poor circulation (cold hands and feet).
- Contractures once bedbound.

- Skin breakdown, pressure injuries.
- Infections that become resistant to treatment with antibiotics.
- Sepsis.

Heads up 7.2. Pain assessment in people with dementia

Assessment of symptoms in people with end-stage dementia can be challenging. The patient may be nonverbal or unable to communicate their needs to others. It is not surprising, then, that pain is undertreated in this population. Pain may be related to comorbid disease, inactivity, arthritis, poorly fitting clothes or dentures, uncomfortable shoes, or emotional suffering such as loneliness, grief, or fear.

Touch therapists should be aware of the following indications of distress. The PAINAD scale is used in some settings to rank these behaviors on a 10-point scoring system (Warden et al., 2003).

Change in facial expression (grimace, frown, furrowed brow, clenched teeth).

Vocalizations (moaning, crying out, shouting).

Rigid, tense body.

Physical restlessness (shifting in bed, inability to settle).

Resistance to being touched or moved.

Refusal to cooperate with activities such as getting dressed, bathing, or transfers.

Irritability. Physical or verbal aggression.

Touching or rubbing an affected part of the body.

Increased respirations, heart rate, blood pressure, and/or sweating.

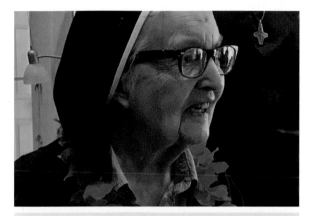

Figure 7.5
Sister Mary Michael is living with dementia in a religious community of nuns from around the world who have taken vows of simplicity and service. The women are a diverse group, including artists, musicians, published authors, activists, and a former rodeo queen. Failing eyesight has made it difficult for Sister to continuing playing and teaching piano, but at 97 years of age she recently joined a group of children singing Christmas carols, remembering every word of every song. The nuns age and eventually die in the community, providing hands-on care for one another.

(Photo provided by the Sisters of St. Mary of Namur.)

Adapting the massage session

Massage for people with dementia can be a poignant and rewarding experience. It is important, however, to be sensitive to any indication from the recipient that touch is unwanted. A desire not to be touched may be temporary or may reflect that the patient is not a good candidate for massage. This can happen even with a patient who has previously enjoyed gentle touch. Any hour of any day may be different, though some people with dementia have predictable highs and lows. Therapists might inquire when scheduling if there is a time of day when the patient might be most receptive to the session. Routine and consistency in verbal and environmental cues for massage may also be helpful.

Family members and hired caregivers who know the patient can assist the therapist to interpret and respond to the patient's needs, along with providing helpful background. It must be remembered that the person with dementia has likes and dislikes, along with a history that likely included work, raising a family, hobbies, accomplishments, and a unique personality, all of which may or may not resemble present reality. Knowledge of the person's life prior to illness can help us to appreciate and connect more deeply to the client.

Other recommendations for adapting the massage session appear below.

- Short session (15–30 minutes, depending on patient response) with focus on one or two body parts.

- Level 1 or 2 pressure. Holds can be very nice.

- Get on the patient's eye level when communicating.

- Keep communication simple and specific, repeating as necessary: "I'd like to put some lotion on your hands" rather than "Would you like a massage?"

- Avoid questions, which can place demand on the client to form a response. Look for nonverbal clues to assess response to gentle touch.

- Some people with anxiety may feel better when familiar people are close by; in such cases, providing the session where others are present can be comforting.

- Incorporate basic care into the session, such as brushing the hair or wiping face or hands with a damp washcloth (Simard, 2013).

- Music can be a way to enrich the massage session, especially when the patient's preferences are known.

Some may be receptive to gentle movement or range of motion (ROM) to music, as if dancing (Simard, 2013).

- Give the patient something to hold if hands are "busy," preferably a soft object such as a blanket.

- Be sensitive to feedback that the patient does not want to be touched, and honor that preference.

- Seek assistance from staff or family as needed. If the patient is anxious, check to see if glasses or hearing aids are worn and functioning properly.

Touching story 7.3. The unexpected gift

As I entered Mrs. M's space for the first time, she looked up from her wheelchair to acknowledge me. I sat down beside her and explained my purpose. "I'm here to put some lotion on your hands," I said. She was unable to speak and looked a little puzzled. I took her hands in mine and sat with her, smiling and nodding as we gazed into each other's eyes. I put lotion on my hands and slowly began massaging hers. She smiled back at me.

After a few minutes, Mrs. M pulled her hand away. I thought she might be telling me that she'd had enough. But then she took my hand in hers and began to gently massage my palm and fingers. Every week after that, Mrs. M reached her hands to me as I entered her space.

LMT Susan Gee, US

Lung disease

The primary feature of lung disease is the distressing sensation of shortness of breath, or dyspnea. Some lung conditions, including pulmonary fibrosis and lung cancer, typically involve a rapid decline. Chronic obstructive pulmonary disease (COPD) tends to have a longer progression. Lung disease is considered end-stage when the patient experiences disabling dyspnea at rest. End-stage patients may endure episodic breathing crises, recurrent infections, and related trips to the emergency room (Ross and Sanchez-Reilly, 2018). There may be fear of a death that involves "suffocating." Fluid overload and fatigue can be extreme.

Given the symptom burden and related anxiety that these patients experience, palliative care would be ideal at an early stage of disease. Many palliative and hospice care teams include a respiratory therapist to assist with symptoms. Medical support often includes supplemental oxygen, which is helpful to some people but less helpful to others. Breathing treatments and inhalers may be used to dilate the airway and to deliver steroid medications which reduce inflammation. Fluids might be managed with diuretics or with procedures such as thoracentesis and paracentesis (see p. 176). Small doses of opioids are often used to palliate the sensation of air hunger.

Common symptoms

Symptoms experienced by people with lung disease are due to poor oxygenation, fluid overload, the labor of breathing, and side effects of treatment. The skin, lips, and fingernails may have a bluish tint (described as cyanotic) from lack of oxygen. Fingers and toes may appear rounded or clubbed. Coughing in some cases is severe enough to result in rib fractures that may be asymptomatic or quite painful. Side effects of treatment are common, including insomnia, agitation, tremors, reduced immune function, and thinning skin over time. Below is a summary of these and other common symptoms.

- Dyspnea.
- Coughing, wheezing.
- Impaired sleep due to insomnia from steroid use and inability to lie flat.
- Fatigue that severely limits activity.
- Frequent respiratory infections.
- Pain in the accessory muscles including pectorals (chest), scalenes (neck), trapezius (back), intercostals (between the ribs), and arms.

- Ascites and/or edema in the lower extremities.

- Easy bruising, skin tears, and poor wound healing.

- Change in appetite, weight loss, cachexia.

- Possible confusion from low O_2, also known as hypoxia.

- "Jitters" or tremors during or immediately following breathing treatments.

- Anxiety. Agitation.

- Depression.

Adapting the massage session

There are a number of nonmedical approaches to shortness of breath that the touch therapist can support. A small fan directed at the face triggers O_2 receptors in the forehead and cheeks. Cool room air and energy conservation (avoiding unnecessary exertion, such as relocating for massage) are ways to reduce respiratory demands. Patients are often taught the "pursed breathing technique," which involves inhaling slowly through the nose for a count of two, then exhaling for a longer count through puckered lips, as if blowing out a candle. Sitting upright or leaning forward expands the diaphragm, which decreases the work of breathing. Any therapy that reduces anxiety, including massage, will have a beneficial impact on dyspnea.

Recommended adjustments for the session include:

- Shorter length of session, based on the client's energy level.

- Level 1 or 2 pressure, depending on the patient's condition.

- Upright position as desired by the patient: seated, with HOB elevated, or leaning forward over a bed tray to increase lung volume (see Figures 4.10 and 4.1, pp. 61–2).

- Patients often prefer cool air and to be uncovered.

- Energy conservation according to activities that cause shortness of breath. May include limited transfers and reduced conversation.

- Gentle massage to accessory muscles, including pectorals (chest) and intercostals (between ribs).

- Gentle tapotement to the posterior torso, maximum level 2 pressure. See Tip 7.1 below on the relief of lung congestion.

- For oxygen-dependent patients, gentle fingertip massage around the head, face, and neck for relief from mask, straps, and O_2 tubing may be very much appreciated.

- Strokes should be directed toward the heart. The intent is to provide comfort, *not* to move fluid.

- See recommendations for dyspnea, pp. 102–3.

- While people on supplemental oxygen are strongly advised not to smoke, some of them do. See p. 41 regarding O_2 safety.

Tip 7.1. Tapotement for the relief of lung congestion

Tapotement is a percussive massage stroke that is rarely used in end-of-life massage, due to the potentially forceful nature of this technique. Modified appropriately, however, tapotement has value for some patients with lung disease who find that gentle, rhythmic tapping can be comforting. The therapist can apply light taps with the fingertips across the patient's back (see Figure 6.7 on p. 103). Patient feedback is crucial to ensure that the technique feels relaxing rather than aggressively "therapeutic." A maximum of level 2 pressure should be used, keeping in mind that many lung patients are on medications that make them prone to bruising.

hardening and scarring that eventually cause organ failure. This scarring is called cirrhosis. Cirrhosis interferes with the liver's ability to filter toxins, metabolize fats, clot the blood, and regulate blood sugar. While liver failure typically occurs over a long period of time, cirrhosis represents damage that is advanced, irreversible, and eventually fatal.

The most common causes of liver disease are heavy alcohol use (see p. 139) and hepatitis C. Other causes include hepatitis B, autoimmune disorders, diabetes, and heart disease. Being overweight or having diabetes can cause nonalcoholic cirrhosis, known as nonalcoholic steatohepatitis, or NASH. Many people with cirrhosis have more than one related condition. There is a strong corollary between hepatitis C and liver cancer, for example. The liver is a common site of metastatic disease from other cancers, including colon, lung, pancreas, stomach, and breast. Liver cancer and metastatic cancer to the liver produce many of the same symptoms as end-stage liver disease.

Common complications

Common complications of ESLD include hepatocellular (liver) cancer, kidney failure, and infections (including peritoneal bacterial infections), in addition to the following:

Esophageal varices, or variceal hemorrhage, occurs when cirrhosis causes blood to collect in the blood vessels surrounding the esophagus. Because the vessels in this area are small with thin walls, they sometimes rupture. Symptoms include pale skin, severe fatigue, shortness of breath, black or tarry stools, bright red blood in stool, and bright red blood in vomit (Sissons, 2020).

Hepatic encephalopathy is a common result of the accumulation of ammonia in the body when the liver begins to fail. Hepatic encephalopathy causes personality changes, decreased level of arousal, and cognitive impairment, which may render the patient dependent on a surrogate decision maker for end-of-life decisions

(Cox-North et al., 2013). Signs of hepatic encephalopathy are observed in nearly 70% of patients with cirrhosis, and symptoms may be debilitating in a significant number of these (Wolf, 2020). Any disease that impacts the liver, including cancer that has metastasized to the liver from elsewhere, can cause hepatic encephalopathy.

Common symptoms

- Ascites, often the earliest symptom (Potosek et al., 2014).

- Edema in the lower extremities.

- Dyspnea.

- Reduced appetite, weight loss, cachexia.

- Muscle wasting.

- Weakness, fatigue.

- Easy bruising, bleeding risk (nosebleeds, etc.)

- Confusion.

- Jaundiced skin and sclera (whites of the eyes). Color may be yellow, orange, or brown. In darker skin, jaundice might be observed in the sclera, palms of the hands, and soles of the feet.

- Extremely dry skin.

- Itching.

- Depression.

- Anxiety.

Adapting the massage session

- Adjust the length of the session to patient's energy and condition.

- Level 1 or 2 pressure.

- Positioning will likely be semi-reclining supine due to ascites.

- Gentle strokes toward the heart on edematous limbs.

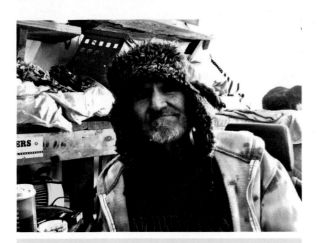

Figure 7.7
A decorated Marine with several tours in Vietnam, Dan was a lively conversationist who shared aspects of his dying year with frank honesty and colorful humor. I will never forget some of our conversations, or the tenderness he revealed to me under his tough exterior. He died of liver disease at age 67.

(Photo by author.)

- Itching is systemic but lubrication of the skin may help.

- Given the high incidence of comorbid hepatitis C and likelihood of skin breakdown at the end of life, the use of gloves is reasonable for all patients with ESLD, including primary liver cancer (see pp. 40–1.)

Brain disorders and injuries

Any time blood flow and oxygen to the brain are disrupted, brain damage can occur. The cause can be a traumatic injury such as a fall, car accident, or other violent impact. Internal events, such as cancer or a viral illness, can damage the brain, as can a cerebrovascular issue (blood clot, bleeding, or aneurysm), known as a cerebrovascular accident or stroke. Brain injuries can also be caused by exposure to toxins, including drugs or alcohol.

The results of brain damage vary widely, depending on the area of the brain that is impacted and the extent of the injury. Damage to the parts of the brain that control respiration or the ability to eat will be fatal without sustained artificial interventions. Damage that is less severe can result in a range of disabilities that impact quality of life and lead to long-term care needs. Some people live for many years with debilities, such as paralysis or inability to communicate.

The loved ones of these patients are faced with difficult decisions regarding life support: namely, mechanical ventilation and feeding. These decisions are often made without the benefit of knowing whether meaningful recovery is possible. Once life-sustaining interventions are initiated, the decision to withdraw those interventions can be terribly difficult. A palliative care team, working in collaboration with other medical providers, can assist the family to develop goals of care, which may change over time, along with providing them with support to work towards achieving these goals.

Chart talk 7.4. Terms related to brain injuries

Therapists may encounter the following terms and abbreviations in the medical chart, all indicating different names for disorders or injuries to the brain:

acquired brain injury (ABI) – an injury occurring after birth that is not degenerative; may be traumatic or nontraumatic.

anoxic brain injury – injury caused by disruption of oxygen to the brain.

cerebrovascular accident (CVA) – medical term for a stroke.

intracerebral hemorrhage (ICH) – bleeding inside the brain.

ischemic stroke – occurs from blockage in the artery that supplies blood to the brain.

subarachnoid hemorrhage (SAH) – bleeding into the space between the brain and surrounding membrane.

traumatic brain injury (TBI) – caused by an external event, such as a fall, collision, or assault.

Common symptoms

People with brain disorders or injuries may experience any of the following.

- Difficulty with communication, understanding, or expression. Speech may be slurred or unintelligible (dysphasia) or there may be no speech at all (aphasia).

- Numbness, weakness, or inability to move, typically on one side of the body. May be minor to severe weakness (hemiparesis) or involve complete loss of strength with paralysis (hemiplegia).

- Headaches (patient may touch head, grimace, or otherwise indicate pain).

- Personality changes, impulsivity.

- Memory loss, problems with concentration.

- Fatigue.

- Nausea, vomiting.

- Seizures.

- Rigidity, spasticity.

- Agitation, delirium.

- Depression, anxiety, and other mental health issues.

- Visual changes, hearing loss.

- Skin breakdown, if mobility is impacted over a long period.

- Contractures, if bedbound for an extended period.

Adapting the massage session

There is debate among experts regarding whether people with impaired consciousness are "aware." Regardless of whether the patient appears to be responsive, touch therapists are encouraged to recognize the intrinsic value of the person they are touching, and the possibility that awareness may occur on many levels that we can't understand. For this reason, it is recommended that the therapist speak and behave as if communication is happening, even if a response is not likely.

- Tell the patient who you are and the purpose of your visit.

- Use the person's preferred name.

- Speak slowly, clearly, and with normal volume. Present one idea at a time and allow the person time to absorb what you are saying and to respond as able.

- Level 1 or 2 pressure in whatever position the patient is found.

- Gentle ROM if the patient does not resist or express pain (see p. 193).

- Do not attempt to "straighten" contractures if there is resistance.

- Rolled washcloths are sometimes placed gently in the hands to cushion contracted fingers.

- If the patient opens their eyes, smile and say hello.

- Music, if the patient or family is able to provide input regarding preferences.

- See additional suggestions for communication on pp. 168–9.

Neurodegenerative diseases

Included in this section are Parkinson's disease, amyotrophic lateral sclerosis (ALS, also known as Lou Gehrig's or motor neuron disease), Huntington's disease, and multiple sclerosis (MS). Though each of these diseases has a distinct trajectory, they all involve the gradual destruction of neurons that control motor function. Other functions may also be affected, including memory, cognition, personality, behavior, communication, and the ability to feed and care for oneself.

The degree of impairment and rate of progression of these diseases vary widely, but symptoms eventually impact every aspect of life. As with dementia and brain injury, the burden on the caregiver is high, given multiple disabilities that may be present over a long period of time. People with neurodegenerative disease are eligible for hospice care when they experience impaired breathing at rest, critical nutritional impairment, or life-threatening complications such as infection or skin breakdown (Ross and Sanchez-Reilly, 2018). Until such parameters are met, these patients and their families can benefit from the support of palliative care to manage symptoms, access caregiver respite, and assist with ongoing decisions related to the care plan.

Parkinson's disease

Parkinson's is the most common movement disorder. There are many types of Parkinson's, each presenting differently. Common symptoms include tremor, rigidity, and a slow shuffling gait called bradykinesia. In general, the disease progresses slowly. Loss of mobility and impaired nutrition lead to weakness, falls, infection, and ultimately to death. Symptoms may include:

- Tremors.
- Muscle rigidity.
- Muscle cramps, pain.
- Impaired communication, slurred or monotone speech, or nonverbal.
- Sensory deficits, such as visual impairment (Hughes, 2019).

- May have impaired mental function, such as memory loss and confusion.
- Bowel and bladder issues, including incontinence and constipation.
- Depression.
- Anxiety.

Suggested adjustments to the massage session are offered on pp. 136–7.

Amyotrophic lateral sclerosis (ALS)

The prognosis for ALS is typically three to five years, though some patients experience more rapid progression than others. Survival can be longer with aggressive measures. Symptoms typically start in the extremities; if symptoms begin in the upper extremities, the dominant arm is usually affected first. A minority of patients experience a bulbar presentation (referring to the bulb of the medulla oblongata at the base of the brain stem), with symptoms first affecting swallowing and speech. Progressive paralysis results in loss of mobility, use of the hands, and ability to swallow. Collapse of the respiratory system follows and is typically the cause of death.

Technological advances allow people with ALS to maintain aspects of daily function, including multifunctional wheelchairs and communication devices. Part of working with these individuals is learning about the equipment they use, which varies widely from patient to patient. People with ALS live longer with tube feedings and mechanical ventilation (BiPAP or tracheostomy, see Chapter 9), though some patients with ALS choose to forego these measures. In end-stage disease, ALS patients have trouble clearing secretions and may need mechanical suction. This disease requires intensive caregiving, with dependence on caregivers to assist with total care.

A summary of ALS symptoms includes:

- Limb weakness or paralysis.
- Muscle cramps and/or muscle rigidity.

- Pain.

- Dyspnea.

- Difficulty swallowing, weight loss.

- Impaired communication.

- Inability to clear secretions.

- Fatigue.

- May or may not have cognitive impairment.

- Depression.

- Anxiety.

Suggested adjustments to the massage session are offered in the opposite column.

Huntington's disease

Huntington's disease, also known as Huntington's chorea, is the most common inherited neurological disease, affecting movement, cognition, and personality. It has been described as simultaneously having ALS, Parkinson's, and dementia (HDSA, 2020). A child born to a parent with Huntington's has a 50% chance of developing the disease. Testing for the genetic marker is very accurate, but most people choose not to be tested; participants in a recent study cited lack of treatment and the burden of certainty that they will die from the disease (Georgetown University, 2019). Huntington's has a long trajectory, 10–25 years, that ends with pneumonia, heart failure, or other fatal complication.

Symptoms may include:

- Personality changes.

- Mood swings, depression, anxiety.

- Memory loss.

- Impaired judgment.

- Unsteady gait.

- Involuntary movements (chorea).

- Pain.

- Slurred speech.

- Difficulty swallowing, weight loss.

Suggested adjustments to the massage session are offered below.

Multiple sclerosis (MS)

People with multiple sclerosis (MS) often have a normal lifespan, with symptoms that vary from mild to severe. In end-stage MS, symptoms result in loss of mobility, impaired nutritional intake, infections, and respiratory issues. Complications from these symptoms or a comorbid chronic disease are usually the cause of death.

Symptoms may include:

- Limb weakness or paralysis.

- Mental confusion or disorientation.

- Dyspnea.

- Difficulty swallowing.

- Difficulty managing respiratory secretions.

- Pain.

- Depression.

- Anxiety.

Suggested adjustments to massage for Parkinson's disease, ALS, Huntington's disease, MS, and other neuromotor diseases appear below.

Adapting the massage session

One common adjustment for people with motor issues is extra time for patients who wish to be repositioned or transferred prior to the session. An example would be a patient who is sitting in a wheelchair but prefers to be in bed for massage. Patients may also need to be suctioned for comfort or need extra time for communication, which may be labored. Additional adjustments include the following.

- Match the length of the session to the patient's energy level.

- Level 1 or 2 pressure.

- Some patients may desire and tolerate very limited and skilled use of level 3 pressure on specific areas of the body.

- Positioning will be highly variable. Some may be able to enjoy a full-body massage in side-lying position, turning midsession to the other side. Others will need to be semi-reclining with their head elevated and supported. Allow the patient or family to determine preferred positioning.

- Some patients will enjoy frequent repositioning, gentle stretches, or range of motion; others will not.

- Do not attempt to straighten contractures or "fix" rigidity.

- Muscle spasm and tremors may respond well to slow, rhythmic, and predictable massage strokes.

- In the event of labored breathing, gently work the scalenes, pectorals, and other respiratory muscles, if desired by the patient.

- Focus on gently working muscles that are overcompensating for others, such as a hand used to operate an assistive communication device.

- Application of heat may help sore muscles. Many people with MS have sensitivity to temperature extremes, either heat or cold. Check in with the patient so that you are aware of these preferences.

HIV/AIDS

For those with access to care, HIV infection has changed dramatically since the introduction of combined antiretroviral therapy (ART) in 1996. Many affected people now achieve normal lifespans, resulting in an aging group of individuals who are prone to the same diseases as the general population.

Several studies describe "premature aging" linked to the virus (Goodkin et al., 2018; Yen et al., 2019). Conditions that appear to be accelerated in people with HIV include

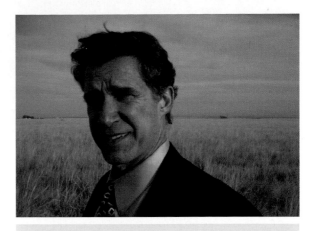

Figure 7.8
Dr. W was a physician, inventor, author, and outdoor enthusiast who wrote "cowboy poetry" as a hobby. After a near-death experience as a young man, he discovered Eastern philosophy. He began a practice of fasting and meditation, which he continued until his death from a neurodegenerative disease at the age of 68.

(Photo by David Spence.)

dementia, liver disease, heart disease, renal disease, lung disease (tuberculosis, COPD, and lung cancer), and a number of other cancers including lymphoma, multiple myeloma, leukemia, and cancers of the liver, prostate, colon, rectum, and reproductive system (Pahuja et al., 2015). People with HIV/AIDS are considered to have reached end-stage when they develop lymphoma, wasting of greater than 33% of lean body mass, renal failure without dialysis, or opportunistic infections that are resistant to treatment (Ross and Sanchez-Reilly, 2018).

While ART has reduced the spread of HIV and improved both longevity and quality of life for compliant users, long-term side effects of ART are still coming to light. Comorbid conditions at the end of life appear to increase the risk of adverse ART events, and some antiretroviral medications can worsen comorbidities (HIV.gov, 2021). There are currently no guidelines to inform patients and their doctors about whether or when to stop ART for these patients at the end of life.

Psychosocial needs can be profound for this group. Numerous studies document links between HIV infection and mental illness, poverty, housing and food insecurity, and substance abuse, all of which can complicate and hasten disease progression (Pahuja et al., 2015; Merlin et al., 2020; Remien et al., 2019). Due to ongoing stigma, some individuals elect not to disclose their HIV status to others (Chan and Chung, 2020). This can present difficulties at the end of life when family members may be involved in care without understanding the patient's decline. Healthcare providers, including touch therapists, must take care as always to protect patient privacy.

Touching story 7.4. Kayla

Sometimes it is difficult to resist having "favorite patients." One of my favorites was a 39-year-old woman with HIV/AIDS. Her comorbidities included vulvovaginal cancer and hepatitis C. She had extensive vaginal wounds and severe neuropathy from chemotherapy. She was bedbound and unable to move her legs. Other wounds included pressure ulcers on both trochanters. At 5'7" tall and weighing 85 pounds, the circumference of her calves was about the same as my wrists.

In spite of her physical frailty and suffering, Kayla was feisty and impish. With a disarming smile that revealed a number of missing teeth, she accessorized her hospital gown with outrageously colorful hats, scarves, and socks. She typically had a lot to say, and countless questions about my life. On days when she was too tired to visit, Kayla stared deeply into my eyes, sometimes for the entire session. Her only child, a son, celebrated his 21st birthday during her stay at the IPU. Kayla held on for this important milestone and passed away the next morning.

Common symptoms

Comorbid conditions in HIV infection cause most of the symptoms that the patient experiences, including the following:

- Pain.
- Peripheral neuropathy.
- Insomnia.
- Fatigue.
- Nausea.
- Depression.
- Anxiety.
- Anorexia, cachexia, "wasting."
- Risk of fractures.
- Dyspnea.
- Dry mouth.
- Cough.
- Bleeding risk.
- Ascites.

Adapting the massage session

Whether a terminal diagnosis or a secondary diagnosis for another terminal condition such as cancer, positive HIV status invites a gentle approach to the massage session. For individuals who have lacked adequate social support, nonjudgmental touch may be a welcome component of the care plan.

Although HIV is a fragile virus that is not transmitted through casual contact, there are a number of infections, including hepatitis C, that may accompany advanced disease. Because immunity and skin integrity are severely compromised at the end of life, it is recommended that touch therapists use gloves while providing massage to a person with end-stage HIV infection. This will protect the patient who is vulnerable, while allowing the therapist to relax and be present in a deeply caring way.

Additional recommendations include the following:

- Adapt duration of session to the patient's energy level.

- Level 1 or 2 pressure, depending on patient's condition.

- Positioning according to patient comfort.

- Thorough hand hygiene, even if gloves are used.

- Maintain one hand's width distance from open skin.

Additional conditions and complications

There are a number of common complications at the end of life that are general rather than related to a specific diagnosis. Several of these are described below.

Addiction, also known as substance use disorder, is a condition that causes untold suffering for the affected individual and that person's loved ones. While many people with substance-related problems work hard to make meaningful recoveries, active addiction can complicate the end of life in numerous ways, impacting symptom management and other aspects of care. Falls and other injuries, hepatitis, HIV infection, mental illness, and history of trauma or abuse have all been linked to substance abuse (Marie Curie, 2019; NIDA, 2020).

When a person in active addiction is no longer able to access and consume their drug of choice, there may be suffering related to withdrawal. Symptoms of withdrawal may be mild to severe, including headache, tremor, sweating, irritability, anxiety, rapid heart rate, high blood pressure, agitation, confusion, seizures, hallucinations, and fever. Nicotine and caffeine withdrawal can likewise contribute to distress at the end of life, potentially causing vomiting, delirium, headache, irritability, anxiety, and restlessness. Management of these symptoms can ease the complications of withdrawal during the dying process.

Substance use disorder is common worldwide, requiring palliative and hospice care providers to recognize the complex needs of the people who are affected. The combined efforts of the team may be needed, starting with medical management of pain and other symptoms in a safe, humane, and ethical manner. Social workers and chaplains can support patient goals for self-determination and reconciliation of important relationships (Reisfelt et al., 2015). Massage can be a comforting expression of nonjudgmental care.

Amputation and limb differences are not uncommon, and touch therapists will likely encounter this diversity at the end of life. Some people are born with limb differences; others lose limbs to disease, injury, or surgery. Common conditions associated with limb loss include diabetes, peripheral vascular disease, advanced DVT, end-stage renal failure, infection, and cancer. Amputations may involve the loss of one or more digits or extremities.

Amputation can represent an improvement in wellbeing for some people, but there can also be difficulties. Challenges may include mobility issues, loss or change of livelihood, loss or change in independence, change in self-image, pain, and grief related to any of these factors. In addition to phantom pain (the perception of pain in a missing limb), there may be pain in joints and muscles used to compensate for changes in biomechanics and posture. Many of these issues are most acute in the immediate aftermath of limb loss, but recovery is highly individual and may be a long process.

Pain following the loss of a limb may be described as burning, aching, cramping, itching, pressure, tingling, numbness, sharp, or shooting. Medications to address pain include nonopioid pain relievers, opioids, muscle relaxants, anticonvulsants, antidepressants, and beta blockers. Many people experience relief from massage to the residual limb (or stump) and compensatory muscles. Below are suggestions for working with affected individuals:

- People use different words to refer to their amputations and may or may not consider themselves to be "disabled." Follow their lead.

Chapter 7

- If patient-preferred language is unknown, the therapist can simply refer to "your legs" or "your arms."

- Propping for the residual limb is highly individual. For some, placement of the remaining limb on pillows is most comfortable. For others, propping can cause discomfort.

- Phantom limb pain often has triggers that are individual. Therapists should be aware that two common triggers are touch and exposure to cold. Ask about triggers prior to providing massage.

Chart talk 7.5. Terms related to amputations

Therapists may encounter these abbreviations in the chart that indicate the location of amputations:

AKA – above-the-knee amputation.

BKA – below-the-knee amputation.

AEA – above-the-elbow amputation.

BEA – below-the-elbow amputation.

Aspiration pneumonia is a common end-of-life complication that occurs when a foreign substance is inhaled into the lungs, typically food, drink, vomit, or the patient's secretions. Symptoms tend to be sudden and uncomfortable, including fever, fatigue, shortness of breath, chest pain, and productive cough (sputum may be foul-smelling or contain blood or pus). Aspiration pneumonia can be prevented by adapting the patient's diet to swallowing difficulties as needed. Palliative care for aspiration pneumonia includes support for respiratory symptoms. Antibiotics may or may not be attempted, depending on goals of care.

Gout is a painful form of inflammatory arthritis that results from hyperuricemia, or too much uric acid in the body. Uric acid crystals in the joints can cause intense pain, swelling, redness, and heat. Gout usually affects one joint at a time, often the large toe, fingers, foot, ankle, or knee. Episodes may be sudden and severe, indicated in nonverbal patients by sudden protectiveness of one hand, or limping (Kilgore, 2011). Gout is primarily linked to heart and kidney disease, along with long-term use of diuretics, aspirin, and some medications used for Parkinson's (Werner, 2019).

Patients with gout will not tolerate touch to the affected area. They may need the bed linen to be "tented" over an affected toe. Cushioned, elevated propping can be helpful. An ice pack (frozen peas or crushed ice wrapped in a pillowcase or tea towel) may provide relief, applied several times per day for up to 20 minutes at a time.

Mental illness is another potential complication at the end of life. Chronic mental illness may have been undiagnosed, untreated, undertreated, or "self-medicated" with drugs or alcohol. Even when the condition has been well managed, symptoms may become destabilized during the dying process.

Mental illness affects a staggering 792 million people in the world, an estimate thought to be low due to under-reporting in all countries (Dattani et al., 2018). In order of prevalence, the most common disorders include anxiety, depression, bipolar disorder, and schizophrenia. Symptoms may include despondency, withdrawal, avoidance, anxiety, fear, mood swings, paranoia, refusal of some aspects of care (being examined, bathing, changing soiled clothes), and lack of compliance with medications.

People with mental illness are at risk of atypical presentations of common end-of-life symptoms, such as pain. Pain is underreported in this group. Some medications used to treat end-of-life symptoms are known to interact with psychiatric drugs and vice versa. Psychiatric care providers do not typically have expertise in end-of-life care, nor do most palliative care providers have psychiatric expertise. Cross-disciplinary collaboration is therefore ideal to help affected people and their loved ones (Shalev et al., 2017).

For patients with mental illness who are open to being touched, a nondemanding massage provided by a caring therapist can facilitate trust and enhance relaxation, providing temporary respite from distressing symptoms. As always, every effort should be made to respect patient autonomy, choice, and dignity. The therapist should seek the support of multidisciplinary palliative or hospice care team members as needed for help with symptoms that are outside the therapist's scope of practice. See pp. 96–7 for additional suggestions to address anxiety.

Pleural effusions or ***pulmonary effusions***, also known as "water on the lungs," involve excess fluid in the thoracic cavity, which may cause sharp chest pain (worse with cough or deep breath), dry cough, fever, chills, and shortness of breath (Medline Plus, 2020). Pleural effusions may be caused by heart failure, cirrhosis, renal disease, pneumonia, or cancer, including but not limited to breast cancer, lung cancer, ovarian cancer, and lymphoma (Thai and Damant, 2015). The goal of palliative treatment is to remove fluid for patient comfort. If the fluid is due to heart failure, diuretics will likely be used. If due to infection, a course of antibiotics may be given. In the case of infection or cancer, fluid may be removed by thoracentesis (see p. 176) or placement of a permanent chest tube. Positioning for massage will need to accommodate both symptoms and interventions. The patient will most likely be comfortable in high Fowler's position with supportive pillows under the head and arms.

Sepsis. People with end-stage disease are vulnerable to sepsis, the body's overwhelming and life-threatening response to infection, which can lead to tissue damage, organ failure, and death (Sepsis Alliance, 2020). The most common sites for sepsis to originate are the bloodstream, lungs, brain, urinary tract, abdominal organs, and skin (Rhee et al., 2019). While bacterial infections are more commonly associated with sepsis, viral sepsis can occur with specific infections including the flu and COVID-19. Decisions regarding treatment versus comfort care depend on the patient's overall health, comorbid disease status, and

goals of care. Even with aggressive intervention, sepsis is often fatal.

People with sepsis may experience fever, chills, pale clammy skin, pain, increased heart rate, decreased blood

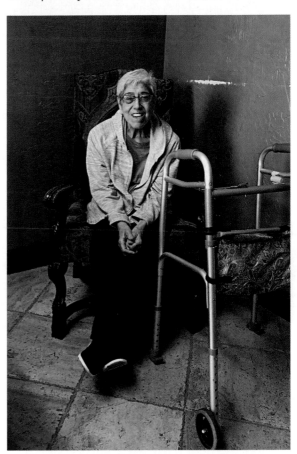

Figure 7.9
Julia was a rugged survivor, one of six children born and raised in an abandoned boxcar, which she deemed "a pretty good childhood" despite extraordinary hardships. A compassionate schoolteacher bought her a dress, shoes, and doll; she treasured the doll for the remainder of her life. Julia was a wonderful cook, with a gift for creating feasts out of random ingredients. Described by her daughter as quiet, humble, and kind, Julia discovered late in life that she loved music. She died at the age of 88 from complications of COVID-19 and dementia.

(Photo courtesy of Lisa Castillo.)

141

pressure, shortness of breath, and changes in mental status including confusion or delirium. A short session using level 1 pressure on a limited area of the body may be comforting, such as caress to the head and forehead, with or without a cool, wet washcloth if fever is present. Gentle holds or Reiki may also be appropriate. Sepsis is not contagious, but standard precautions apply to working with these patients.

**Trauma and PTSD** can occur as a result of serious illness, a terminal diagnosis, invasive medical procedures, or the dying process. Medical trauma can also trigger preexisting trauma for individuals who have experienced military combat, violence, emotional or physical abuse, sexual trauma, a serious accident, natural disaster, poverty, racial or ethnic trauma, abandonment, or neglect. These experiences, which patients may or may not choose to reveal to us, can complicate the dying process by creating a persistent inner perception of feeling unsafe.

Trauma-informed care places the patient in control of their body and their environment. A description of the touch session (including areas of the body that the therapist might touch), patient consent, respect for boundaries and defenses, and ongoing assessment of the patient's responses are all required, along with a willingness to stay present in a nonthreatening way.

Patients who consent to massage should be assured that they can request to end the session at any time they wish to. Touch therapists can support the patient's needs by remaining alert for nonverbal signals that suggest discomfort.

Conclusion

This chapter is intended to introduce touch therapists to the medical conditions they are most likely to encounter in end-of-life work. Ongoing clinical curiosity and the learning that results can help touch therapists to engage with their medical colleagues, to anticipate some of the issues with which the patient might be coping, and to develop competencies in responding to these needs. It is important, however, to hold loosely to assumptions based on any disease profile that may or may not fit the patient's actual experience. An educated mind can also be an open mind, allowing the people we serve to guide our care for them.

References

American Society of Clinical Oncology (ASCO), 2020. _Superior vena cava syndrome._ [online] Available at: <https://www.cancer.net/coping-with-cancer/physical-emotional-and-social-effects-cancer/managing-physical-side-effects/superior-vena-cava-syndrome>.

Canadian Cancer Society (CCS), 2020. _Bowel obstruction._ [online] Available at: <https://www.cancer.ca/en/cancer-information/diagnosis-and-treatment/managing-side-effects/bowel-obstruction/?region=on>.

Castro, M., 2019. Conservative management for patients with chronic kidney disease refusing dialysis. _Jornal Brasileiro de Nefrologia,_ [e-journal] 41(1), pp. 95–102. Available at: <http://doi.org/10.1590/2175-8239-JBN-2018-0028>.

Chan, I. and Chung, R., 2020. _Meeting psychosocial needs of HIV patients._ [online] Available at: <www.aids.gov.hk/pdf/g190htm/05.htm>.

Cox-North, P. et al., 2013. The transition to end-of-life care in end-stage liver disease. _Journal of Hospice & Palliative Nursing,_ [e-journal] 15(4), pp. 209–215. Available at: <https://doi.org/10.1097/NJH.0b013e318289f4b0>.

Damron, T. et al., 2020. _Evaluation and management of complete and impending pathologic fractures in patients with metastatic bone disease, multiple myeloma, and lymphoma._ [online] Available at: <https://www.uptodate.com/contents/clinical-presentation-and-evaluation-of-complete-and-impending-pathologic-fractures-in-patients-with-metastatic-bone-disease-multiple-myeloma-and-lymphoma>.

Dattani, S. et al., 2018. _Mental health._ [online] Available at: <https://ourworldindata.org/mental-health>.

Georgetown University Medical Center, 2019. _Why adults at risk for Huntington's choose not to learn if they_ *inherited deadly gene.* [online] Available at: <https://www.sciencedaily.com/releases/2019/05/190516103715.htm>.

Goodkin, K. et al., 2018. End-of-life care and bereavement issues in HIV/AIDS. *Nursing Clinics of North America,* [e-journal] 53(1), pp. 123–135. Available at: <http://dx.doi.org/10.1016/j.cnur.2017.10.010>.

HIV.gov, 2021. *Guidelines for the use of antiretroviral agents in adults and adolescents with HIV.* [online] Available at: <https://clinicalinfo.hiv.gov/en/guidelines/adult-and-adolescent-arv/adverse-effects-antiretroviral-agents>.

Hughes, S., 2019. *Visual dysfunction: an underrecognized symptom of Parkinson's?* [online] Available at: <https://www.medscape.com/viewarticle/920438>.

Huntington's Disease Society of America (HDSA), 2020. *Overview of Huntington's disease.* [online] Available at: <https://hdsa.org/what-is-hd/overview-of-huntingtons-disease>.

Kilgore, C., 2011. Gout deserves tender treatment in elderly. *Caring for the Ages,* [e-journal] 12(7), pp. 20-21. Available at: <https://doi.org/10.1016/S1526-4114(11)60200-X>.

Kolonko, C., 2012. *Why is peritoneal dialysis underutilized in the US compared to hemodialysis?* [online] Available at: <https://www.hcplive.com/view/why-is-peritoneal-dialysis-underutilized-in-the-us-compared-to-hemodialysis->.

Komatsubara, K. and Diuguid, D., 2016. *Clotting and bleeding in oncology patients.* [online] Available at: <https://www.cancernetwork.com/view/clotting-and-bleeding-oncology-patients-clinical-scenarios-and-challenges>.

MacDonald, G., 2014. *Medicine hands, massage therapy for people with cancer.* 3rd ed. Forres, Scotland: Findhorn Press.

Marie Curie, 2019. *Caring for someone with substance abuse problems at the end of life.* [online] Available at: <https://www.mariecurie.org.uk/professionals/palliative-care-knowledge-zone/equality-diversity/people-with-substance-use>.

Mastnardo, D. et al., 2016. Intradialytic massage for leg cramps among hemodialysis patients: a pilot randomized controlled trial. *International Journal of Therapeutic Massage & Bodywork*, [e-journal] 9(2), pp. 3–8. Available at: <https://www.ncbi.nlm.nih.gov/pmc/articles/PMC4868507>.

Medline Plus, 2020. *Pleural effusion.* [online] Available at: <https://medlineplus.gov/ency/article/000086.htm>.

Merlin, J. et al., 2020. *Issues in HIV/AIDS in adults in palliative care.* [online] Available at: <https://www.uptodate.com/contents/issues-in-hiv-aids-in-adults-in-palliative-care>.

National Hospice and Palliative Care Organization (NHPCO), 2020. *Hospice facts and figures.* [online] Available at: <www.nhpco.org/factsfigures>.

National Institute on Drug Abuse (NIDA), 2020. *Part 3: the connection between substance use disorders and HIV.* [online] Available at: <https://www.drugabuse.gov/publications/research-reports/common-comorbidities-substance-use-disorders/part-3-connection-between-substance-use-disorders-hiv>.

Naughton, B., 2020. *Weird wounds part 2: calciphylaxis, the heart attack of the skin.* [online] Available at: <https://www.woundsource.com/blog/weird-wounds-part-2-calciphylaxis-heart-attack-skin>.

Pahuja, M. et al., 2015. HIV/AIDS. In: Cherny, N., ed. 2015. *Oxford textbook of palliative medicine.* Oxford: Oxford University Press. Ch. 15.1.

Pennington, B. M. and Howell, C. M., 2019. *End-stage renal disease, hyperkalemia, and dialysis.* [online] Available at: <https://www.reliasmedia.com/articles/144679-end-stage-renal-disease-hyperkalemia-and-dialysis>.

Potosek, J. et al., 2014. Integration of palliative care in end-stage liver disease and liver transplantation. *Journal of Palliative Medicine,* [e-journal] 17(11), pp. 1271–1277. Available at: <https://doi.org/10.1089/jpm.2013.0167>.

Reisberg, B., 1984. *Functional Assessment Staging (FAST).* [pdf] Available at: <https://www.elderguru.com/wp-content/uploads/2021/07/Functional-Assessment-Staging-FAST-Scale.pdf>.

Reisfelt, G. et al., 2015. *Substance use disorders in the palliative care patient.* Fast Fact #127. [online] Available at: <https://www.mypcnow.org/fast-fact/substance-use-disorders-in-the-palliative-care-patient>.

Remien, R. et al., 2019. Mental health and HIV/AIDS: the need for an integrated response. *AIDS 2019*, [e-journal] 33(9), pp. 1411–1420. Available at: <https://doi.org/10.1097/QAD.0000000000002227>.

Rhee, C. et al., 2019. Prevalence, underlying causes and preventability of sepsis-associated mortality in US acute care hospitals. *JAMA Network Open*, [e-journal] 2(2), e187571. Available at: <https://doi.org/10.1001/jamanetworkopen.2018.7571>.

Robson, P., 2014. Metastatic spinal cord compression: a rare but important complication of cancer. *Clinical Medicine (London)*, [e-journal] 14(5), pp. 542–545. Available at: <https://dx.doi.org/10.7861%2Fclinmedicine.14-5-542>.

Ross, J. and Sanchez-Reilly, S., 2018. *Hospice criteria card.* [pdf] Available at: <https://cdn.ymaws.com/www.nmnpc.org/resource/resmgr/2018_annual_conf-_presentations-handouts/6_johnson/Hospice_Card__JSR_SSR_JMH_20.pdf>.

Sepsis Alliance, 2020. *Bacterial sepsis versus viral sepsis.* [online] Available at: <https://www.sepsis.org/news/covid-19-and-viral-sepsis>.

Shah, A. and Aeddula, N. R., 2021. *Renal osteodystrophy.* [online] Available at: <https://www.ncbi.nlm.nih.gov/books/NBK560742>.

Shalev, D. et al., 2017. A staggered edge: end-of-life care in patients with severe mental illness. *General Hospice Psychiatry*, [e-journal] 44(1), pp. 1–3. Available at: <https://dx.doi.org/10.1016/j.genhosppsych.2016.10.004>.

Siddiqui, F. and Weissman, D., 2015. *Hypercalcemia of malignancy.* [pdf] Available at: <https://www.mypcnow.org/wp-content/uploads/2019/02/FF-151-Hypercalcemia-of-malignancy.-3rd-Ed.pdf>.

Simard, J., 2013. *Namaste care, the end-of-life program for people with dementia.* Baltimore: Health Professions Press.

Sissons, C., 2020. *Everything you need to know about esophageal varices.* [online] Available at: <https://www.medicalnewstoday.com/articles/esophageal-varices>.

Thai, V. and Damant, R., 2015. *Malignant pleural effusions, interventional management.* Fast Fact #157. [online] Available at: <https://www.mypcnow.org/fast-fact/malignant-pleural-effusions-interventional-management>.

Warden, V. et al., 2003. Development and psychometric evaluation of the Pain Assessment in Advanced Dementia (PAINAD) scale. *Journal of the American Medical Directors Association* [e-journal] 4(1), pp. 9–15. Available at: <http://dementiapathways.ie/_filecache/04a/ddd/98-painad.pdf>.

Werner, R., 2019. *A massage therapist's guide to pathology.* Boulder, CO: Books of Discovery.

Wolf, D., 2020. *Hepatic encephalopathy.* [online] Available at: <emedicine.medscape.com/article/186101-overview>.

WHO, 2017. *Cardiovascular diseases.* [online] Available at: <https://www.who.int/health-topics/cardiovascular-diseases#tab=tab_1>.

WHO, 2018. *Cancer.* [online] Available at: <https://www.who.int/news-room/fact-sheets/detail/cancer>.

WHO, 2019. *Dementia.* [online] Available at: <https://www.who.int/news-room/fact-sheets/detail/dementia>.

Yen, Y. et al., 2019. *Human immunodeficiency virus increases the risk of incident heart failure.* [online] Available at: <https://www.medscape.com/viewarticle/909181>.

Additional resources

Rice, D., 2020. Discussions of common conditions, symptoms, and medications. [conversations in person, via Zoom and telephone] (Personal communication, 12 August 2020, 23 September 2020, 25 September 2020, 7 October 2020, 22 October 2020).

I never expected … the most meaningful experiences I'd have as a doctor – and really, as a human being – would come from helping others deal with what medicine cannot do as well as what it can.

–Atul Gawande

In 1967, Cicely Saunders created a single sheet of paper titled *Drugs Most Commonly Used at St. Christopher's Hospice*, a humble document that contained "the single most important advance in end-of-life care that has ever been made" (Baines, 2011). The principles reflected in that document – revolutionary at the time – continue to guide the palliative use of medications to this day. A modern version of Saunders's list, created by the International Association for Hospice and Palliative Care (IAHPC), includes 33 medications deemed to be essential in addressing 21 symptoms of advanced disease (IAHPC, 2007). The use of these drugs by knowledgeable clinicians working alongside an interdisciplinary team is the cornerstone of palliative care.

Chapter 8 describes the most common medications used in the last six months of life, their intended effects, potential side effects, and how the massage session must be adjusted accordingly for comfort and safety. A summary for quick reference of these drugs is provided on pp. 158–60. This information, as important as it is, exists in the context of several larger issues that shape and sometimes complicate the choices made by patients and their prescribing providers. Touch therapists will benefit from a broader understanding of this context, including why some medications are stopped and others are started, drug delivery methods and how these are adapted to the dying process, common off-label uses of palliative medicines, and fears about addiction. The use of marijuana to treat end-of-life symptoms will also be addressed.

Most touch therapists enter end-of-life work without a medical background, but the subjects of this chapter become familiar over time, including the names of medications that frequently appear in the medical chart. Also reassuring is the fact that the adjustments to massage that are warranted from a medication standpoint have likely already been made, based on the client's declining condition. In short, lighter pressure, fall risk precautions, and avoidance of contact with medications applied to skin are the primary safety measures. Awareness of the bigger picture will help touch therapists to become informed members of the care team, with deeper appreciation for the tensions that often accompany end-of-life pharmacology. Our role, as always, is to provide knowledgeable, neutral support for patients while adhering to our scope of practice.

As noted by MacDonald and Tague, touch therapists practicing in clinical settings will likely have access to expertise from teammates regarding medications and their potential impact on massage (MacDonald and Tague, 2021). My trusted resources on this subject include palliative care nurse practitioner Deb Rice, hospice nurse Jeanna Thompson, and hospice physician Dr. Stephen Hines, who together provided most of the information in this chapter. While there are countless online resources on medications, there is no substitute for a personal ally who can help make sense of the vast and sometimes conflicting information available. Touch therapists in end-of-life care are urged to develop professional alliances modeled on the team approach to palliative care. Such alliances help to ensure that therapists are supported in their understanding and application of clinical information as this knowledge pertains to the practical aspects of massage.

Fears and other barriers to symptom management

It is not unusual for people to have undertreated symptoms at the end of life. This is hard to reconcile with the fact that patients are admitted to hospice on an average of

15.7 different prescription drugs (Sera et al., 2013). One reason for this paradox – poor symptom control despite high pill count – is that the focus of treating or preventing disease has little to do with how the patient feels. A palliative approach is one that balances the goals of treatment and well-being, while hospice aims to prioritize the quality of a person's remaining time without attempting to extend it. The goals of medication in this context become quite simple, and yet the reality can be complex.

One barrier to good symptom management at the end of life is that doctors may fail to recognize or communicate to their patients that they are dying (Rice, 2020). Chronic disease trajectories can be unpredictable, and many physicians admit that they are reluctant to destroy hope for their patients or that they don't know how to broach the subject. Dr. Anna Beck of the Huntsman Cancer Institute refers to typical conversations about end-of-life care as "too little, too late, and not great" (Beck, 2019). Initiatives around the world are seeking to address this problem with training and resources for doctors to enable them to answer the "surprise question": would you be surprised if the patient died in the next 12 months? If the answer is no, it is time to discuss end-of-life care (Bailey, 2018). Early conversations about prognosis are consistently linked to more timely enrollment in comfort-oriented care, better quality of life, and higher rates of patient satisfaction (Enzinger et al., 2015; Temel et al., 2010).

Another barrier to effective symptom management is fear of opioid addiction or death from overdose. These worries are widespread among patients, families, and many doctors in nonpalliative specialties, often reinforced by stories of someone they knew who died shortly after starting morphine. While there is no question that the misuse of opioids is a tragedy of global proportion, this concern requires fundamental reframing in the context of the dying experience. Opioid doses used by hospice and palliative care teams are carefully controlled and well below the threshold for hastening death; in fact, Saunders determined that patients whose symptoms are appropriately managed with medication are often more alert, more active, and better able to enjoy their daily activities (Baines,

2011). A large body of research reveals that substance abuse in terminal patients is extremely rare (Price et al., 2015; Fallon and Cherny, 2015).

A related concern that may cause patients and families to delay the use of medication for comfort is fear of drug tolerance, where higher doses of medication are required over time to achieve relief. The worry is that there will come a time when no amount of medicine will be enough. It is true that the body adjusts to medications; this is why side effects often subside over time. But there is consistent agreement in the palliative care community that medication should correspond to the timing and severity of symptoms, without undue concern for the issue of drug tolerance (Rice, 2020). When terminal patients experience the need for increasing doses of medication due to disease progression, the team will diversify the medication profile as needed. For the vast majority of patients with limited lifespans, symptoms can be controlled with negligible risk of addiction and tolerance. Even in palliative care settings where patients are expected to live for many years, opioids can be managed safely and effectively, with proper expertise (Price et al., 2015).

Terminal patients with past or current substance abuse problems present a more complicated scenario. In the case of individuals who are abstinent as part of their recoveries, there may be a conflation of the use of pain medication with "relapse." Those who are living with active addiction can present other kinds of challenges to the care team, including drug interactions, possible abuse of prescribed medications, and drug diversion, where medications are taken or sold by people other than the patient. Despite these difficulties, a fundamental principle of palliative care is that *everyone* has the right to a dignified death without undue suffering. Ethical and compassionate approaches to caring for individuals with substance abuse issues may include the use of nonopioid analgesics when appropriate, use of extended-release or abuse-deterrent formulations, small amounts of opioids prescribed at frequent intervals, and increased support to address the psychosocial dimensions of suffering (O'Neill et al., 2017; Gaertner et al., 2019).

Heads up 8.1. The importance of keeping count

Many years ago, I was providing a massage for a patient in the hospital. On my way out of the room, I glanced down to see a small yellow object on the floor. When I picked it up, I realized it was a pill. Ignorant of what medication it might be, I took it to the nurses' station. The nurse's eyes widened, and she said, "Thank you for finding this!" The pill was oxycodone, a controlled narcotic.

Whether in the home environment or hospital, every agency follows strict guidelines for the storing and dispersing of controlled substances. These medications are carefully counted and recorded at each home visit or shift change. After a patient dies, agencies typically have specific protocols for safely disposing of or "wasting" remaining medications. These steps are designed to prevent diversion and misuse of these drugs and are taken very seriously, as they should be.

Touch therapists working in home or inpatient settings can support this effort by immediately reporting misplaced medications or situations that seem irregular. The inpatient unit where I currently work has instructed all staff to refrain from interrupting nurses while they are counting, drawing up, dispensing , or wasting medications. As part of the hospice or palliative care team, touch therapists share responsibility for patient safety.

Another barrier to symptom management is the issue of access. In some locations, restrictive regulation of narcotics is an impediment to obtaining palliative medications. Additional challenges include cost and episodic shortages of drugs. Disruptions of the supply chain can occur during incidents of natural disaster, conflict between countries, or disease, requiring providers to be skilled in making drug substitutions when necessary.

Medications that are discontinued or used with care at the end of life

There often comes a point in the dying process when the burdens and risks of some drugs outweigh their benefits. As dying impacts nutritional status, organ function, and metabolism, the potential for drug interactions and adverse effects increases. Medications that require frequent monitoring may create impossible demands on patients and caregivers, and drugs to address goals that exceed projected lifespan lose their relevance. While the risk-versus-benefit threshold is highly individual, it is common practice at the end of life to discontinue medications that are potentially unsafe or inconsistent with short-term well-being. The process of identifying and stopping harmful or unhelpful medications is known as deprescribing. The goal of deprescribing is to reduce the problem of polypharmacy, a term for the use of multiple medications without due regard for benefit versus harm.

The benefits of deprescribing include enhanced safety and comfort, improved functional status, and convenience. But this does not mean that deprescribing is always easy. While some patients are pleased to simplify their medications, others feel attached to medicines that have helped them in the past; in the patient's or loved one's mind, stopping these can seem like "giving up." Changes to the medication regimen must be handled with sensitivity and skill by the medical team, prioritizing trust, open communication, education, and shared decision making. As always, optimal quality of life is ultimately defined by the patient or surrogate decision maker.

Medications that are commonly discontinued

Medications that may be discontinued at the end of life include drugs to manage chronic conditions (high cholesterol, blood pressure, and diabetes). Cholesterol medications, known as statins, have no short-term benefit and often cause GI problems, musculoskeletal pain, insomnia, and upper respiratory irritation, especially in people with liver or kidney problems. Blood pressure medications, or antihypertensives, may become unsafe, creating a risk of falls as blood pressure naturally decreases at the end of life (Delgado et al., 2017). Diuretics to manage edema and ascites must be used with care that blood pressure does not fall too low. The management of diabetes must also be adapted at the end of life. As patients eat less, they are at risk of potentially dangerous *low* blood sugar. For most type 2 diabetics, it becomes safer to discontinue insulin; type 1 diabetics may need ongoing monitoring to adjust insulin doses for safety (Niznik et al., 2020).

Anticoagulants are another group of drugs that must be reevaluated, as the patient's risk of bleeding needs to be weighed against the risk of clotting (Huisman et al., 2021). Dementia medications may be discontinued as their benefits decrease over time; these medications can cause nausea, diarrhea, insomnia, and other side effects that are not well tolerated in people with end-stage disease (Mitchell, 2015). Vitamins are usually left to patient preference; some people feel better or more energetic when taking supplements; others experience GI side effects. Whether or not to use antibiotics is addressed on a case-by-case basis, depending on goals of care, patient comfort, and tolerance of side effects like GI upset, nausea, and diarrhea.

A final group of medications that warrant mention are vasopressors and inotropes, cardiovascular medications that are delivered through continuous IV infusion. These drugs, typically dobutamine, dopamine, and milrinone, are often initiated in the intensive care unit (ICU) to resuscitate patients in acute heart failure. Some studies indicate that long-term use is associated with accelerated decline, sepsis, and life-threatening arrhythmias, problems which often require monitoring in an intensive care setting (Overgaard and Džavík, 2008). Patients with a hospice mindset may opt to discontinue "pressors" and "drips." Many hospices, in fact, lack the resources and training to care for people on these medications (Ciuksza et al., 2015).

Some medications can be stopped abruptly with no adverse effect. Others must be tapered gradually for patient comfort and safety. In the case of IV vasopressors and inotropes, withdrawal requires palliative support. As always, the patient's goals and preferences should guide decisions, with help as needed from the care team. It is the job of the physician or nurse practitioner to explain the risks and benefits of each medication in the context of the patient's changing condition. Additional team members may be involved in providing emotional support as the patient and family adjust to comfort-oriented strategies that optimize the quality of the patient's remaining time.

The Beers list

The Beers criteria is a list of nearly 100 medications that have been determined to be potentially harmful to adults aged 65 and older. Created in 1991 by Dr. Mark Beers, the list is frequently revised to reflect updated evidence regarding medications to be avoided or used with care. An example of a class of medications on the Beers list is anticholinergic drugs, which may cause pronounced side effects in older people, including sedation, blurred vision, dizziness, confusion, delirium, hallucinations, fall risk, and urinary retention. Long-term use of anticholinergic drugs (three years or more) has been linked to a higher risk for the development of dementia. Risk is compounded when two or more anticholinergic drugs are used together, or when one or more anticholinergic medications are used in combination with an opioid for pain (Fixen, 2019).

Medications with anticholinergic properties have been used for many decades to treat numerous conditions, including COPD and Parkinson's disease. Some anticholinergics are commonly used in hospice and palliative care to manage terminal secretions (atropine and scopolamine), bowel obstructions (metoclopramide), and itching (diphenhydramine, or Benadryl). Other drugs on the Beers list have value to address end-of-life depression, anxiety, agitation, and fluid overload.

The Beers warnings are evaluated carefully by the palliative care or hospice team in the context of the patient's symptom burden and expected lifespan. As always, potential benefits must be weighed against potential risk at each phase of the patient's decline, avoiding the use of any medication that is not necessary to reduce suffering. At the end of life, long-term consequences are often secondary to the relief of short-term distress.

Approaches to prescribing

Just as some medications are eliminated from the care plan to improve comfort at the end of life, others will be added. Drugs are frequently prescribed to manage pain, shortness of breath, constipation, anxiety, fluid retention, nausea, vomiting, itching, seizures, and secretions. Some medications address more than one symptom, and some symptoms require more than one drug. Responses vary from person to person; thus, each care plan is highly individual.

While there are common trends in palliative prescribing practices, specific protocols differ from agency to agency. Each hospice, hospital, or palliative care practice will have its own formulary, an inventory of medications that are utilized by that organization. Physicians and nurse practitioners develop personal preferences that influence drug choices. In some settings with an onsite pharmacy, providers may do their own compounding. An example of this practice is the topical use of metronidazole (Flagyl), an antibiotic typically taken by mouth for infection. Our medical team often applies the contents of a metronidazole capsule to a wound for odor control; opioids can likewise be compounded into topical creams or gels for painful skin ulcers. One physician I worked with created a custom "cocktail" of liquid medications that were delivered in mist form through a nebulizer. It is not uncommon for hospices to make effective use of medications in a way that is considered off label or unlicensed.

Just as providers have preferences, patients and caregivers do, too. Patient preferences may be based on past experience, positive or negative. Patients have values and

goals that must be heard and honored, even as the medical team educates and empowers the patient to consider new approaches. The addition of medications to control symptoms can cause new side effects (drowsiness or itching, for example), which are bothersome but often resolve after the first 48 hours. If patients and their loved ones are informed in advance of a likely scenario, they are in a better position to evaluate each change to the care plan.

Heads up 8.2. Preparing families for what might happen

A common sequence of events at the hospice inpatient unit is that a patient arrives in crisis with a symptom such as pain or vomiting. The patient may not have slept in days due to the severity of the symptom. The medical team initiates effective symptom management, and the weary patient feels such relief that they sleep for 24 hours. The family may blame the medication for making the patient sleepy. This may be true in part, as some medications do cause drowsiness. It is just as true, however, that an exhausted patient desperately needs rest, and the right medication can make this rest possible.

Our medical team tries to prepare the family for this scenario, but also for the possibility that the patient may "let go" once they are comfortable. When this happens, it is not that the medication hastened death, but rather that the patient was very close to dying while struggling in a way that was prolonging the dying process. We tend to see two possible outcomes of good symptom management. The patient may get more comfortable and summon the will to fight for more time with better quality of life. But the patient may also get comfortable enough to surrender to a peaceful death.

The general approach to prescribing and dosing is to "start low and go slow," using a step ladder approach endorsed by the World Health Organization (Anekar and Cascella, 2020). Mild pain, a score of 1–3 on the Edmonton scale, is addressed with mild analgesics, such as acetaminophen (paracetamol) or ibuprofen. Moderate pain with a score of 4–6 may warrant adding a small dose of a mild, short-acting opioid. The dose can be increased, or other medications added, if symptoms persist or become severe, indicated by a score of 7–10. If symptoms are continuous or occur often, the patient may be switched to a routine extended-release or long-acting medication to provide coverage for 12 hours, 24 hours, or longer. The care plan often includes a combination of routine medications and *pro re nata* (PRN, as needed) "rescue doses" of short-acting drugs. A multimodal approach includes different categories of drugs to increase effectiveness and decrease side effects.

Anticipatory prescribing is another approach to medications at the end of life. Because distressing symptoms can develop quickly and without warning, the hospice team prepares patients and their families by making medications available in advance of a crisis. The comfort kit, or "just-in-case box," is a small supply of medications kept in the patient's home, typically in the refrigerator. Instructions for use are kept with the kit, along with emergency phone numbers for 24-hour telephone support. While the comfort kit might never be used, it can relieve anxiety for patients and their loved ones to know it's there if needed.

Heads up 8.3. The comfort kit

A 79-year-old woman with COPD was referred for massage therapy. The woman lived alone, with a son who lived nearby. I arrived in the home and was alarmed by the woman's shortness of breath, which I hoped would improve with massage. That did not happen, however. In the span of 20 minutes, the woman became increasingly anxious, which exacerbated her dyspnea. I tried having her lean forward, to no avail. The woman provided me with her son's phone number, but he did not answer. I called the hospice agency, described the situation, and was immediately patched through to a nurse.

The nurse advised me to go to the woman's refrigerator where she told me to look for the comfort kit; she had to describe to me what it looked like. The nurse had me put her on speaker so that she could coach me through locating a small vial of liquid morphine. With shaking hands, I opened the vial and used the oral syringe to draw up a small amount as directed by the nurse. I emptied the syringe into the patient's mouth, and she swallowed the medication. The nurse had me stand in front of the patient and place the patient's hands on my shoulders so that they were raised. With the nurse remaining on the line, and the patient positioned with maximum lung capacity, the patient's dyspnea slowly decreased.

For me, this was a frightening experience that taught me the following lessons:

- Therapists should clarify emergency procedures with their supervisors, including who should be called in the event of an unexpected crisis. Phone numbers should be easily accessible. If a patient is on hospice, the call should go to the designated caregiver or the hospice agency, not to 911.

- Patients with poorly controlled symptoms may not be good candidates for massage, unless there is adequate onsite support from a caregiver or staff member.

- Therapists should become familiar with the contents and use of the comfort kit, hoping they will never be in a position to use it but being prepared in case they are.

- If you depend on reading glasses, keep them accessible at all times. Labels on the medications are tiny, as are the lines on the syringes.

A final strategy used in prescribing medications is a time-limited trial, or TLT. When it is not clear whether a disease process might be reversible, the clinical team may recommend a trial period to evaluate the results of an intervention. This concept can be applied by palliative care providers to a potentially life-sustaining therapy when more time and clarity are needed to make a difficult decision (Siropaides and Arnold, 2020). A TLT can also help discern the success or failure of an intervention to address a distressing symptom in hospice care. An example would be a trial of medication, or conversely, a trial of *reduced* medication. The patient and loved ones can then evaluate for themselves whether the medication is helpful.

Delivery systems and dosing

Medications may be delivered to the body through a variety of routes. The oral route is generally preferred (abbreviated as PO, short for *per os*, which is Latin for "through the mouth"). Oral medications are easy, noninvasive, and inexpensive, though they do require an average of 30 minutes to an hour to be effective. PO medications may not be an option for people with swallowing difficulties, including seizures, head and neck cancer, or reduced level of consciousness. Patients with nausea, vomiting, and other GI problems may be unable to tolerate anything by mouth. In such cases, the delivery system may change to sublingual (under the tongue) or buccal (between the gums and the cheek), where medication is absorbed through the mucous membranes. Sublingual and buccal drugs may come in a dissolving pill form, film, or spray. These drugs bypass the liver and stomach and achieve the desired effect much faster than oral medications.

Rectal or vaginal suppositories likewise bypass the stomach with a higher and faster absorption rate but are more invasive, making them less appealing to some people. A common use of suppositories at the end of life is acetaminophen, or paracetamol, for terminal fever. Our team has had success with lowering fever by placing the acetaminophen suppository under the patient's armpit, where it is absorbed through the skin. This takes a little longer to be effective but is less invasive.

Transdermal patches, containing medication designed to be absorbed through the skin into the bloodstream, may be used for pain (fentanyl and lidocaine), agitation (clonidine), or secretions (scopolamine). Medication via transdermal patch often takes 12–24 hours to reach therapeutic dose, so other medications may be used to control symptoms in the meantime. Patches vary in how long they last and how effective they are. They require a layer of adipose tissue for dispersal throughout the body, making them less effective for cachectic patients.

Unlike the medications described thus far, which are systemic, topical medications applied to the skin can be used to target a specific site in the body. This can be ideal for a localized symptom. Topical products include lotions, ointments, and gels such as ketoprofen, diclofenac, and lidocaine for pain. Many of them come in preloaded syringes so that the dosing is exact. Depending on local guidelines, touch therapists may or may not be permitted to apply these products under medical supervision. Nonprescription analgesics containing menthol, camphor, and capsaicin are covered on p. 110. Medications delivered subcutaneously, intravenously, or via inhalation are addressed in Chapter 9.

Regarding dosing, palliative care and hospice patients are generally advised that it is better to stay ahead of pain than to "chase it." The timing for routine medications to reach peak effect is intended to provide a baseline level of around-the-clock comfort. If rescue doses are frequently needed, the clinical team may opt to increase the routine or basal dose to provide better coverage. Some patients perceive and report that the relief they receive from massage helps them to sleep longer or keeps them from needing PRN medication for breakthrough pain. This is wonderful when it happens, but massage is not intended to replace medication. Routine medications should be provided on schedule, even if the massage session must be interrupted.

A patient may request to decrease or even forego a scheduled medication in order to be more alert for a specific occasion. The occasion might involve legal documents that need to be signed, or a visit from family, friends, a member of the clergy, or funeral home. On the other hand, extra medication is sometimes given in anticipation of an event that may cause or exacerbate pain, shortness of breath, or anxiety. Examples of these activities include repositioning, a shower or bed bath, wound care, or vehicular transport from one location to another. Physician orders are typically created in a way that allows for flexibility in responding to the patient's goals and needs as they vary from day to day and hour to hour.

Chart Talk 8.1. Types of effects

In addition to their intended effects, medications can cause side effects, adverse effects, paradoxical effects, or any combination thereof. Sometimes medications are used off label for their known side effects, in which case side effects are considered to be therapeutic, as described below.

Side effect – any result of a drug that occurs in addition to the intended effect (McGraw-Hill, 2002b). Side effects are typically predictable and may be either therapeutic or undesirable. When undesirable, they can often be managed. An example is constipation caused by opioids; laxatives and opioids are often initiated at the same time as an opioid to address this predictable problem.

Adverse effect – an unwanted reaction to a drug which can sometimes but not always be predicted. Adverse effects can be extreme and dangerous (McGraw-Hill, 2002a). Examples include gastric bleeding from prolonged use of NSAIDS, or allergic reactions that are highly individual.

Paradoxical effect – a response that is the opposite of the expected or desired result. An example is the occasional person who becomes extremely agitated on a medication for anxiety (Thompson, 2021).

Essential and common medications

The World Health Organization (WHO) defines essential medicines as those required to meet the basic healthcare needs of the population. At the request of the WHO, the International Association for Hospice and Palliative Care (IAHPC) developed a list of essential medicines for palliative care in 2007, based on the consensus of palliative care experts around the world. The IAHPC list is intended to guide palliative and hospice care providers to develop their own best practices according to local resources.

According to one large study, the six drugs used most frequently in hospice care are acetaminophen, morphine, haloperidol, lorazepam, prochlorperazine (Compazine), and atropine (Sera et al., 2013). These medications, listed alphabetically in the chart beginning on p. 158, address at least nine common symptoms, including pain, dyspnea, anxiety, agitation, delirium, nausea, vomiting, hiccups, and secretions. All but atropine for secretions are included on the IAHPC list. These and other common palliative medications are grouped by symptom below.

Medications for pain

There are two broad categories of pain medications: opioids, which dull pain sensation, and adjuvant analgesics, or "helper" medications, which may be used by themselves or in combination with opioids. Adjuvants are also used to target specific types of pain as described on the following page. Adjuvant medications include acetaminophen (Tylenol), also known as paracetamol or by the abbreviation APAP; NSAIDs such as ibuprofen (Motrin or Advil), aspirin, diclofenac, naproxen, or ketorolac; steroids; certain antidepressants; and anticonvulsants. Acetaminophen is sometimes added to opioids as a combination pill, making acetaminophen the most common medication used at the end of life (Sera et al., 2013).

Medications for nociceptive pain

Nociceptive pain, described in greater detail on p. 109, is the most common type of pain, involving unpleasant stimuli detected by pain receptors, known as nociceptors. Mild nociceptive pain may respond well to APAP or NSAIDS, though NSAIDS must be avoided or used with care in people with renal impairment, gastric disease, or risk of bleeding (UPMC, 2021). Both APAP and NSAIDS are used sparingly or not at all in patients with liver impairment.

For nociceptive pain that requires a stronger analgesic, the medical team will likely prescribe an opioid. The opioid of choice in hospice care is morphine sulfate (Roxanol), which is also used to alleviate shortness of breath. Morphine is effective, inexpensive, and easy to convert to a variety of delivery methods as needed. Immediate release tablets and liquid morphine can be placed under the tongue or in the cheek if the patient is unable to swallow. Other common opioids used for nociceptive pain at the end of life include codeine, hydrocodone (Norco, Lortab, Vicodin), oxycodone (Percocet, OxyContin), hydromorphone (Dilaudid), and fentanyl patches. Antianxiety drugs such as diazepam (Valium), lorazepam (Ativan), or midazolam (Versed) are sometimes added to enhance pain control, if needed. Side effects for opioids and antianxiety drugs may include sedation, confusion, nausea, and itching, which often resolve or improve after a few days of use. Fall risk must be monitored while sedation and confusion are present; constipation will require ongoing management as described on p. 154.

Medications for bone pain and neuropathic pain

Bone pain and neuropathic pain are treated differently than nociceptive pain, often with adjuvant drugs (acetaminophen or ibuprofen) or drugs that are used off label. Specifically for neuropathic pain, an anticonvulsant such as gabapentin (Neurontin) or carbamazepine (Tegretol) might be used, or an antidepressant such as nortriptyline (Pamelor), amitriptyline (Elavil), venlafaxine (Effexor), or duloxetine (Cymbalta). Care must be taken when using these drugs in patients with renal insufficiency.

The only opioid that specifically targets neuropathic pain and bone pain is methadone. Methadone must be gradually titrated under careful supervision by an experienced provider. Because methadone does not produce euphoria, it is sometimes used with patients at risk of substance abuse. Sedation and dizziness are common side effects warranting fall precautions. Methadone is not as likely as opioids to cause constipation; however, amitriptyline sometimes can (Hines, 2022).

Corticosteroids such as dexamethasone (Decadron) are another class of drugs sometimes used for bone or nerve pain. "Dex" is also used to decrease cranial pressure (nausea, vomiting, and seizures) in people with brain cancer, stroke, and head injuries. It has the benefit of increasing appetite, decreasing fatigue, and promoting a sense of well-being in some people. Undesirable side effects may include insomnia, easy bruising, increased risk of infection, and impaired wound healing. Over time, dexamethasone may cause the skin to become extremely dry and thin, leading to persistent skin tears. Some people experience mood changes such as agitation or aggression and are unable to tolerate dex.

> ### Personal note to the reader 8.1. It's not always about the medication
>
> Early in my career, I had a much harder time being with pain. With the many medications available to treat symptoms, I did not understand why anyone would need to suffer. As I matured as a therapist, I came to understand that there are many reasons for suffering at the end of life. A pain level that might not feel acceptable to me might be acceptable to another person. Some patients are willing to endure discomfort in order to be more present with their suffering and more awake with their loved ones. There is always a trade-off, and the patient needs to be in charge of finding their preferred balance. Now when I ask about a patient's pain level, my follow-up question is "Are you satisfied with your pain level, or would you like to see if we can make you more comfortable?"

Depending on the answer, I can support the patient in addressing the symptom with the medical team.

A second thing I've observed firsthand is the concept of total suffering. Pain that is emotional or spiritual is no less real than physical pain and is often felt in the body as a distressing symptom. I am grateful to work with an interdisciplinary team of professionals who bring diverse perspectives to approaching pain. Medication is typically a necessary but small part of the solution.

Perhaps the most difficult scenario is one where a patient can't make their needs known and the surrogate decision maker refuses medications that the staff feels are necessary for patient comfort. This situation is typically complicated by issues of mistrust, misunderstanding, and fear, where the family might worry that the patient has been or will be overmedicated. There is much that a skilled palliative or hospice team can do to address these issues. Ultimately, though, the provider must abide by the decisions of the appointed spokesperson. Being with this situation can be extremely difficult, but I can't think of a more important time for calm, caring presence.

Medications for constipation

A bowel regimen to prevent or treat constipation usually includes one or more of the following medications. The most common side effects are bloating, gas, cramping, and diarrhea.

- Docusate sodium (Colace).
- Sodium picosulfate (Lactulose).
- Bisacodyl (Dulcolax).
- Polyethylene glycol (Miralax).
- Magnesium hydroxide (Milk of Magnesia).

- Magnesium citrate.
- Senna.

Medications for anxiety and agitation

Hospice patients are often treated for anxiety or restlessness with sedatives known as benzodiazepines, or benzos, a class of drugs which one doctor I know refers to as "wine in a pill." Two of the most common benzos, both included on the IAHPC list of essential medicines, are diazepam (Valium) and lorazepam (Ativan). The latter has been noted at our inpatient unit to occasionally cause the paradoxical effect of extreme agitation (Thompson, 2021). Benzodiazepine tablets can be placed under the tongue, in the cheek, or dissolved in a small amount of warm water if the patient has difficulty swallowing.

Midazolam (Versed) is another drug on the IAHPC list which may be used at the end of life for anxiety, agitation, and delirium. Midazolam provides a stronger level of sedation when other benzos have been ineffective. Additional benzos used by some hospices include alprazolam (Xanax) which is often effective for shortness of breath, and clonazepam (Klonopin) which is more long-acting (Thompson, 2021). Benzodiazepines can cause sedation, confusion, disorientation, dizziness, and increased risk of falls. These side effects are compounded when benzos are used with other common drugs at the end of life, particularly opioids.

Haloperidol (Haldol) is the common medication for terminal agitation, delirium, and hallucinations. It is also given off label for nausea. Haloperidol side effects include dizziness, light headedness, and sedation, all contributing to fall risk. Risperidone may also be used to address delirium. In some patients, these drugs can paradoxically cause or worsen delirium.

Medications for depression

Antidepressants are selected at the end of life based on the potential for side effects, drug interactions, secondary benefits, and what has worked for the patient in the past.

Expected lifespan must also be considered. Patients in the last weeks of life may not gain any benefit from an antidepressant that requires time to reach therapeutic effect. Based on the above criteria, providers may prescribe citalopram (Celexa), fluoxetine (Prozac), nortriptyline (Pamelor), or trazodone, all on the IAHPC list of essential medications. Other antidepressants used by some hospice providers include escitalopram (Lexapro), sertraline (Zoloft), paroxetine (Paxil), venlafaxine (Effexor), duloxetine (Cymbalta), methylphenidate (Ritalin), and doxepin. Side effects vary by antidepressant, but often include sedation, dry mouth, and GI problems. Citalopram and fluoxetine can also cause paradoxical hyperactivity (Hines, 2022).

Medications for shortness of breath

The first-line therapy for shortness of breath is a small dose of an opioid, typically morphine. The dose is lower than when morphine is given for pain. In addition to morphine, dexamethasone is often used. Benzodiazepines are sometimes added to relieve anxiety related to shortness of breath, including diazepam (Valium), lorazepam (Ativan), and alprazolam (Xanax). As noted above, opioids and benzodiazepines can cause sedation and dexamethasone may cause easy bruising and thinning of the skin. Drugs delivered by inhalation for symptoms related to shortness of breath are discussed on pp. 175–6.

Medications for nausea and vomiting

Drugs for nausea and vomiting depend on the probable cause of these symptoms. Essential medications for nausea and vomiting include metoclopramide (Reglan), haloperidol (Haldol), and lorazepam (Ativan). The team may also try olanzapine (Zyprexa), procholorperazine (Compazine), ondansetron (Zofran), promethazine (Phenergan), or diphenhydramine (Benadryl). All drugs used for nausea and vomiting may cause sedation with increased risk of falls.

Medications for fluid retention

Furosemide (Lasix) is commonly used in hospice care for fluid overload, though it is not considered an essential

medication by the IAHPC. Furosemide must be used with care due to the potential for it to cause low potassium. Spironolactone (Aldactone) may be used as a potassium-sparing alternative (Thompson, 2021). Side effects for furosemide, spironolactone, and other diuretics may include GI symptoms, in addition to low blood pressure and dizziness, which contribute to fall risk.

Medications for itching and hiccups

Medications that may be used for itching at the end of life include diphenhydramine (Benadryl), doxepin, and chlorpromazine (Thorazine). Of these, only diphenhydramine is considered to be an essential drug. Chlorpromazine may also be used for chronic hiccups, though haloperidol is more common. Dizziness and sedation are side effects for all these medications. Triamcinolone cream applied to the skin may provide temporary relief of itching, though this symptom often requires a systemic approach.

Medications for seizures

Lorazepam (Ativan) and diazepam (Valium), both considered to be essential medications, are commonly used to control seizures. Levetiracetam (Keppra) or midazolam (Versed) may also be used. Dizziness and sedation are the main side effects of these drugs. Both seizures and the medications to treat them increase the risk of falls.

Medications for oral secretions

When accompanied by signs of distress, or if terminal secretions are disturbing for the family, the medical team may try one or more of the following medications for secretions:

- Scopolamine transdermal patch. May cause sedation. Delirium is a possible adverse effect.

- Diphenhydramine (Benadryl). May cause drowsiness.

- Hyoscyamine (Levsin). May cause dizziness, drowsiness, dry mouth, urinary retention, and GI problems.

- Atropine eye drops, placed in the mouth or under the tongue. May cause dry mouth, alleviated with sips of water or ice chips. Not used by every hospice, due to cost.

Medications for wounds

As described in Chapter 6, wound healing is not always possible at the end of life. Interventions are aimed at containment, infection control, pain relief, and odor management for patient comfort and dignity. Strategies include:

- Analgesics for pain, which may cause sedation.
- Metronidazole (Flagyl) capsule or solid pill, opened or crushed and placed in the wound bed for odor, especially for fungating tumors.
- For cancer wounds, wound gel or salve mixed with sublingual Roxanol is sometimes applied directly to the wound.
- Activated charcoal dressings for odor control.

Antibiotics

Antibiotics, sometimes abbreviated ABX, may be used to treat bacterial infections at the end of life, including respiratory infections, pneumonia, urinary tract infections (UTIs), and cellulitis. While antibiotics are not considered essential medications by the IAHPC, they may be justified for infections that cause distressing symptoms, such as confusion and delirium, which are common with UTI. Pneumonia may or may not be treated at the end of life, depending on the patient's comfort, overall condition, and the goals of care. The most common antibiotics used at the end of life include:

- Sulfamethoxazole/trimethoprim (Bactrim).
- Penicillin (amoxicillin).
- Levofloxacin (Levaquin).
- Ceftriazone (Rocephin Injectable).

Side effects may include rash, stomach pain, diarrhea, nausea, and vomiting (WebMD, 2021).

A note on marijuana use in hospice and palliative care

The medical use of cannabinoids or marijuana is legal in many parts of the world, but restricted or forbidden in others. Of the two species of cannabis, *Cannabis indica* is used more frequently for relief of pain, nausea, and vomiting (UPMC, 2021). Delivery routes for medical cannabinoids include pills, topical forms, tinctures, liquids, and dry leaf formulations for vaporization and nebulization.

The list of medical conditions for which medical marijuana may be useful is constantly being updated, based on studies of varying quality. Cannabis may play a helpful role in several terminal conditions including stroke, Parkinson's, ALS, MS, Huntington's, and HIV (UPMC, 2021). The American Academy of Neurology supports the following in regard to MS: "Oral cannabis extract and synthetic THC, the active ingredient in marijuana, are probably effective for reducing patient-reported symptoms of spasticity and pain" (Hamid, 2019). To date, however, evidence for other applications is considered inconclusive. In studies on cannabis for people with Parkinson's and nausea or vomiting, central nervous system and psychiatric side effects were reported with high concentrations of THC, including sedation, agitation, hallucinations, and sleep disturbances (Häuser et al., 2017). While adverse effects appear to be dose-related, lack of standardized potencies is one obstacle to meaningful research (Brody, 2021).

Studies indicate more promising results for the use of cannabis for neuropathic pain, with results comparable to those achieved with codeine. Topical application of THC may likewise have benefit for localized neuropathic pain (Hamid, 2019). Cannabis is not included in the hospice benefit in the US, nor in the IAHPC list of essential medicines. Hospice and palliative care providers will need ongoing education to respond to consumer interest in the medical use of cannabinoids at the end of life, along with quality research to explore potential risks and benefits.

Commercially available cannabis for medical use includes:

- Dronabinol (Marinol, Syndros).

- Nabilone (Cesamet).

- Nabiximols (Sativex, not available in the US).

- Cannabidiol (Epidiolex).

Palliative sedation as a last resort

In very rare circumstances, the efforts of the palliative or hospice team fail to relieve suffering at the end of life. When severe symptoms persist despite the care team's best efforts, palliative sedation may be considered as a last resort. Palliative sedation is defined by the American Academy of Hospice and Palliative Medicine as the "intentional lowering of awareness towards, and including, unconsciousness for patients with severe and refractory symptoms" (AAHPM, 2014). This option is used not to hasten death, but to provide relief while allowing death to take its natural course.

The participation of the patient or patient's proxies in the decision to use palliative sedation is paramount. Degree of sedation must be carefully managed to correspond to the patient's degree of distress and can be reduced if the target symptoms are thought to be temporary. Comfort care is continued to ensure the dignity of the sedated person. This care may include level 1 massage with an emollient lotion or cream to moisturize the skin and as a means to convey caring presence.

A summary of what touch therapists need to know

While most people at the end of life will experience at least some of the side effects, adverse effects, and paradoxical effects described in this chapter, individual responses are quite variable. An "opioid-naïve patient," defined as someone who has not taken opioid medication in a certain time frame – 30 days, for example (Pino and Wakeman, 2021) – is more likely to experience sedation and other side effects. Patients whose doses are stable over time typically become acclimated to their medications in a way that allows them to function more normally. Studies suggest that patients on chronic opioids with no dose change in the past week are at no greater risk of automobile accidents than the general population (Schisler et al., 2015). But it is just as true that conditions in people at the end of life can change abruptly and without warning. Therapists must remain alert to possible effects of medication and end-stage disease, respecting each patient's highest and safest degree of function while addressing questions and concerns to the clinical team as needed.

Adapting the massage session for medications at the end of life

- Refer to clinical teammates and Table 8.1 as needed, until the names of common medications become familiar. The table contains an alphabetical list by generic name of common medications used at the end of life.

- Opioids, benzodiazepines, and many other medications can cause impaired perception and feedback. Massage pressure for people on these medications should be confined to levels 1 or 2, depending on level of arousal and responsiveness.

- Patients on anticoagulants and steroids such as dexamethasone require a maximum of level 2 pressure, or level 1 if widespread bruising is present. Anticoagulants include aspirin, warfarin (Coumadin), clopidogrel (Plavix), rivaroxaban (Xarelto), and apixaban (Eliquis). Figure 8.1 on p. 161 demonstrates how easily bruising can occur.

- Due to the number of medications that cause sedation, fall risk precautions should be considered for every patient at the end of life. Safety measures include returning the hospital bed to the lowest position; placing objects the patient might need within reach, including the call light; using bedrails if customary;

Table 8.1 Common medications in palliative care

Generic name	Brand name	Uses	Risks and precautions
Acetaminophen (Paracetamol)*	Tylenol	Mild pain, bone or neuropathic pain, fever	GI reactions
Alprazolam	Xanax	Anxiety, agitation	Sedation, fall risk
Amitriptyline	Elavil	Depression, neuropathic pain	Drowsiness, dizziness, fall risk
Atropine ophthalmic drops		Secretions	Eye irritation, dry mouth
Bisacodyl*	Dulcolax	Constipation	GI reactions
Carbamazepine*	Tegretol	Neuropathic pain	Drowsiness, dizziness, fall risk
Citalopram*	Celexa	Depression	Drowsiness, fall risk
Clonazepam	Klonopin	Anxiety	Drowsiness, dizziness, fall risk
Chlorpromazine	Thorazine	Itching, hiccups, nausea	Drowsiness, dizziness, fall risk
Codeine		Moderate to severe pain	Sedation, fall risk
Dexamethasone*	Decadron	Bone pain, nerve pain, dyspnea, nausea/vomiting	Bruising, thinning skin, pressure risk
Diazepam*	Valium	Anxiety, agitation, seizures	Sedation, fall risk
Diclofenac	Voltaren	Mild to moderate pain	GI reactions
Diphenhydramine*	Benadryl	Itching, nausea/vomiting	Sedation, fall risk
Docusate sodium	Colace	Constipation	GI reactions
Doxepin		Itching, depression	Drowsiness, fall risk
Fentanyl (transdermal patch)*		Moderate to severe pain	Sedation, fall risk, avoid site
Fluoxetine	Prozac	Depression	Drowsiness, fall risk

Generic name	Brand name	Uses	Risks and precautions
Furosemide	Lasix	Fluid retention, edema, ascites	Low BP, fall risk, urinary urgency
Gabapentin*	Neurontin	Bone pain, nerve pain	Drowsiness, dizziness, fall risk
Haloperidol*	Haldol	Agitation, delirium, nausea/vomiting, hiccups	Sedation, fall risk
Hydrocodone	Norco, Lortab, Vicodin	Moderate to severe pain	Sedation, fall risk
Hydromorphone	Dilaudid	Moderate to severe pain, dyspnea	Sedation, fall risk
Hyoscine butylbromide*	Scopolamine, Buscopan	Secretions, nausea	Drowsiness, dizziness, fall risk
Hyoscyamine	Levsin	Secretions	Drowsiness, dizziness, fall risk
Ibuprofen*		Mild to moderate pain	GI reactions
Lactulose		Constipation, hepatic encephalopathy	GI reactions
Levetiracetam	Keppra	Seizures	Drowsiness, fall risk
Levomepromazine*	Nozinan	Nausea/vomiting, terminal agitation, pain	Drowsiness, fall risk
Loperamide*	Imodium	Diarrhea	GI reactions
Lorazepam*	Ativan	Anxiety, agitation, nausea/vomiting, seizures	Sedation, fall risk
Megestrol acetate*	Megace	Loss of appetite	DVT, pressure risk (Bolen et al., 2000)
Methadone*		Bone pain, nerve pain	Sedation, fall risk
Metoclopramide*	Reglan	Nausea/vomiting	Sedation, fall risk
Midazolam*	Versed	Seizures, agitation	Sedation, fall risk
Morphine*	Roxanol	Moderate to severe pain, dyspnea	Sedation, fall risk

continued

Table 8.1 *continued*

Generic name	Brand name	Uses	Risks and precautions
Nortriptyine	Pamelor	Depression, nerve pain	Drowsiness, dizziness, fall risk
Octreotide*		Diarrhea, nausea, vomiting	Dizziness, fall risk
Ondansetron	Zofran	Nausea, vomiting	Sedation, fall risk
Oxycodone*	Percocet, OxyContin	Moderate to severe pain, dyspnea	Sedation, fall risk
Polyethylene glycol	Miralax	Constipation	GI reactions
Prednisolone*		Loss of appetite, inflammation	Bruising, thinning skin, pressure risk
Prochlorperazine	Compazine	Nausea/vomiting	Mild sedation, fall risk
Promethazine	Phenergan	Nausea/vomiting, constipation	Sedation, fall risk
Senna*	Senokot	Constipation	GI reactions
Sodium picosulfate		Constipation	GI reactions
Tramadol*		Mild to moderate pain	Sedation, fall risk
Trazodone		Insomnia, depression	Sedation, fall risk
Zolpidem*	Ambien	Insomnia	Sedation, fall risk

Information in this chart was provided by Stephen Lee Hines, MD, FACP (2022); Deborah Rice, RN, MSN, GNP-BC (2020); and Jeanna Thompson, RN (2021).

*Denotes medications appearing on the IAHPC Essential Medicines for Palliative Care (IAHPC, 2007).

avoiding unassisted patient transfers; and reporting concerns about unsafe situations in the home.

- Orthostatic hypotension (dizziness upon standing) is common at the end of life, due to patient condition and medications such as diuretics, insulin, medicines for high blood pressure, and tricyclic antidepressants (Thompson, 2021). Follow fall precautions as described above, especially regarding unassisted patient transfers.

- Avoid contact with transdermal patches. If a patch detaches from the patient's skin, don gloves before handling. The patch should be given immediately to a nurse rather than thrown away. Deaths have occurred

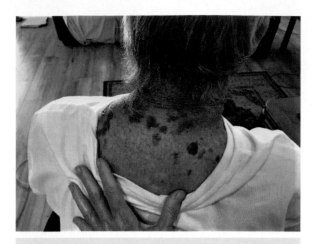

Figure 8.1
The patient in this photo acquired widespread bruising from long-term steroids to manage shortness of breath. These appeared after he wore a collared shirt, indicating how easily bruising can occur. I provided massage for this patient over a period of eight months and never used more than level 1 pressure, which he loved.

(Photo by author.)

in children who find used patches that were not disposed of properly.

- Heat increases the absorption of transdermal medications. Do not use a heating pad or any other source of heat over a skin patch.

- Use gloves when applying topical analgesics or other products with active ingredients.

- Medications for constipation, including bisacodyl (Dulcolax), lactulose, polyethyleneglycol (Miralax), and senna (Senokot), can cause a sudden urge to defecate. Be alert for signs of agitation or discomfort that may indicate the patient needs to access a bed pan, bedside commode, toilet, or change of clothing (Hines, 2022).

- Furosemide (Lasix) likewise causes urinary urgency. This will not be an issue for patients who use a Foley catheter, but therapists should be sensitive to the needs of those who may need quick access to a urinal, bedside commode, toilet, or dry brief.

Conclusion

What Saunders recognized more than four decades ago, and what hospice and palliative care providers continue to recognize, is that the dying process demands unique approaches to the use of medications. Drugs are selected or discontinued based on whether they are likely to improve or impair comfort, and are delivered in the safest, least invasive manner possible. The goal is to use the minimal amount of medication necessary to achieve quality of life, while supporting the patient to remain as functional and comfortable as possible. Long-term concerns may become irrelevant or secondary to short-term goals.

While the care team has expertise in the anticipated effects of the medications used at the end of life, it must be remembered that reactions to medications are extremely individual. Side effects most likely to impact the massage session include dizziness, confusion, sedation, bruising, and deterioration of the skin. These same symptoms can be caused or exacerbated by advanced disease and the dying process. A practical approach is to assume that massage for *all* people with advanced illness must be adapted, whether for the side effects of medication *or* the impact of disease, by adjusting massage pressure, remaining alert to the risk of falls, and being mindful of the presence of transdermal patches. Learning all we can about common drugs used at the end of life, combined with common sense and consultation with clinical colleagues, will ensure that gentle touch is a safe and welcome complement to medicine.

References

AAHPM, 2014. *Statement on palliative sedation.* [online] Available at: <http://aahpm.org/positions/palliative-sedation>.

Anekar, A. A. and Cascella, M., 2020. *WHO Analgesic Ladder.* [online] Available at: <https://www.ncbi.nlm.nih.gov/books/NBK554435>.

Bailey, M., 2018. *Doctors learning how to have end-of-life conversations.* [online] Available at: <https://www.

physicianleaders.org/news/doctors-learning-how-to-have-end-of-life-conversations>.

Baines, M., 2011. Pioneering days of palliative care. *European Journal of Palliative Care,* [e-journal] 18(5), pp. 223–227. Available at: <https://www.stchristophers.org.uk/wp-content/uploads/2015/09/EJPC_18_5_Baines.pdf>.

Beck, A., 2019. *Serious illness conversation guide.* [pdf] Available at: <http://www.instituteforhumancaring.org/documents/Providers/Serious-Illness-Guide-old.pdf>.

Bolen, J. C. et al., 2000. Deep vein thrombosis as a complication of megestrol acetate therapy among nursing home residents. *Journal of the American Medical Directors Association,* [e-journal] 1(6), pp. 248–252. Available at: <https://pubmed.ncbi.nlm.nih.gov/12812608>.

Brody, J. E., 2021. *Medical marijuana is not regulated as most medicines are.* [online] Available at: <https://www.nytimes.com/2021/03/08/well/live/medical-marijuana.html>.

Ciuksza, M. S. et al., 2015. *Use of home inotropes in patients near the end of life.* Fast Fact #283. [online] Available at: <https://www.mypcnow.org/fast-fact/use-of-home-inotropes-in-patients-near-the-end-of-life>.

Delgado, J. et al., 2017. Blood pressure trajectories in the 20 years before death. *JAMA Internal Medicine,* [e-journal] 71(1), pp. 93–99. Available at: <https://doi.org/doi:10.1001/jamainternmed.2017.7023>.

Enzinger, A. et al., 2015. Outcomes of prognostic disclosure. *Journal of Clinical Oncology,* [e-journal] 33(32), pp. 3809–3817. Available at: <https://www.ncbi.nlm.nih.gov/pmc/articles/PMC4737862/pdf/zlj3809.pdf>.

Fallon, M. T. and Cherny, N. I., 2015. Opioid therapy: optimizing analgesic outcomes. In: Cherny, N. I. *Oxford textbook of palliative medicine.* 5th ed. Oxford: Oxford University Press. Ch. 9.4.

Fixen, D. R., 2019. 2019 AGS Beers Criteria for older adults. *Pharmacy Today,* [e-journal] 25(11), pp. 42–54. Available at: <https://www.pharmacytoday.org/article/S1042-0991(19)31235-6/fulltext>.

Gaertner, J. et al., 2019. Early palliative care and the opioid crisis: ten pragmatic steps towards a more rational use of opioids. *Annals of Palliative Med,* [e-journal] 8(4), pp. 490–497. Available at: <https://doi.org/10.21037/apm.2019.08.01>.

Hamid, K., 2019. *The use of medical marijuana in hospice and palliative care.* [pdf] Available at: <http://cchospice.org/wp-content/uploads/2019/09/K.-Hamid-F1-Carolinas-Conference-Medical-Marijuana-2019-Presentation-Kiran-Hamid-1.pdf>.

Häuser, W. et al., 2017. Cannabinoids in pain management and palliative medicine: an overview of systematic reviews and prospective observational studies. *Deutsches Ärtzteblatt International,* [e-journal] 114(38), pp. 627–634. Available at: <https://www.ncbi.nlm.nih.gov/pmc/articles/PMC5645627/pdf/Dtsch_Arztebl_Int-114-0627.pdf>.

Hines, S., 2022. Discussion of medications. [conversation via telephone] (Personal communication, 18 January 2022).

Huisman, B. A. et al., 2021. Physicians' opinions on anticoagulant therapy in patients with limited life expectancy. *Seminars in Thrombosis and Hemostasis,* [e-journal] 47(6), pp. 735-744. Available at: <https://pubmed.ncbi.nlm.nih.gov/33971680>.

IAHPC, 2007. *List of essential medicines for palliative care.* [pdf] Available at: <https://hospicecare.com/uploads/2011/8/iahpc-essential-meds-en.pdf>.

MacDonald, G. and Tague, C., 2021. *Hands in health care: massage therapy for the adult hospital patient.* 2nd ed. Edinburgh: Handspring Publishing.

McGraw-Hill Concise Dictionary of Modern Medicine, 2002a. *Adverse effect.* [online] Available at: <https://medical-dictionary.thefreedictionary.com/adverse+effect>.

McGraw-Hill Concise Dictionary of Modern Medicine, 2002b. *Side effects.* [online] Available at: <https://medical-dictionary.thefreedictionary.com/side+effects>.

Mitchell, S. L., 2015. Advanced dementia. *North England Journal of Medicine,* [e-journal] 372(26), pp. 2533–2540.

Available at: <https://doi.org/10.1056/NEJMcp1412652>.

Niznik, J. et al., 2020. Deintensification of diabetes medications among veterans at the end of life in VA nursing homes. *Journal of American Geriatrics*, [e-journal] 68(4), pp. 736–745. Available at: <https://doi.org/10.1111/jgs.16360>.

O'Neill, R. et al., 2017. *Abuse-deterrent opioid formulations*. Fact Fact #329. [online] Available at: <https://www.mypcnow.org/fast-fact/abuse-deterrent-opioid-formulations>.

Overgaard, C. B. and Džavík, V., 2008. Inotropes and vasopressors. *Circulation*, [e-journal] 118(10), pp. 1047–1056. Available at: <https://www.ahajournals.org/doi/epub/10.1161/CIRCULATIONAHA.107.728840>.

Pino, C. A. and Wakeman, S. E., 2021. *Prescription of opioids for acute pain in opioid naïve patients*. [online] Available at: <https://www.uptodate.com/contents/prescription-of-opioids-for-acute-pain-in-opioid-naive-patients>.

Price, J. R. et al., 2015. Opioid therapy: managing risks of abuse, addiction, and diversion. In: Cherny, N.I., 2015. *Oxford textbook of palliative medicine*. 5th ed. Oxford: Oxford University Press. Ch. 9.5.

Rice, D., 2020. Discussions of common conditions, symptoms, and medications. [Conversations in person, via Zoom and telephone] (Personal communication, 12 August 2020, 23 September 2020, 25 September 2020, 7 October 2020, 22 October 2020).

Schisler, R. E. et al., 2015. *Counseling patients on side effects and driving when starting opioids*. Fast Fact #248. [online] Available at: <https://www.mypcnow.org/fast-fact/counseling-patients-on-side-effects-and-driving-when-starting-opioids>.

Sera, L. et al., 2013. Commonly prescribed medication in a population of hospice patients. *American Journal of Hospice and Palliative Medicine*. [e-journal] 31(2), pp. 126–131. Available at: <https://doi.org/10.1177/1049909113476132>.

Siropaides, C. H. and Arnold, R., 2020. *Time-limited trials for serious illness*. Fast Fact #401. [online] Available at: <https://www.mypcnow.org/fast-fact/time-limited-trials-for-serious-illness>.

Temel, J. S. et al., 2010. Early palliative care for patients with metastatic non-small-cell lung cancer. *North England Journal of Medicine*, [e-journal] 363(8), pp. 733–742. Available at: <https://www.nejm.org/doi/pdf/10.1056/NEJMoa1000678>.

Thompson, J., 2021. Discussion of medications. [Conversation] (Personal communication, 2 December 2021).

UPMC Palliative and Supportive Institute, 2021. *Palliative care symptom guide*. [online] Available at: <https://www.upmc.com/-/media/upmc/services/palliative-and-supportive-institute/documents/palliativecaresymptomguide.pdf?la=en>.

WebMD, 2021. *What are antibiotics?* [online] Available at: <https://www.webmd.com/a-to-z-guides/what-are-antibiotics>.

Additional resources

Benzodiazepine Information Coalition, 2021. *Paradoxical reactions*. [online] Available at: <https://www.benzo-info.com/paradoxical-reactions>.

Fuentes, A. V. et al., (2018). Comprehension of top 200 prescribed drugs in the US as a resource for pharmacy teaching, training and practice. *Pharmacy (Basel, Switzerland)*, [e-journal] 6(2), p. 43. Available at: <https://doi.org/10.3390/pharmacy6020043>.

MacCallum, C. A. et al., 2021. Is medical cannabis safe for my patients? A practical review of cannabis safety considerations. *European Journal of Internal Medicine*, [e-journal] 89(1), pp. 10–18. Available at: <https://doi.org/10.1016/j.ejim.2021.05.002>.

Swallowing is difficult, use G-tube. Six ounces of water with one bag of formula, shaken, not stirred.

—Instructions from a patient with a feeding tube

People often arrive at the end of life with a lot of gear. There is a wide array of equipment, known in healthcare as durable medical equipment (DME), to help people maintain capacity and independence, and to aid their helpers in providing care for them. There are tubes to deliver nutrition or medications to the body and drains to relieve the body of fluids and wastes. There are even machines, sometimes implanted in a person's body, that support failing organs to perform their functions. There is no question that medical technology can extend and improve life.

Assistive technologies have drawbacks, however, including side effects that often become more burdensome as the body declines. Interventions that prolong life can be especially problematic when they conflict with an individual's goals for a peaceful death. A person's right to choose or refuse treatment is endorsed by the World Health Organization as "the right to control one's health and body" and to "be free from interference . . . [including] nonconsensual medical treatment" (WHO, 2017). When a person can no longer speak for themselves, a surrogate decision maker will speak on that person's behalf, ideally remaining true to the person's expressed wishes. Decisions can be spiritually and emotionally charged, forcing questions to the surface about what it is to live a meaningful life. Clinicians, including touch therapists, are likely to have their own opinions about this, which may or may not align with the choices of patients and their proxies.

This chapter will address common interventions during the last six months of life, including suggestions for adapting massage to accommodate both the presence and the withdrawal of these measures. Regardless of the choices made, patients and families should never feel abandoned. In collaboration with an interdisciplinary team, touch therapists have the opportunity to embrace patient autonomy and dignity in a way that affirms life, even as life comes to an end.

Touching story 9.1. A patient educates our team

Janette, affectionately known as Janie, was 44 years old with two teenage sons when she was diagnosed with a motor neuron disease. She and her husband, Rick, worked as industrial engineers, designing distribution centers for large retailers across the country. Janie loved music, gardening, friends, and family. Among her large social circle, she was famous for creating music playlists for every occasion, sometimes very silly ones. She grew vegetables in the backyard, which the family enjoyed each summer.

By the time I met Janie, the symptoms of her disease were already advanced. In keeping with her engineering background, Janie created a detailed document to educate our team about her care during respite stays at the hospice inpatient unit. The stories in this chapter include excerpts from these instructions.

What I've observed with Janie and countless other patients is that people are amazingly resilient in coming to terms with changes in their health, and the interventions needed to support these changes. There may be initial resistance to measures which represent tangible evidence of disease progression, along with grief for lost abilities, changing roles, and dependence on medical assistance. But there can also be a sense of liberation and improved quality of life, both with decisions to initiate interventions and, when appropriate, to discontinue them.

Equipment

Two of the most common types of DME that touch therapists will encounter in end-of-life care are mobility devices and hospital beds. This section will also address appliances to assist people with vision, hearing, and communication.

Mobility devices

Dying usually involves a transition from independent mobility to lack of mobility, with a number of steps in between. Some diseases, like ALS and Parkinson's, actually *target* mobility; for these patients, loss of mobility may come early in the dying process. For others, there is a gradual decline in strength and stamina, which eventually requires the use of mobility aids and assistance from others. People may start with a cane, and progress to a walker or rollator with wheels to support balance and weight bearing. With increasing weakness, many people transition to a wheelchair. During the final stages of dying, most are confined to bed.

Heads up 9.1. When people lose their mobility

Loss of independent mobility at the end of life is a game changer, with physical, social, and psychological consequences. Dignity issues arise when the patient needs help with bathing and toileting. The patient may grieve a loss of privacy or an increasing sense of isolation as their world becomes smaller. Physical complications of immobility include increased risk of constipation, blood clots, pneumonia, urinary tract infections (UTIs), skin breakdown, slow wound healing, muscle pain, and contractures. Some patients are understandably resistant to giving up their mobility and may persist in attempting to walk even after it becomes unsafe. Falls and injuries are a frequent outcome.

Wheelchairs allow people at the end of life to access spaces and experiences which would otherwise be unavailable due to fatigue or debility. There is great variety in types and sizes of wheelchairs, from simple manual designs to sophisticated electric models that adjust for standing, sitting, or reclining. Electric or battery-powered wheelchairs can be operated with a control stick, by voice, or by exhalation. Over time, patients and their carers develop expertise and proficiency in the use of their chairs to accomplish everyday activities.

Another specialized device is a geri chair (or geriatric recliner), often available in facilities. Geri chairs are larger and less portable than wheelchairs, but they do have castors so that they can be moved. Covered in vinyl which is easily sanitized, they provide the option of reclining or sitting upright with or without a tray table, using a bar or lever to make manual adjustments. Geri chairs are intended to be comfortable for longer periods of sitting, allowing an alternative for patients who are confined to bed. Some patients make good use of a geri chair, but others prefer the familiarity, comfort, and ease of their own wheelchair.

Adapting the massage session

- Slow the pace of everything. Allow time for transfers or provide massage wherever the patient is found. Tips for positioning in wheelchairs and geri chairs are found on p. 62.

- Keep transfers safe. If a patient requests to be moved for massage, ask staff or family members for help as needed.

- Patients and caregivers are experts on their equipment and have likely adapted their own ways of doing things. Be respectful of the patient's independence and allow them to do as much as they safely can for themselves.

- At the conclusion of the session, make sure any items that have been moved are placed back in the person's reach.

- Share concerns with the family or medical team. You may be the first person to notice an unsafe situation.

- Assure patients and families that massage can be adapted for their needs in the weeks or months ahead. Sample script: "There may come a time when you want to spend more time in bed. We can easily do your massage wherever you're most comfortable on a given day."

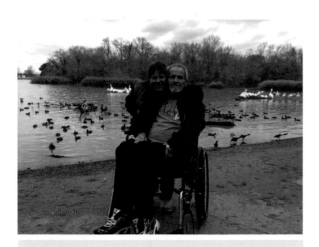

Figure 9.1
A wheelchair can assist patients and their loved ones to continue enjoying activities together. This was Daniel's last outing with Cici two weeks prior to his death.

(Photo courtesy of patient's family.)

Hospital beds

Hospital beds have wheels and are designed to raise and lower, making it easier for patients to get in and out of bed and for others to provide care for them without stooping. The head of the bed can be raised to ease breathing and the foot can be raised to help reduce edema. Hospital beds are narrow and can be placed in an area of the home that is high or low traffic, depending on preference. Larger individuals may be more comfortable in a bariatric bed, which is wider and built to support more weight. Rails are a common accessory, spanning the entire length or part of the bed. Rails can be raised or lowered, providing protection and a grab bar for repositioning. An overbed tray table is another common accessory. Hospital beds, rails, and tray tables are typically provided by hospice, but families may be expected to provide their own linens. Most standard-size hospital beds require extra-long twin sheets. Sheets for bariatric beds will likely need to be purchased from a medical supply store.

Mattress options, including gel, air, and memory or reflex foam toppers, are an evolving technology. Some beds have a pressurized mattress for the prevention of skin breakdown. Even with these options, many people find a hospital bed to be less comfortable than a standard bed. Hospital beds may disrupt the closeness that couples feel when they sleep together, which can represent a loss for both parties. Staff at our IPU routinely support partners, children, and parents who wish to lie beside their loved one. I once provided a massage for a patient and her teenaged daughter who was curled up next to her, using one hand to caress the mother and the other to caress the daughter while they fell asleep in each other's arms.

Adapting the massage session

- Massage can easily be provided in a hospital bed, as described on p. 63.

- The hospital bed can be raised for massage with advance notice provided to the patient, but must be lowered and wheels locked at the conclusion of the session.

- Bedrails, if used, should be returned to the upright position following the session. Take care with tubing when raising or lowering bedrails.

- Be aware that bed alarms and cameras are sometimes used to monitor patient safety. Some alarms attach to the patient's gown or clothing and can be activated during repositioning. The alarms are very loud and startling!

- A tray table, cane, walker, TV remote, cell phone, or any other personal belongings moved for massage should be returned to their original locations. Reaching is a common cause of patient falls.

Communication and visual devices

Touch therapists specializing in end-of-life care may encounter a variety of assistive technologies to support impaired sight, hearing, and communication. These include low-tech appliances such as eyeglasses, hearing aids, magnifiers, amplifiers, dry-erase boards, writing tablets, and alphabet boards. Alphabet boards, some of them digital, allow the user to point or gaze at words, letters, symbols, and pictures.

Phones, tablets, and computers have revolutionized communication for those with access. There are apps that generate sound, either from text or from previously recorded messages. The technology of voice banking allows people to record their own voices while they can still speak, allowing them to personalize phrases such as "Thank you," "I love you," and the names of loved ones. Even inside jokes can be recorded for later use (Your ALS Guide, 2021).

Because these technologies are changing so rapidly, we must look to patients, their caregivers, and our colleagues to educate us. Once introductions and consent have been navigated, the universal language of touch will likely reduce the need for communication during the session. It remains important, however, for patients to be able to express feedback and to make their needs known to the fullest extent possible.

Touching story 9.2. Janie's equipment

What I first noticed about Janie when I entered her room was not her equipment, but the bold streak of purple dye in her silky gray hair. She was seated in her electric wheelchair, which was bright green with all-terrain tires. The wheelchair, like Janie's hair, was downright sporty.

Instructions in Janie's medical chart, authored by Janie, included photos of her preferred configuration of pillows for optimal support. "Please prop my feet," she had written, "so they don't flop forward." The instructions emphasized that Janie needed good neck support. Her notes read, "If my neck isn't supported, it is painful, and I am unable to see to type on my phone."

At our first meeting, I introduced myself and described the massage services available at the inpatient unit. Janie raised her eyebrows and slowly began typing her response, using a text display app. I observed that she had good use of her left hand and partial use of the right. It took Janie a while to type each letter, but finally the message displayed: "Where have you been all my life?"

Adapting the massage session for a person with impaired hearing or communication

- Slow down. Communication will take longer than usual. Offer pauses to allow time for the patient to respond (Happ, 2020).

- Don't shout. Speak as you normally would, using adult vocabulary. The patient or caregiver will let you know if you need to raise your volume.

- People may hear better from one ear than the other. Inquire about this and position yourself accordingly.

- Moving closer to the patient's ear may reduce the need to speak at high volume.

- People sometimes have shortcuts for single-word responses, such as a thumbs up for "yes" and thumbs down for "no." They may be able to blink once or twice to indicate responses to questions. Ask staff or family if there is anything you should know to better communicate with the patient.

- Use pointing and gestures as needed (Happ, 2020).

- A patient's equipment should be treated as an extension of their body (Rossen et al., 2012). Do not touch or move equipment without permission.

Adapting the massage session for a person with impaired sight

- Announce your presence and movements verbally. Tell the person before you touch them. Tell them when you are moving to another area of the room or to another area of the body, and when you are leaving the room.

- Touch therapists may be tempted to dim the lights for a more relaxing ambiance. Keep in mind that people with visual impairment may need bright light.

- Ask before moving any object at the bedside, and return the item to its previous location when the session is complete.

- Make sure that glasses are accessible if they were removed for massage.

- In the inpatient setting, make sure the person can access the call light. One option is to place the call light in the person's hand.

Cardiac devices

Pacemakers and implanted defibrillators

A pacemaker is surgically implanted below the skin, typically on the left side of the body. It may be close to the skin surface and visible as a round raised area, roughly the size of a pocket watch. Others are buried more deeply and may go unnoticed by the touch therapist. Pacemakers use electrical signals to synchronize heart rhythm with subtle pulses that are rarely felt by the patient. They may improve energy and shortness of breath.

An implanted defibrillator, known as an automatic implanted cardiovertor defibrillator (AICD) or simply an implanted cardiovertor defibrillator (ICD), is slightly larger than a pacemaker and may be visible beneath the skin. ICDs are usually placed below the left clavicle, in the abdomen, or on the side of the chest under the armpit. These devices are designed to shock the heart back into rhythm and may be experienced as a strong thump to the chest, which can be startling and uncomfortable. The risk of pacemakers and ICDs is low but can include an increased chance of infection and DVT.

Left ventricular assist devices (LVADs)

A left ventricular assist device, or LVAD, is a surgically implanted heart pump. The LVAD is sutured into the front of the patient's chest or abdomen, with a hose that connects to a battery pack outside the body. The battery must be recharged nightly. LVADs were originally intended to keep patients alive while waiting for heart transplant. Though this is still one purpose of this device, its use has expanded as a "destination therapy" for people who are not candidates for heart transplant. LVADs improve well-being and extend survival for some people with advanced heart disease, but the surgery is invasive with a high risk of complications. Repeat hospitalizations are common for infection, bleeding, DVT, and stroke. People with LVADs are unable to bathe or swim, as the external components must remain dry.

Adapting the massage session

- Due to DVT risk, use a maximum of level 2 pressure to the upper body and upper extremities of people with pacemakers and ICDs. An LVAD device is more invasive and calls for level 1 pressure to the entire body.

- If a pacemaker or ICD is new (eight weeks or less), it is best to avoid the affected quadrant, including chest, shoulder, back, and arm, until the incision is well healed. This scenario will be rare in our work, since these devices are usually not implanted in the last six months of life.

- Patients with an LVAD will need to be positioned for comfort, generally semi-reclining or high Fowler's position.

- Avoid the area of the chest or abdomen where the LVAD hose is inserted.

- See p. 118 regarding additional adjustments to massage for people with heart disease.

Respiratory devices

A number of oxygen delivery systems are available for people with conditions that impact lung function, such as COPD, heart failure, pulmonary fibrosis, ALS, lung cancer, and cancer that has spread to the lungs from elsewhere in the body. Each type of device requires a way to store the oxygen (in liquid or gas form), a way to deliver the oxygen, and an interface that connects the system to the user. The system chosen will depend on how much lung function remains, how much oxygen is needed for comfort, and the patient's goals for longer life versus quality of life.

Nasal cannulas and nasal pillows

A nasal cannula is the least invasive and most common method of oxygen delivery, used to provide low-flow oxygen for patients who are unable to breathe adequately on their own. The cannula typically wraps around the patient's ears, with soft rubber prongs that rest inside the nostrils. A long tube connects the cannula to an oxygen concentrator or portable tank in the home, or to an O_2 wall unit in an inpatient environment. Side effects are typically minor, including nasal dryness and skin irritation at points of contact with tubing, primarily the ears. Soft padding can be used to cushion the ears and cheeks. A water-based gel can soothe dry nasal passages.

When lungs are more severely damaged, the patient may need an oxygen flow rate that exceeds the capacity of a nasal cannula. In these cases, there are systems that can deliver higher-flow oxygen through a larger cannula or nasal pillow (soft plugs that seal the nostrils). These higher-flow systems use humidified oxygen and are still relatively comfortable for patients.

Noninvasive ventilation (NIV)

The next level of oxygen support, noninvasive ventilation (NIV), includes BiPAP and CPAP. Both use pressurized air delivered through a facemask that fits over the nose and mouth. CPAP stands for continuous positive airway pressure and is often used at night for sleep apnea to ensure steady inhalation. BiPAP, or bilevel positive airway pressure, is a more complex device with two airway settings – one for the inhalation and one for the exhalation. BiPAP may be used by people with ALS, COPD, or congestive heart failure. Some people need BiPAP only at night; others use it during waking hours as well.

NIV can help some people sleep better, allowing more energy and better quality of life during the day. But NIV is also noisy and uncomfortable, especially when used continuously. Patients will be unable to communicate, eat, or drink while wearing the mask. Some people experience claustrophobia. The air pressure can be great enough to cause facial bruising. For these reasons, efforts may be made at the end of life to wean patients off NIV and onto a more comfortable alternative. NIV will continue to blow air into the body after the heart stops beating, so BiPAP must be turned off at the time of death.

Intubation

The most invasive type of respiratory support is intubation, involving use of a ventilator that mechanically moves air into and out of the lungs. The ventilator connects to the patient's respiratory system through a tube which is placed down the throat (endotracheal intubation) or via tracheostomy (a hole or stoma through the neck into the trachea). A patient who is intubated may need to be suctioned frequently to keep the airway free of mucus. Forced breathing will continue at death, until mechanical ventilation is turned off.

For some people, intubation is an emergency procedure after a catastrophic injury or illness, when it may not be known whether meaningful recovery will be possible. Strokes and COVID-19 are examples. For others, whether to be "trached and vented" is a premeditated decision that accompanies a chronic disease known to result in respiratory failure, such as ALS. The decision is consequential, regardless of how it is made. Once trached and vented, the patient will likely be unable to speak. They will require tube feeding and 24/7 caregiving. Some people choose intubation so that they can live longer, spend more time with loved ones, or accomplish a work or legacy-related goal. Whether these aspirations outweigh the limitations of life on a ventilator is a very personal decision.

Adapting the massage session

- Use caution not to step on or pull O_2 tubing.

- Any stoma, including tracheostomy, is vulnerable to contamination. Avoid the area.

- Ventilated patients may be sedated or have limited arousal. As always, use level 1 pressure if the patient is unable to communicate.

- A patient on a ventilator may open their eyes when touched or spoken to. Eye contact, a smile, and letting the patient know what you are about to do can be reassuring. Watch carefully for nonverbal feedback.

- It may feel good to work on the posterior neck underneath the intubation band, around the head straps of a BiPAP, or behind the ears where O_2 tubing can cause tenderness, as shown in Figure 9.2.

- Use of noise-cancelling ear buds with patient-preferred music can be a way for patients to escape the sound of a BiPAP or respirator. This can be especially nice during a massage.

- See p. 129 regarding additional adjustments to massage for people with lung disease.

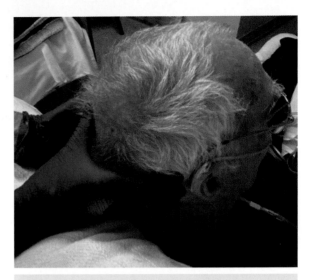

Figure 9.2
Skin breakdown can occur from contact with oxygen tubing. In this photo, the therapist is applying gentle circular massage to the surrounding area. The patient created the padding seen over the right ear.

(Photo by Beth Giniewicz.)

Devices for nutrition and hydration

There are two types of artificial nutrition and hydration, the enteral route and the parenteral route. The enteral route uses an alternate pathway to the GI system. An example is a nasogastric tube (or NG tube), inserted through the nose into the stomach. NG tubes can be used to provide nutrition, hydration, and medication. They may also be used to suction stomach contents or GI secretions to alleviate nausea or vomiting, or to promote bowel rest in a patient with bowel obstruction or GI bleeding. NG tubes are uncomfortable for most patients and are typically used for a short period, two weeks or less. They may cause sore throat, increased mucus at the back of the throat, breathing issues, and nasal irritation. Patients may exhibit restlessness and agitation and have been known to pull their NG tubes out.

Another enteral feeding tube is a percutaneous endoscopic gastrostomy (PEG), a tube which is surgically inserted through the skin into the stomach. Alternately, a tube can be placed in the intestines, called a jejunal tube, or J tube. These devices bypass the mouth and esophagus, delivering nutrition, fluids, or medication directly to the lower GI tract. Like the NG tube, a PEG or J tube can be used with suction for drainage if needed. A PEG or J tube is more comfortable than an NG tube and therefore more appropriate for longer-term use. Another longer-term option is TPN, total parenteral nutrition. TPN bypasses the GI tract entirely, delivering nutrition directly to the bloodstream through an IV in the lower arm or chest.

Some people use a feeding tube for most of their calories but are safely able to indulge in small amounts of food by mouth. Otherwise, artificial nutrition and hydration should not be confused with the enjoyable or social aspects we associate with eating. Tube feedings consist of a liquid diet; J tubes allow the option of pureed foods. These foods are not tasted since the tongue is bypassed. Hospice endorses careful hand feeding when tolerated for pleasure and social contact, along with thickened liquids or ice chips by mouth.

Adapting the massage session

- Treat a feeding tube as you would any other indwelling device. Avoid the immediate area and use a maximum of level 2 pressure.

- Position the patient for comfort. This may be especially important immediately following tube feeding.

- Leakage and skin irritation at the tube site should be reported to the nurse.

Bowel and urinary tract devices

Bowel and bladder problems are common for people with advanced diseases. An example is colorectal or abdominal cancer, or surgery for one of these cancers, that has damaged or blocked the normal pathways for urine or feces. When this happens, waste products may be surgically rerouted to a new opening in the body. A flexible catheter may be used to connect this new opening to the

skin, or a tube may be created from a piece of the person's intestines. What appears on the outside of the body is a fleshy ring of red, moist tissue called a stoma.

Chart talk 9.1. Types of stomas

The most common stomas include the following.

Colostomy – an opening in the colon.

Ileostomy – an opening in the small intestine.

Cystostomy – an opening in the bladder.

Nephrostomy – an opening in the kidney.

Colostomies, ileostomies, and cystostomies involve a stoma on the lower abdomen, often on the right side. Nephrostomies exit the body on the back side close to the kidneys. The catheter or stoma is connected to a bag outside the body that must be emptied or changed by the patient or caregiver. The patient typically cannot control how quickly the bag fills, or how often it must be changed. Leaking is common and may result in skin irritation, fungus, odor, and potential embarrassment for the patient. Ground coffee is sometimes placed under the patient's bed to absorb odors. As with any indwelling device, there is a risk of infection.

Incontinence, or loss of bladder or bowel control, is another problem at the end of life. Incontinence may be caused by a number of diseases, spinal injuries, or by the dying process itself. Wounds, pressure ulcers, pain, inability to get in and out of bed, and several end-of-life medications can also interfere with bowel and bladder function. Approaches might include the use of a bedside commode, bedpan, urinal, or incontinence garments, also known as disposable briefs or adult diapers. For regular ongoing incontinence of urine, the use of a urinary catheter may be helpful. Urinary catheters are also used for urinary retention when a person is unable to pass urine. Urinary retention is extremely uncomfortable and may cause agitation.

A catheter uses a flexible tube to drain urine from the body into a collection bag. The most common type of catheter is the Foley catheter, which is inserted into the urethra and held in place by a tiny balloon. Sometimes a suprapubic catheter is used, in which a small hole is made in the abdomen to reach the bladder. A condom catheter is an external device that can be worn over the tip of the penis by men with incontinence. A condom catheter is connected to a drainage bag and must be changed daily.

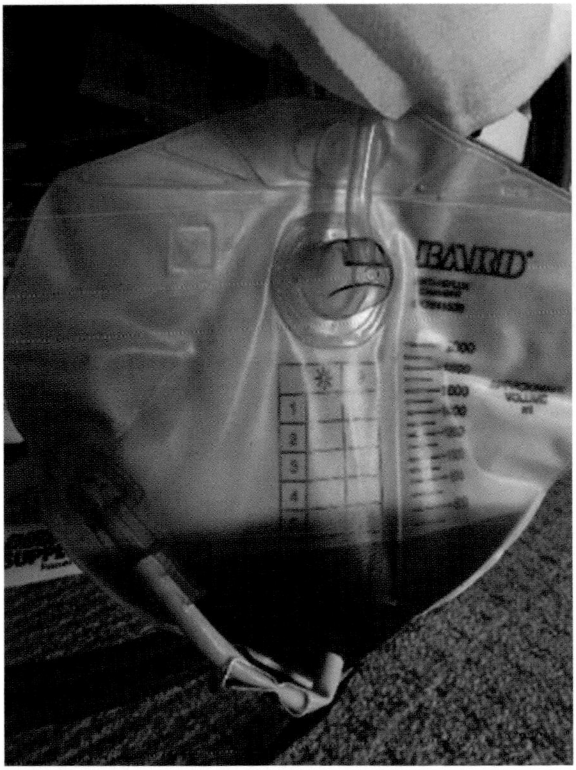

Figure 9.3
A Foley bag hangs from the patient's bed below the level of the bladder for good drainage. The dark color of the urine is typical during the later stages of dying. It is also not unusual for there to be blood or sediment in the urine.

(Photo by author.)

Touching story 9.3. Continent care at the end of life

Other than brief respite stays at the hospice inpatient unit, Janie was cared for at home, where she required assistance to use a bedside commode. She wrote the following in her care notes. "Potty transfer requires three people: one to carry under arms, one to carry legs, and one person to manage ventilator." When she came to the IPU for her final days, she consented to a Foley catheter.

I often wondered why we put Foleys in so many of our patients. To me, it seemed invasive and a risk for infection. What I've come to understand is how difficult it is to keep patients clean and dry, and how vulnerable the skin becomes when it is exposed even for a short time to concentrated urine. Patients may experience pain when they have to be moved to clean the perineum, change the bedlinen, and put on a dry brief. When this care takes place in the home, the burden on caretakers can be overwhelming.

Though I have come to see the benefit of urinary catheters, some patients experience discomfort or anxiety when having them inserted. Patients are premedicated and massage can be used prior to or during the catheter insertion to help calm patients. Once the catheter is inserted, most people don't seem bothered. But I have seen patients become agitated by the urge to urinate, even when they have a Foley. We remind them, "It's okay, you can just let go." But it remains a struggle for many people to lose control of their bladder and bowels.

Adapting the massage session

- Be sensitive to a patient's need to urinate, defecate, or have their collection bag emptied or changed. These needs should be addressed prior to massage so that the patient can truly relax.

- Positioning will need to accommodate bowel and bladder devices, according to what is comfortable for the patient.

- Take care with tubing and collection bags when lowering or raising beds and bedrails, or assisting patients to reposition.

- Leakage should be reported promptly to the nurse.

- A sudden increase in agitation, confusion, or restlessness may indicate a UTI and should be reported to the nurse.

Pain control devices

Subcutaneous

People with nausea, vomiting, intestinal obstruction, or difficulty swallowing may be unable to swallow medication. In such cases, a needle may be used to provide medicines needed for comfort. A subcutaneous (sub-Q) needle is the least invasive of these methods, involving a needle placed just under the skin into the fatty tissue between the skin and muscle. The patient must have enough body fat for good dispersal of the medication. Typical sites for sub-Q injection are the upper arm, upper leg, hips, chest, or abdomen. Dosing may be provided by repeat injections, or a needle that is held in place with tape for repeat access. The latter must be changed every few days. Sub-Q needles are small and usually not painful.

An application of the sub-Q route that is common in the UK and Australia is the syringe driver, a battery-driven portable device used to deliver a continuous infusion of medication over a 24-hour period. While syringe drivers have not been universally adopted, they are con-

sidered to be an essential component of British palliative care (Graham and Clark, 2005). Ronna Moore shares that volunteers at her palliative care agency make cloth holders for the drivers, which can then be carried like a purse (Moore, 2021). Moore points out that this is one way to reduce visible medical technology, which is important to some patients.

Subcutaneous drugs are absorbed slowly, which may reduce the side effects from some medications. Slow absorption can be a drawback when symptoms are severe, however. Only small doses of medication can be provided via sub-Q, which is an additional limitation. The syringe driver must be refilled every 24 hours, using a locked box to control dosage.

Intravenous

When pain is severe and difficult to control, large doses of pain medications can be delivered very quickly via IV, taking effect in 5–15 minutes. The IV is placed in one of three places, depending on the length of time the IV will

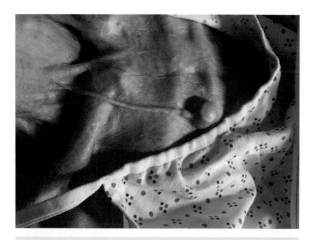

Figure 9.4
Ports used to deliver chemotherapy are a type of intravenous central line, typically located on one side of the clavicle. In the hospice setting, they can be used for palliative medications.

(Photo by author.)

be needed. For short duration (two to three days), a small vein in the thumb, large toe (also known as the great toe), or female breast may be used. For up to eight weeks, a midline might be placed, typically in the arm. A midline goes into the vein about 20 cm (8 inches), but not all the way to the heart. For longer-term IV access, a central line may be preferred. Central lines may be in the jugular or other central vein, or in the leg or arm (a peripherally inserted central catheter, or PICC line).

Some IVs are attached to a patient-controlled analgesia (or PCA) pump, which allows the patient to access IV medication as needed with the push of a button. The dose is controlled by machine. Patients with PCA pumps who are unable to manage this by themselves can be assisted by family or care staff who can push the button for them when they exhibit signs of distress. The dose is controlled by computer program so that it is not possible to exceed the prescribed amount. A dose delivered by PCA pump is called a bolus. Once placed, these systems are typically painless for the patient, but they do present risk of infection and DVT.

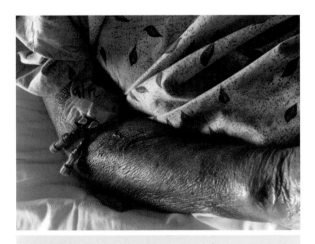

Figure 9.5
A PICC line with a double lumen is another type of central venous access, commonly used in inpatient environments to help control severe symptoms.

(Photo by author, first appeared in *Hands in health care*.)

Adapting the massage session

- Avoid insertion sites, due to risk of infection.

- Level 1 pressure in a limb with a PICC or midline, due to risk of DVT.

- Take care when repositioning the patient not to dislodge the device (Moore, 2021).

Procedures

Dialysis

Dialysis, or hemodialysis, is an artificial means to "clean" the blood of wastes and excess fluid in people with kidney problems. The machine, called a dialyzer, is sometimes described as an artificial kidney. An access point is surgically created for dialysis using a vein in the body; there are different types, including arteriovenous fistulas, percutaneous fistulas, arteriovenous grafts, or central venous catheters. Once the blood is cleansed of toxins, it is returned to the bloodstream.

Dialysis is an intensive intervention requiring several hours per treatment, multiple times per week. Burdens include risk of infection, risk of DVT, discomfort during access, travel to and from the appointments, and time devoted to the procedure. There is a type of dialysis that can be performed at home, called peritoneal dialysis, a system which is implanted in the abdomen. But peritoneal dialysis also has complications, including risk of infection and inability to bathe or swim. Peritoneal dialysis must be performed several times per day.

Breathing treatments

Breathing treatments are often provided at the end of life to ease symptoms such as swelling of the airway, shortness of breath, coughing, congestion, constriction, and wheezing from COPD and other chronic lung diseases. These involve medications delivered in the form of vapor through a device called a nebulizer. Nebulizers use compressed air to turn liquid medicine into mist, which the patient breathes through a mask worn over the nose and mouth. The treatment takes 15–20 minutes.

People often experience fast relief from a breathing treatment. But the medications delivered via nebulizer can cause shaking, nervousness, headache, or irritability. Massage can be provided as a comfort during or after a breathing treatment. See p. 103 for adjustments to massage for shortness of breath.

Paracentesis, thoracentesis, and wound drains

Paracentesis and thoracentesis, also called "taps," are sometimes used in advanced disease to remove excess fluid from the body. Paracentesis removes fluid from the abdominal cavity, called ascites. Thoracentesis removes fluid from the space between the lungs and the chest wall, known as pleural effusion. In both procedures, a hollow needle or tube is inserted through the skin into the affected body cavity. A local anesthetic is provided to lessen discomfort from the needle.

People typically experience immediate relief of dyspnea and other symptoms after a pleural or abdominal tap. The fluid will likely return, however, given that the cause – cirrhosis, heart disease, kidney disease, or cancer – is often incurable. If frequent taps are needed for comfort, a permanent catheter can be placed in the body to drain ascites or pleural fluid as needed, weekly or even daily (see Figure 9.6). Touch therapists can offer gentle massage to relax and distract patients during paracentesis and thoracentesis. The therapist will need to work around these tubes and their insertion sites when encountered. Drains and stents used to prevent infection of wounds should likewise be avoided.

Decisions to forego or withdraw life-prolonging therapies

Whether to initiate, continue, or withdraw life-prolonging therapies can be one of the most difficult decisions a person will ever make. Deliberations are typically muddied with strong emotions, including the feelings of loved

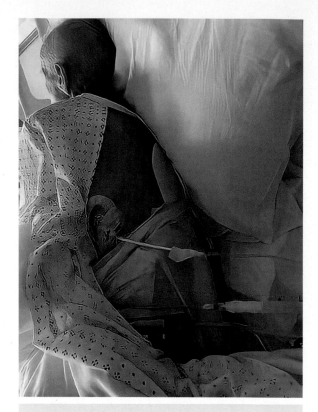

Figure 9.6
Patients often have multiple devices. The woman above has a Foley catheter and bilateral chest tubes to relieve chronic pleural effusion. She also has a port-a-cath which is not visible in the photo. She was nonetheless able to roll onto her right side in a high Fowler's position for massage to her head, neck, and shoulders.

(Photo by author.)

ones, which complicate the choices. Patients are urged to document their wishes long before it is time to make such decisions, but risks and benefits are abstract concepts, until they're not. People deserve boundless compassion as they navigate this complex and agonizing terrain where there is no pain-free outcome.

The interventions that people most frequently decline or discontinue at the end of life include cardiopulmonary resuscitation, dialysis, artificial nutrition and hydration, cardiac devices (ICDs and LVADs), and mechanical ventilation, each described below. Ideally, a hospice or palliative care team is available to assist with information, decision making, symptom management for the patient, and emotional support for the family. Some interventions can be discontinued in a supportive home setting; others may require an inpatient level of care. Sometimes there are multiple interventions to be discontinued, requiring medical support with sequencing.

CPR and DNR

Cardiopulmonary resuscitation, or CPR, may involve forceful chest compressions, electric shocks to the heart, or a tube placed down the throat for mechanical ventilation in the event that a person's heart or breathing stops. These interventions are provided by emergency personnel by default, unless they are aware that the patient has created a DNR, or "do not resuscitate" order. The acceptance of the concept of DNR, also known as DNAR or "do not attempt resuscitation," varies by country, state, or province, as does the process for documentation.

The DNR was created to protect people in their last months of life from receiving aggressive measures that may result in suffering and prove to be futile. CPR for people with terminal conditions is generally associated with poor outcomes, as cardiac arrest in these scenarios is often due to advanced illness rather than a reversible cause (Ramenofsky and Weissman, 2015). The line between recovery and nonrecovery can be vague and subject to interpretation, however. Each person has a right to decide under what conditions they would want to be resuscitated.

Many people assume that hospice requires patients to sign a DNR, but that is not the case. One large US study determined that 12.9% of hospice enrollees elect full code status including CPR, a choice primarily associated with male gender, younger age, nonwhite race, home setting of care, and cancer diagnosis (Ankuda et al., 2017). Once emergency medical services are set into motion, the patient will likely be discharged from hospice services in order to pursue aggressive care.

Discontinuing dialysis

Some people endure dialysis for many years until decline is well advanced. Discontinuation typically occurs when the patient becomes too weak or blood pressure falls too low to withstand the rigors of treatment. From the last day of dialysis, death can be expected within days or up to two or three weeks, depending on remaining kidney function. Dying for these patients may include symptoms caused by uremia, or excess of urea, creatinine, and nitrogen (see p. 130 regarding end-stage kidney disease). These symptoms can include confusion, sedation, fluid overload, nausea, and itching, which can be managed by the palliative or hospice care team. Touch therapists may play a role in providing lubrication to the dry skin that often accompanies renal failure.

Discontinuing tube feedings and IV fluids

The topic of artificial nutrition and hydration can trigger deep emotion and conflict for people. Families may wish to initiate or continue tube feedings or IV fluids because they fear their loved one will die of dehydration or starvation. While supplemental feeding has clear benefits in the early stages of some diseases, benefit at the end of life is less clear. Some studies suggest that supplemental feeding can actually hasten death in people with cancer (Sihra and Kinzbrunner, 2011). As the body loses its ability to absorb and metabolize food, patients with feeding tubes often develop diarrhea, bloating, nausea, and vomiting. Fluid overload from IV hydration can cause edema, shortness of breath, and excess secretions. Aspiration pneumonia is a risk with any feeding tube. TPN carries an additional risk of infection and DVT.

When risks and burdens outweigh benefits, patients and families may choose a comfort-oriented approach to tapering or stopping artificial nutrition and fluids. The feeding tube can be left in place while the decision is evaluated. Hunger is rarely a problem, but patients do sometimes experience thirst, which can be alleviated with ice chips, sips of water as tolerated, and oral lubricants such as Biotene. Massage with an emollient cream can help dehydrated skin. It can take two or more weeks for a person to die without nutrition or fluids, but this natural progression is consistent with a more comfortable dying process. As always, symptoms of the underlying terminal disease will be managed as needed by the care team.

Deactivation of implanted defibrillators

Pacemakers do not prolong or impact the dying process. The device simply stops working when the patient dies. Pacemakers are removed from the body prior to cremation because they can explode at high heat. An implanted defibrillator, on the other hand, must be turned off by the manufacturer in order to prevent distressing shocks to the heart during active dying. Some newer ICDs function as both defibrillator and pacemaker; the defibrillator function can be disabled in these models without affecting the function of the pacemaker (Kinzbrunner, 2011). Deactivation of an ICD is painless and there is little risk of immediate death. If the care team is unable to access the manufacturer for an imminent patient, a magnet may be taped over the device to inhibit the sensor.

LVAD deactivation

A left ventricular assist device presents a more complicated scenario at the end of life. LVAD patients typically die of stroke, infection, or multiorgan failure. Most choose to have their LVADs deactivated in order to avoid a prolonged death in which heart function is artificially preserved as the rest of the body is dying (Dunlay et al., 2016). The LVAD deactivation protocol should be clearly explained to patients and their families, with ample opportunity to ask questions and explore concerns. The discussion should include the care team's plan for managing anticipated symptoms, which can include dyspnea, anxiety, agitation, and secretions.

While most deactivations occur in the ICU, a growing number of hospice inpatient units are able to provide holistic support for this experience, which may allow for the presence of loved ones and pets, music, massage, and spiritual support. After deactivation, most people die within one hour (Dunlay et al., 2016). From the care team's standpoint, LVAD deactivation must be carefully orchestrated to safeguard the comfort and dignity of the patient and family, with a plan in place for post-death care and bereavement support. Team members can also benefit from an opportunity to process the experience, once family has been taken care of.

Withdrawal of mechanical ventilation

Like LVAD withdrawal, the withdrawal of mechanical ventilation must be medically supervised and carefully planned. "Compassionate extubation" is often provided in the hospital or hospice inpatient setting where a full team, including a respiratory therapist, can be present to support both patient and family. Everyone at the bedside should understand the sequence of steps. Alarms connected to the device are silenced in order to create the most peaceful environment possible. Medications to prevent shortness of breath and other distress are given via IV so that symptoms are well managed. Death may occur within minutes, or the patient may breathe on their own for hours or days. Ongoing comfort care, family support, and bereavement services are available as needed. Touch therapists can play a vital role in this support.

Touching story 9.4. Janie's death

Janie and Rick had talked at length about her wish for a peaceful death. She had chosen to sign a DNR shortly after her hospice admission. As her disease progressed, she became more fatigued. Her tube feedings began to cause nausea, making it hard to tolerate them. One of her lungs collapsed, increasing the work of breathing and adding to her anxiety. Her pain also increased, requiring stronger medications. She slept almost continuously, but it was not a restful sleep. There was nothing peaceful about the way she was dying.

Janie requested to come to the hospice inpatient unit to have her artificial ventilation discontinued. The clinical team met with the couple and extended family members over several days to review Janie's wishes and to discuss in detail what a vent withdrawal would involve. The family asked that the chaplain, music therapist, and massage therapist be present. It was decided that these visits would be staggered to avoid a large group at once.

On the morning of Janie's vent withdrawal, the care team met to review the protocol. The massage therapist entered Janie's room just as the aide was completing her bath. The therapist brushed Janie's purple hair one last time, then set up a small stool at the foot of the bed and began to massage Janie's feet with warm lotion. Extended family trickled in, greeting one another, stroking Janie's face, and holding her hands. The day was warm, and someone opened the patio door. The respiratory therapist turned off the vent alarm. The sound of birds filled the room.

The chaplain arrived, and the massage therapist gently held Janie's feet while a prayer was offered. The family told stories about Janie, sometimes crying and sometimes laughing. Janie slept, finally appearing relaxed and comfortable, and the therapist slipped out of the room as the music therapist arrived to sing Janie's favorite songs. The massage therapist brought additional chairs into the room for family who were standing at the bedside.

The respiratory therapist gradually reduced the settings on the ventilator. The nurse stood by with additional medications to prevent respiratory distress. Janie rested comfortably throughout. After the ventilator was turned off, the room became quiet.

Liberated from the machine, Janie breathed on her own for a little while, as her family whispered loving words to her. Her respirations slowed. And then, without effort or struggle, Janie's breathing stopped. The team stood by for a silent moment, then departed quietly to provide privacy for the grieving family.

Adapting the massage session

The day of the withdrawal procedure will be emotional for all concerned. It is therefore ideal to explore the patient's or family's wishes regarding massage in the days prior, including whether massage is wanted and, if so, when – prior to the procedure, during, or both. As a precursor to the withdrawal protocol, gentle touch can help to relax and honor the dying person. If they have enjoyed massage previously, and if the therapist has an established relationship with patient and family, all the better. I have attended compassionate extubations and LVAD withdrawals where a large family group was present, where I felt my role should be minimal and unobtrusive. But I have also been present when a primary caregiver was alone for this momentous occasion, and they seemed glad for me to remain in the room.

Below are specific suggestions for touch therapists to support withdrawals of life-prolonging measures.

- The room may be crowded. Take a small portable stool or be prepared to stand. Find a way to be unintrusive and show deference to loved ones at the bedside.

- Assist in making loved ones feel physically comfortable and supported. This may involve making sure they have a chair or placing pillows behind the back or under the arms.

- Make sure tissues are at hand.

- Stopping an intervention that has kept a person alive is an emotionally intense experience. Take time to settle your nervous system prior to and after the experience. Process with appropriate teammates as needed.

- Therapists may wish to prepare themselves with additional education on the topic of compassionate extubation. A good resource may be found at: https://apmonline.org/wp-content/uploads/2015/02/APM-Guidance-on-Withdrawal-of-Assisted-Ventilation-Consultation-1st-May-2015.pdf.

Conclusion

Janie's last four years of life while living with a motor neuron disease included travel, concerts, and attendance at her sons' soccer games. She took up painting and, with the help of friends, self-published a book of watercolors as a legacy project. She remained connected to friends through Facebook and in-person visits. In the midst of a challenging illness, she had fullness of life which she could not have achieved without the aid of her wheelchair, communication devices, feeding tube, and artificial ventilation. Her last days of life were made more comfortable with a Foley catheter and IV medications. She and her family chose to stop artificial ventilation to allow a peaceful death, with physical, emotional, and spiritual support from the hospice team. Her story demonstrates the benefits of medical interventions, and the benefits of supported withdrawal on a timetable that revolves around the patient's changing needs and goals. The care team's responsibility is to engage with the patient and family in ethically and medically sound decision making, to palliate symptoms as needed, and to offer ongoing support. There can be a role for gentle touch at each step of the way.

References

Ankuda, A. et al., 2017. Electing full code in hospice: patient characteristics and live discharge rates. *Journal of Palliative Medicine*, [e-journal] 21(3), pp. 297–301. Available at: <http://europepmc.org/article/MED/28872978>.

Dunlay, S. M. et al., 2016. Dying with a left ventricular assist device as destination therapy. *Circulation Heart Failure*, [e-journal] 9(10), e003096. Available at: <http://dx.doi.org/10.1161/CIRCHEARTFAILURE.116.003096>.

Graham, F. and Clark, D., 2005. The syringe driver and the subcutaneous route in palliative care: the inventor, the history and the implications. *Journal of Pain and Symptom Management*, [e-journal] 29(1), pp. 32–40. Available at: <https://doi.org/10.1016/j.jpainsymman.2004.08.006>.

Happ, M., 2020. *Communicating with a patient on a ventilator*. [online] Available at: <dailynurse.com/communicating-with-a-patient-on-a-ventilator-tips-from-a-specialist>.

Kinzbrunner, B. M., 2011. Invasive cardiac interventions. In: Kinzbrunner, B. M. and Policzer, J. S., eds. 2011. *End-of-life care: a practical guide*. 2nd ed. New York: McGraw-Hill. Ch. 20.

Moore, R., 2021. Discussion of syringe drivers. [email] (Personal communication, 12 December 2021).

Ramenofsky, D. H. and Weissman, D. E., 2015. *CPR survival in the hospital setting*. [online] Available at: <https://www.mypcnow.org/fast-fact/cpr-survival-in-the-hospital-setting>.

Rossen, C. B. et al., 2012. Everyday life for users of electric wheelchairs: a qualitative interview study. *Disability and Rehabilitation: Assistive Technology*, [e-journal] 7(5), pp. 399–407. Available at: <https://doi.org/10.3109/17483107.2012.665976>.

Sihra, L. and Kinzbrunner, B. M., 2011. Artificial nutrition and hydration. In: Kinzbrunner, B. M. and Policzer, J. S., eds. 2011. *End-of-life care: a practical guide*. 2nd ed. New York: McGraw-Hill. Ch. 24.

WHO, 2017. *Human rights and health*. [online] Available at: <https://www.who.int/news-room/fact-sheets/detail/human-rights-and-health>.

Your ALS Guide, 2021. *ALS Communication Devices*. [online] Available at: <https://www.youralsguide.com/communication.html>.

Additional resources

Arenella, C., n.d. *Artificial nutrition and hydration at the end of life: beneficial or harmful?* [online] Available at: <https://americanhospice.org/caregiving/artificial-nutrition-and-hydration-at-the-end-of-life-beneficial-or-harmful>.

Cancer Research UK, 2020. *Types of tube feeding.* [online] Available at: <https://www.cancerresearchuk.org/about-cancer/coping/physically/diet-problems/managing/drip-or-tube-feeding/types>.

Connor, S. et al., 2020. Introduction. In: Conner, S. R., ed. *Global atlas of palliative care.* 2nd ed. [e-book] London: Worldwide Palliative Care Alliance. Available at: <WHPCA_Global_Atlas_DIGITAL_Compress.pdf> Ch.1.

Dunn, H., 2017. *Hard choices for loving people.* Naples, FL: Quality of Life Publishing Co.

FCA, 2019. *Advanced illness: feeding tubes and ventilators.* [online] Available at: <https://www.caregiver.org/advanced-illness-feeding-tubes-and-ventilators>.

Jacquet, S. and Trinh, E., 2019. The potential burden of home dialysis on patients and caregivers: a narrative review. *Canadian Journal of Kidney Health and Disease,* [e-journal] 6(1), pp. 1–7. Available at: <http://dx.doi.org/10.1177/2054358119893335>.

Kōkua Mau, 2016. *Tube feeding.* [pdf] Available at: <https://kokuamau.org/wp-content/uploads/FEEDING-TUBE-Info-Kokua-Mau.pdf>.

Oneschuk, D. et al., 2018. *Total parenteral nutrition (TPN).* [pdf] Available at: <https://www.albertahealthservices.ca/assets/info/peolc/if-peolc-palliative-care-tips-issue24.pdf>.

Panke, J. T. et al., 2016. Discontinuation of a left ventricular assist device in the home hospice setting. *Journal of Pain and Symptom Management,* [e-journal] 52(2), pp. 313–317. Available at: <https://doi.org/10.1016/j.jpainsymman.2016.02.010>.

Prendergast, T. and Puntillo, K., 2011. Withdrawal of life support: intensive care at the end of life. In: McPhee, S. J. et al., eds. 2011. *Care at the close of life: evidence and experience.* New York: McGraw-Hill. Ch. 38.

Rice, D., 2020. Discussions of common conditions, symptoms, and medications. [conversations in person, via Zoom and telephone] (Personal communication, 12 August 2020, 23 September 2020, 25 September 2020, 7 October 2020, 22 October 2020).

Wachterman, M. et al., 2018. Association between hospice length of stay, health care utilization, and Medicare costs at the end of life among patients who received maintenance hemodialysis. *JAMA Intern Med,* [e-journal] 178(6), pp. 792–799. Available at: <http://dx.doi.org/10.1001/jamainternmed.2018.0256>.

Whitmer et al., 2009. Medical futility: a paradigm as old as Hippocrates. *Dimensions of critical care nursing,* [e-journal] 28(2), pp. 67–21. Available at: <http://dx.doi.org/10.1097/DCC.0b013e318195d43f>.

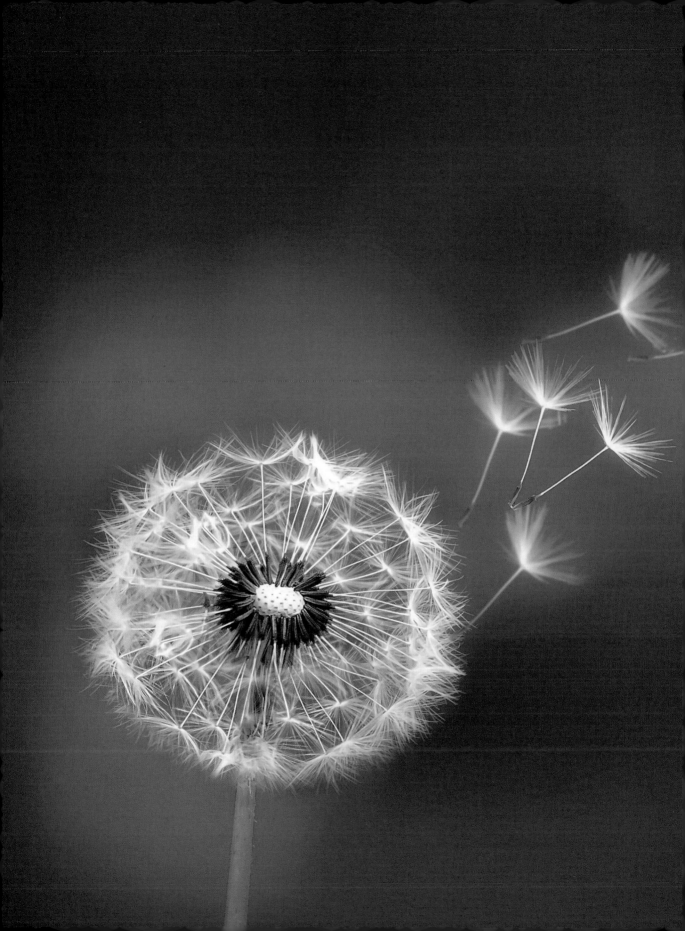

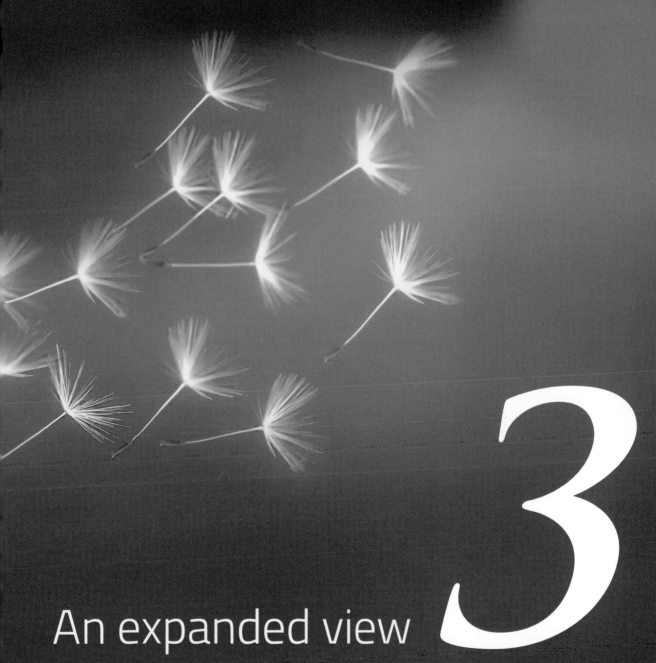

An expanded view 3

Therapies to complement massage   185

Providing inclusive care   199

Epilogue: Parting lessons   213

Appendix: Patient assessment   215

Appendix: Simplified assessment tool   217

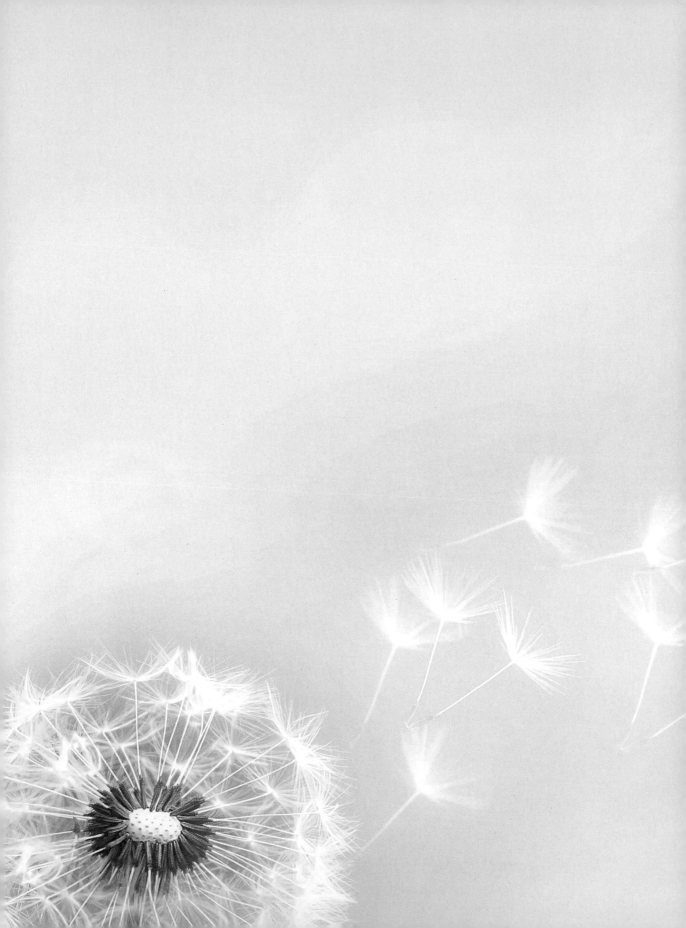

Never underestimate the healing effects of beauty.

–Florence Nightingale

Massage is an extraordinary gift at the end of life. But it is only one of many possible ways to bring comfort and pleasure into a dying person's world. There are numerous therapies that can easily be combined with massage to enhance or complement the experience of touch, including aromatherapy, hydrotherapy, thermal therapy, energy work, music therapy, and pet therapy, to name a few. These therapies may be practiced by specialists with advanced training and credentials, or by massage therapists, end-of-life doulas, and nurses who have training in multiple modalities. There are also simple applications of many modalities that anyone can safely use when a patient is receptive. This chapter will offer ideas for basic applications of several complementary therapies that can be incorporated into the massage session.

Just as massage is "dialed back" to accommodate the demands of dying, any addition to the session must also be dialed back. Touch therapists will need to monitor patient response to assure that the elements of the session, both individually and in combination, do not overwhelm or cause distress. In this spirit, a less-is-more approach is ideal when combining therapies. But there is also an opportunity for creativity and playfulness in expanding our work to gently engage more of the patient's senses – sight, sound, and smell. These tools can be especially useful when the patient's sensitivity to touch is so great that our reach is literally limited. An example is a session in which "massage" might be confined to light energy work or the use of an essential oil.

Therapies to complement massage can be viewed as additional tools in our repertoire to nurture diverse aspects of the human spirit. Exposure to these practices can serve to energize our continual learning and to keep our work fresh. We may also find that integration of these therapies into our work and homelife can be an effective form of self-care. It is my hope that Chapter 10 will open the door to endless possibility.

Using essential oils

Leaves, stems, roots, flowers, and tree resins have been used throughout history for both medicinal and spiritual care of the sick and the dying. The distillation of essential oils (EOs) is a more modern practice, involving the extraction of concentrated active molecules from plants. CO_2 extraction is a related process that results in therapeutic substances used much like EOs. Essential oils and CO_2 extracts may be helpful for symptom relief, to stimulate remembrance and life review, to enhance patient dignity when odors are present, to provide emotional and spiritual support, to anoint at the end of life and after, and to ease the grief of mourners (Godfrey, 2018; Hartman, 2012). These practices are widespread around the world and have the potential to enhance the end-of-life experience for patients and caregivers alike. Multiple studies cite benefits including enhanced sense of well-being (Louis and Kowalski, 2002) and reductions in anxiety (Louis and Kowalski, 2002), depression (Louis and Kowalski, 2002), pain (Lakhan et al., 2016), and nausea and vomiting (Fearrington et al., 2019).

The use of oils through the practice of aromatherapy – or aromacare, a term preferred by renowned expert Madeleine Kerkhof (Kerkhof, 2015) – has increased in clinical settings as the evidence of benefit becomes clearer. Certified Clinical Aromatherapy Practitioners are professionals with expertise in the selection and blending of EOs and CO_2 extracts to address symptoms via inhalation or application to the skin. A less clinical approach to the use of EOs is the myrrophore tradition. With origins in ancient Egypt, this practice involves "myrrh bearers" who use specific sacred oils, chosen for their spiritual qualities (Warner, 2018). Sacred oils are not used for massage, but are diluted and rubbed between the practitioner's hands, which are then held above the recipient's body to support transition through the final stages of dying. The practitioner might also deliver a sacred oil while holding the recipient's hand.

There is much to know and appreciate about EOs and their potential in end-of-life care. Touch therapists with interest in this field are encouraged to pursue additional study or consultation with aromatherapy colleagues. Those of us who lack such education must respect the potency of these oils and use them with care and restraint. Select oils which are known for their safety, use small amounts of oil in appropriate dilutions, and restrict application to the least invasive method possible. These safeguards will be detailed in the following pages.

One of the beauties and one of the complications of using essential oils at the end of life is that it is not only the patient who may be exposed to an oil we use at the bedside. Others who live in close proximity, visitors, care staff, and therapists themselves will be impacted. This can be a positive benefit, assuming all parties are receptive. It is important to be sensitive and circumspect, especially with individuals who are unable to communicate their preferences. In such cases, touch therapists must rely on trusted family members for guidance, along with close observation of the patient's response to determine tolerance or lack thereof. Kerkhof herself advises against the use of essential oils if the therapist has no way to determine the patient's preference regarding scent: "We have seen that a dying patient became very restless upon use [of an oil] and died that way" (Kerkhof, 2022).

Safety with essential oils

One of the guiding principles of EO use is that oils must be properly diluted with a "carrier" rather than used full-strength on the skin. Carrier oils have their own useful properties, including nourishing the skin. Carriers favored by aromatherapists and myrrophores include grapeseed oil, jojoba, and sweet almond oil for those without nut allergies. A 0.5–1% dilution is suggested for use on the skin. This translates to 2–6 drops of essential oil per 30 ml of carrier oil (30 ml is equal to 1 fluid ounce or six teaspoons). For a 10 ml bottle of carrier oil, 1–3 drops of EO will be sufficient.

Topical application is not necessary to achieve benefits, however. Inhalation is simpler and endorsed as safer for people at the end of life whose senses may be heightened (Secretan, 2021). One method for the delivery of EOs by inhalation is a personal aromatherapy inhaler, also called an aromastick. These are small, capped tubes with a cotton insert soaked in 5–10 drops of essential oil. Aromasticks are inexpensive and easy to assemble, and last up to several months. A simpler option is to place a few drops of oil on a tissue, a cotton ball, or a patch designed for this purpose. The oil will evaporate quickly, so these methods will be more short-lived. In addition to being safer, advantages of inhalation over application to skin are that the EO does not need to be diluted and that exposure can be more easily controlled. If the EO is to be used on the skin, tolerance should first be established. A doctor's order may be required for skin application in some settings.

Heads up 10.1. Aromatherapy and fire safety

While essential oils are considered to be flammable, the risk pertaining to a small quantity such as a 5 ml bottle (equivalent to 1.7 fluid ounces) is quite small and would require direct and deliberate contact with an open flame. Given the common presence of supplemental oxygen in palliative care settings, it is unlikely that fire-burning diffusers would be used in these environments. Therapists should be mindful but not overly preoccupied with fire hazards when working with small quantities of EOs and CO_2 extracts (Kerkhof, 2022).

Essential oils are sold in amber or blue glass bottles to protect them from light. They degrade over time and should be stored in a cool, dark place with lids that are tightly sealed. Shelf life varies and expirations should be monitored, starting with the date the bottle is opened. It's important to work with quality essential oils in order to experience their supportive benefits and to avoid adverse reactions. A reputable supplier will provide access to a Certificate of Analysis (COA) for each oil, with characteristics and constituents of the oil or extract, including date of extraction, which will indicate shelf life (Kerkhof, 2022).

Patients with end-stage disease, including respiratory distress or seizures, may be triggered by certain oils in ways that are unexpected. Emotional responses are likewise impossible to predict. Some oils have the potential to interact with medications or medical conditions such as epilepsy; others can irritate fragile skin or mucous membranes. Low body weight and skin thinning can increase absorption rates when oils are applied topically. It is therefore prudent for therapists without advanced training to introduce EOs in the most conservative manner, ideally in such a way that the oil can be removed from the environment if a patient's reaction is unfavorable.

Essential oils for palliative care

The following EOs, used properly, have the potential to safely ease a number of common symptoms at the end of life. These "starter oils" are divided below into those used for aromacare and those used as sacred oils. Botanical or Latin names are the international standard and should be utilized when seeking additional information on each oil.

EOs for aromacare

Lavender (*Lavandula angustifolia*) is a popular EO, known for its balancing, calming, and pain-relieving properties. It is endorsed by Madeleine Kerkhof for addressing neuropathic pain, muscle stiffness, cramps, spasms, and anxiety related to shortness of breath (Kerkhof, 2019). Low doses may be helpful for insomnia, but high doses can cause agitation (Kerkhof, 2015).

Bergamot (*Citrus bergamia*) is a light, refreshing oil that is both uplifting and relaxing. Like other citrus oils, bergamot can reduce depression, irritability, anxiety, and insomnia. It is recommended as an adjuvant oil to reduce the discomfort of dyspnea (Kerkhof, 2019). Avoid use on areas of the skin that might be exposed to sunlight. Keep unopened bergamot in the refrigerator. Once opened, store in a cool place and use within one year (Kerkhof, 2015).

Frankincense (*Boswellia carterii*) has a unique aroma that can be described as warm, rich, and woody. It may improve lung function and anxiety related to dyspnea (Kerkhof, 2019). Frankincense is a spiritual oil conducive for some people to prayer and meditation. It can be used to anoint the body prior to or following death, or for grief support. It is considered to be a sacred oil and is therefore included in the list of sacred oils below.

Ginger CO$_2$-total extract (*Zingiber officinalis*), with its analgesic and anti-inflammatory properties, is Madeleine Kerkhof's first choice for the relief of nausea (Kerkhof, 2019). It can be used by itself but may be more effective as a blend for nausea: 50% ginger CO$_2$-total, 20% peppermint CO$_2$-select or EO, 20% lemon, and 10% lavender (Kerkhof, 2019).

Peppermint EO or CO$_2$-select extract (*Mentha piperita*) can be helpful for nausea as noted above, especially as one ingredient in a blend. It can alleviate pain, particularly nerve pain. Peppermint may provide relief for some people with dyspnea, providing an "instant feeling of free breathing"; for others, however, the menthol component of peppermint can be an irritant for airways (Kerkhof, 2019). It should be used conservatively until tolerance is established.

> ### Ideas for incorporating aromacare into the massage session
>
> - After assessing indications and possible contraindications, place 1–3 drops of essential oil on a tissue or cotton ball. If the patient and others present respond favorably, the tissue or cotton ball can be placed inside a pillowcase, pocket, or fold of the blanket or sheet.

- Once tolerance is established, a 0.5–1% dilution of essential oil in a carrier can be used on a small area of intact skin.

- Avoid the eyes and other mucous membranes. Avoid application of EOs to the hands, since patients may touch or rub their eyes.

- Assessment of response should be ongoing, as response to fragrance can vary from visit to visit.

- Sensitivity to *all* stimuli (visual, auditory, and olfactory) may be heightened during active dying. Even a 0.5–1% dilution of EO can be too much at this stage (Kerkhof, 2022). It is therefore best in the last days and hours of life to err on the side of the lowest dose (one drop) introduced in a manner (on a tissue, for example) that can be removed from the bedside if reaction is unfavorable.

- Essential oils can be a lovely addition to post-mortem care, if consistent with the family's wishes. A 0.5–1% dilution of a favorite oil in a carrier oil can be applied as desired to the entire body. Family can be invited to participate in this ritual as a way to honor the body of their loved one (Hartman, 2012).

Sacred oils

Fragonia (*Agonis fragrans*) is a very new essential oil, described as light and joyful. Fragonia lifts, energizes, and harmonizes the spirit, and so is an excellent oil for transitions and change.

Frankincense (*Boswellia carterii*) is known for aligning spirit with the divine. It is one of the most valued oils of the ancient world. Frankincense is believed to soothe inner chaos, strengthen spiritual connection, and heal "soul wounds" (Warner, 2018). It can also be used to consecrate a sacred space.

Elemi (*Canarium luzonicum*) is good for surrender and letting go. It is an excellent oil to use during a vigil when death is prolonged or fear is present. Elemi is a "threshold oil," helping people to trust in a higher power for guidance (Warner, 2018).

Ideas for using sacred oils

- Place a 1% dilution of EO into your hands, rub hands together, and place them over the crown of the head, the heart, or other desired area of the body.

- In the same manner, the therapist can rub the dilution into their hands and simply hold the patient's hand (Warner, 2018).

Water, heat, and cooling techniques

The therapeutic use of water (hydrotherapy) and temperature (thermal therapy) is another ancient but enduring strategy which can easily be incorporated into massage. Potential benefits include relaxation and pain relief (Sinclair, 2020). Therapists should be aware that some diseases provoke sensitivities to temperature. Other preferences seem to be innate and particular to each person.

Heat therapy

The body responds to heat with the dilation of blood vessels to bring more blood flow and oxygen to the area, which in turn can reduce muscle tension, spasm, and pain (Sinclair, 2020). Heat therapy can be beneficial for musculoskeletal discomforts related to immobility and debility. My personal experience is that many people are comforted by the sensation of heat provided with warm hands, warm lotion, and warm linen. Additional ideas and precautions for the use of heat are provided below.

Ideas for incorporating heat into the massage session

- Use a warmer for lotion prior to massage (see p. 44).

- Warm hands held in place (with or without Reiki or other energy technique) can be very soothing. The therapist's hands can be warmed under warm running water, by briskly rubbing the hands together, or using "hot pocket warmers." Another strategy is to begin the massage over clothing or top sheet until the therapist's hands are warm.

- Some care settings are fortunate to have blanket warmers. Blankets, towels, or washcloths can also be warmed in a clothes dryer.

- Damp heat can be applied as a compress or simply to refresh the face or body. Place a washcloth under warm or hot running water, ring out excess moisture, and gently apply as desired. When damp applications are used, the patient's clothing and linen can be kept dry with a disposable waterproof pad, found in most care settings.

- Electric blankets and heating pads are not ideal for use with people at the end of life due to risk of burns. If clients or families are using electric sources of heat, they should be cautioned not to use them for prolonged periods (even on low settings), or with people who have a reduced level of arousal. Due to the risks involved, inpatient settings typically require a doctor's order before allowing a patient to use a heating pad from home.

- Heat should not be applied to areas of the body with past exposure to radiation (Santiago-Palma and Payne, 2001).

- Hot compresses should not be applied to areas of the body with inflammation, edema, risk of lymphedema, impaired sensory perception, atrophy, poor blood supply, or DVT.

- The skin should be monitored for redness during the session, and heat should be removed if redness occurs. Darker skin may not produce reddening, thus extra care should be taken when using heat on highly pigmented skin.

- For the short duration of a massage on a fully alert person, a homemade "rice sock" can be used. Place several handfuls of rice inside a tube sock and tie a knot at the open end. Warm the sock in a microwave for 20 seconds at a time, shaking the rice well to distribute the heat. Check the temperature by laying the sock on the inside of your arm before use with a patient. A few

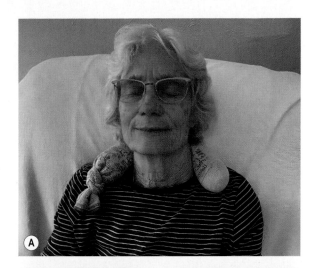

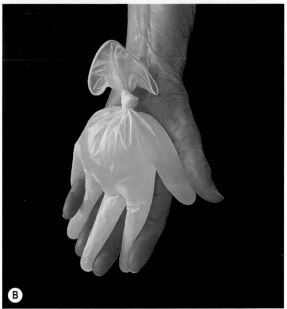

Figure 10.1

Two methods for providing heat therapy. (A) A sock filled with rice can be heated in the microwave. (B) A "glove buddy" filled with warm tap water shapes to the contours of the patient's hand but can be placed anywhere on the body for relief. Use the largest size glove available and fill it with water to just above the finger joints, in order to leave room for the knot.

(Photos by Candice White.)

drops of essential oil can be added to the rice sock after heating.

Cooling techniques

Some conditions or symptoms cause sensitivity to heat, including fever, multiple sclerosis, and lung conditions that inhibit breathing. In people with sensitivity or aversion to warmth, a cooling technique may be more welcome, starting with a cooler air temperature in the room. Cold can reduce inflammation and pain by constricting blood vessels. As always, safety and patient comfort are paramount when offering cold therapies.

Ideas for incorporating cooling techniques into the massage session

- A small fan clipped to the bedrail of a hospital bed can assist with shortness of breath or the discomfort of feeling too hot (see p. 103).

- An open window or door in cool climates can facilitate circulation of cool air.

- A homemade rice sock can be placed in a refrigerator and applied to the body as desired.

- As with heat, extreme cold can injure fragile tissues, especially in people with impaired sensory perception or reduced level of arousal. For this reason, a cool temperature is safer than a freezing temperature.

- Cold packs should not be applied to areas of the body that are atrophied, skin that has been exposed to radiation, or ischemic limbs (Santiago-Palma and Payne, 2001).

- Cold therapy is contraindicated for patients with Raynaud's syndrome (Santiago-Palma and Payne, 2001).

- For a person with fever, see p. 106 regarding cool compresses.

- For a person with nausea, see p. 107 regarding cool compresses.

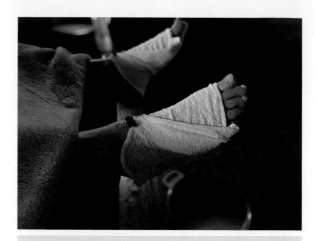

Figure 10.2
Cool or warm compresses are easy to use in any setting, adjusting water temperature for desired effect and patient preference. A waterproof pad can be used to keep bed linen and clothing dry. In this photo, binder clips are used to hold the compress in place.

(Photo by author.)

- While aides provide full bed baths, a damp cool cloth can be used at other times (including during massage) to refresh the face or exposed extremities.

Energy work

Approaching the body from an energetic standpoint is another ancient concept that has stood the test of time. The ancient Chinese identified the body's energy as "chi," the ancient Indians knew it as "prana," and the Japanese called it "ki." Two energy therapies currently used in some palliative and hospice care settings are Therapeutic Touch and Reiki. Therapeutic Touch was introduced in the early 1970s by New York University professor of nursing Dolores Krieger and medical intuitive Dora Kunz. Reiki is thought to have been "rediscovered" by Japanese monk Dr. Mikao Usui in the mid-1800s, with roots that likely precede written language. Both Therapeutic Touch and Reiki involve hand positions on or above the body.

A number of small studies suggest that energy techniques can be beneficial to address pain, anxiety, and

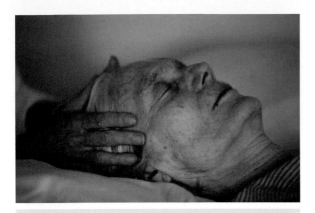

Figure 10.3
Reiki may be used to begin and end a massage session. The crown of the head is one of the standard hand placements.

(Photo by Candice White.)

depression (Baldwin, 2020). Recipients may report a sensation of warmth, tingling, or deep relaxation. Given the potential benefits and noninvasiveness of these approaches, energy work can be a safe and potentially helpful addition to any massage. Therapeutic Touch and Reiki are easy to learn and can be practiced by anyone after only a few hours of training.

Ideas for incorporating energy work into the session

- In my experience, any energy that is transmitted through the therapist's hands during a session will be beneficial, regardless of communication or understanding.

- Some patients, families, and professional colleagues will be open and curious about energy medicine; others will not. Gentle holds incorporated into the massage don't require any more clarification than other techniques used during the session.

- Motivated patients and loved ones can learn energy therapies for their own use.

- Touch therapists and other team members can incorporate energy work into their self-care. I find it very comforting to place my hand over my heart throughout my day and while falling asleep at night.

Music

Music – alone or in combination with massage – has the power to inspire, soothe, and transform. For some people at the end of life, music can be a profound source of reminiscence and comfort, whether enjoyed privately or shared with others. Even patients close to the moment of death have been observed to respond to music, making it an experience that can connect loved ones when language is no longer accessible. One of the most moving encounters I ever witnessed was an elderly woman who died in her husband's arms while the music therapist played a song from their wedding.

The documented benefits of music therapy include significant improvements in pain, anxiety, depression, and shortness of breath (Gallagher et al., 2017). Studies indicate that the positive impact of music on quality of life persists even as illness progresses (Rossi and Arnold, 2015). Music therapists are highly trained professionals who support the dying process with a variety of approaches, including active participation from the patient or family when desired and possible. The patient may sing along or play an instrument. Some instruments, such as the reverie harp, are designed to be played by anyone, regardless of skill. Patients may help assemble a playlist of recorded music that is personally meaningful. They might be assisted by the music therapist to analyze song lyrics or even to compose music as a legacy project. The two music therapists at our hospice agency are sometimes asked to sing at memorial services, often by patients or families who have formed a comforting attachment to these professionals.

Two other approaches to music at the end of life include music thanatology and the use of volunteer singers and musicians. Music thanatology, also referred to as "prescriptive music," involves a harp with or without singing to provide mindfully chosen therapeutic elements (Mendoza,

2019). The tempo is generally slow and meditative, and the experience of the patient and family is one of passive listening. The services of the thanatologist might be paid for by the care facility or hospice, or donated by the musician. Another volunteer effort is provided by Threshold Choirs, which now exist around the globe. These groups consisting of three or four people who sing a cappella at the bedside. The songs are short and repetitive, often composed by Threshold Choir members, with lyrics that focus on love, caring, release, and going home (Mendoza, 2019).

When touch therapists have the opportunity to work with music therapists and other skilled musicians at the bedside, the synergy between massage and live music can be breathtaking. The cadence of massage and music often sync in a way that is extremely relaxing to both the recipients and the practitioners of the session. But music can also provide moments of surprising energy and even humor. One music therapist shared that she sometimes has patients request selections from bawdy musicals or rock bands such as Pink Floyd. Her most unusual request, however, came from an older woman who shyly asked that two songs be played at her memorial service: Ave Maria and Pinkfong's "Baby Shark" (Montes, 2021).

Ideas for incorporating music into the massage session

- Touch therapists may play a role in promoting live music in the settings where they work. Advocating for the hiring of music therapists or accessing a Threshold Choir may be options.

- Where such resources exist, massage and music therapies can be coordinated as desired, provided simultaneously, or staggered such that there is brief overlap of music and massage.

- Touch therapists might find themselves humming or singing quietly while providing massage. Those with gifted voices will be especially appreciated at the bedside!

- Recorded music can be provided by the patient or family to be used during the massage. Recorded music should always be patient-preferred to ensure that associations are positive.

- Listening libraries by genre may be available or developed in facilities with listening devices or smart TVs.

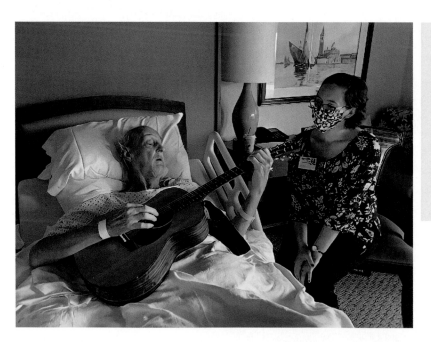

Figure 10.4
Sometimes it is the patients themselves who are the musicians. A patient at the T. Boone Pickens Hospice Inpatient Unit reached for this music therapist's guitar and played with gusto, providing joy to himself, his family, and the therapist.

(Photo courtesy of Kathleen Montes.)

Simple rather than complex music may be better tolerated as dying progresses: a single instrument or a cappella voice, for example, rather than a full symphony of instruments. Tempo should be soothing and consistent throughout each song in the playlist.

Patients should be monitored for signs that music is too stimulating or disturbing. The release of emotions (tears, for example) may be a healthy response when supported by the therapist.

Range of motion

People at the end of life tend to be more sedentary, with loss of muscle tone, strength, and range of motion (ROM). Immobility contributes to musculoskeletal pain, stiffness, and loss of function. Passive movement (in which the therapist supports and moves or stretches parts of the patient's body) can be incorporated into a massage, so long as these movements are slow, gentle, and enjoyed by the patient. When it is the patient or a loved one who requests ROM, it is important to clarify the goals of this desire. A goal for the patient to "get stronger" or to "walk again" should be received with understanding, compassion, and validation of the desire. But the therapist must also distinguish comfort-oriented movement from rehabilitative therapy. As disease progresses, it is likely that activity and function will decrease over time, regardless of efforts to halt or reverse this trajectory. An aggressive approach is likely to be more harmful than helpful.

That said, it can feel very good to an immobilized or bedridden person to experience a session of assisted gentle movement. It is important to provide each stretch in moderation, up to the point of resistance and no further. If the patient experiences pain at any point, the ROM should be scaled back or stopped. Mindful positioning is also essential for the therapist. Smaller joints (wrists and ankles, for example) can be mobilized by a therapist in a seated or standing position with the weight of the limb fully supported by the bed. Larger joints (elbows, knees, shoulders, and hips) will likely require some lifting, which is best accomplished by the therapist in a standing position with the bed height adjusted for the therapist's com-

fort. The relative size and weight of patient and therapist must be considered so that lifting is safe for both parties.

Ideas for incorporating ROM into the massage session

While providing massage to the upper extremities, gently flex and extend the wrists several times as

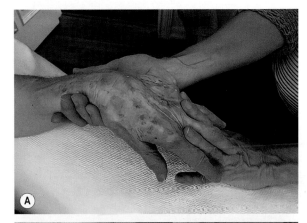

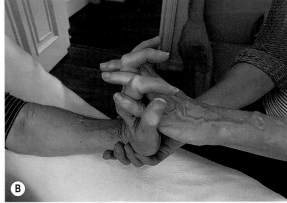

Figure 10.5

Range of motion for the wrist might include (A) flexion by bending the wrist toward the inner arm and (B) extension by bending the wrist toward the top of the forearm. In both cases, movements are slow and gentle, and the wrist is securely supported by the therapist.

(Photos by Candice White.)

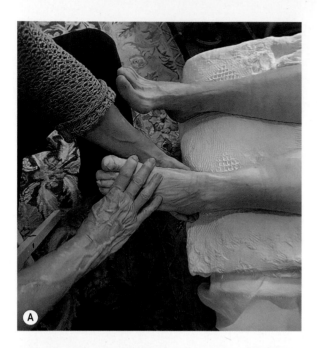

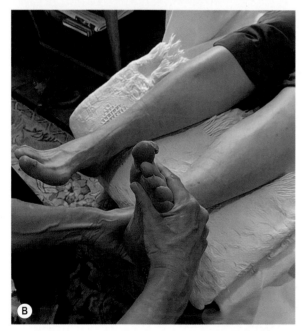

Figure 10.6

(A) Pointing and (B) flexing the foot.

(Photos by Candice White.)

shown in Figure 10.5, then slowly circle the wrists in each direction.

- While providing massage to the lower extremities, support the heel with one hand and use the other to gently point and flex the feet several times as shown in Figure 10.6, then circle the ankles in each direction.

- Explore with the patient supported movements of the joints and limbs that feel good, bending the knees and elbows or circling the hips and shoulders in each direction.

- Safe ROM depends on patient input and should not be performed on patients who are unable to provide feedback.

Animals

Many people have singular and extraordinary relationships with their pets. These relationships may intensify during serious illness, when some animals seem to have an uncanny sensitivity toward human suffering. The bonds of unconditional and mutual affection between species remain a central fact of life for many patients, even as they lie dying. Touch therapists in palliative and hospice care may therefore come in contact with animals in proximity to the people who love them. Dogs and cats are the most common species encountered, but I have also met rabbits, pigs, goats, horses, and birds. These animals are most often present in home settings, but a number of care facilities now welcome pets or offer pet therapy programs. Patients may also be accompanied by service animals who assist them with a variety of needs.

Animals can provide soothing companionship for people at the end of life, easing loneliness, reducing stress, and enhancing well-being. They can also be an asset in the development of rapport between therapists and patients, providing opportunities for conversation and shared interest. At our hospice inpatient unit where volunteers provide pet therapy and patients' pets are welcome, I have observed that staff enjoy the levity that animals can inject into an otherwise intense environment. A bowl of dog treats sits at each nurses' station, and many of us go out of our way to interact with animals when they visit the unit.

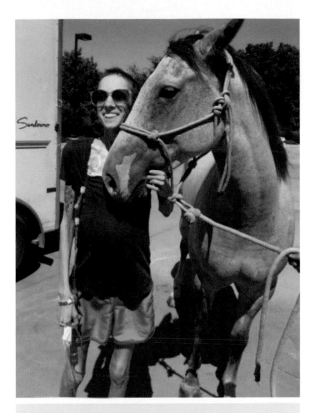

Figure 10.7
This young patient's family and friends brought two of her beloved horses to the inpatient unit parking lot, so that they could see each other one last time. The patient and this horse were champion barrel racers prior to her diagnosis.

(Photo courtesy of patient's family.)

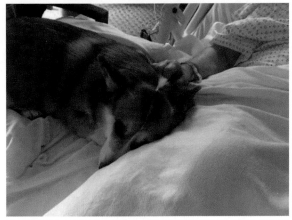

Figure 10.8
This pet was placed in a chair at the patient's bedside, but that was apparently not close enough. She inched her way onto the bed and spent a quiet afternoon at her person's side. It was hard to tell who enjoyed the visit more – the dog, the patient, the patient's family, or the staff who observed this moving encounter.

(Photo by author.)

It must be acknowledged that the special connection between people and their animals can also be a source of grief when the bond is broken. Anyone who has ever lost a pet is painfully familiar with this sorrow, which is no less profound when it is the patient who must leave the relationship. Some people confront this loss when they are no longer able to care for a pet. Others are separated by a change in location when they require a more advanced level of care. Many express concerns about what will happen to their pets, and some require assistance to make arrangements and say goodbyes.

Ideas for supporting the presence of animals

- Some animals are temperamentally suited to navigate delicate environments and situations; others are not. The comfort and safety of people *and* animals are essential.

- Most animals are openly curious and welcoming of extra attention. They may want to be on the owner's lap, beside the owner in bed, or at the feet of the therapist. So long as the animal is comfortable with the therapist and vice versa, it is best to support the patient's wishes.

- Pets who are normally docile may be protective of their owners when they experience the intrusion of numerous caregivers and changes they don't understand. If an animal's behavior seems wary or aggressive, or if the therapist is uncomfortable with the animal's presence, it is appropriate to ask that the animal be confined during the visit.

- Never assume than an animal is or is not a service animal. Working animals may or may not be wearing a special vest or harness. When meeting an animal for the first time, ask before petting, feeding, or addressing the animal.

- Not everyone loves animals. Some people have allergies or a history of a negative experience with an animal that results in lingering fear. Self-compassion, respect for others, and reasonable boundaries may be required.

Nature

Connection with nature is profoundly important to well-being for many people. Patients often relate that what they miss most as they decline are simple pleasures such as taking walks, sitting under a tree, or indulging in outdoor pastimes like fishing or bird watching. Our work may support people to reconnect with some of these experiences. In a radio interview, massage therapist Ronna Moore recounted her work with a palliative care patient confined to bed. "Having worked with him a couple of times, we were able to give him enough comfort to get out of bed and look at his tomatoes outside. He hadn't been able to see his tomatoes for several months. This was a great achievement for him" (Moore, 2012). Touch therapists can also look for opportunities to incorporate contact with nature into the massage session. Sometimes this means taking the session outdoors, and sometimes it means bringing a piece of the natural world to the bedside.

Ideas for incorporating nature into the massage session

- Patients or families often ask at the touch therapist's first visit, "Where should we do this?" If the patient is ambulatory or uses a wheelchair and the weather is pleasant, the therapist might respond with the question, "Would you prefer to have your massage indoors or outdoors?"

- Things to consider in providing a massage outdoors include climate, shade, and ease of access. The patient might require sunglasses, a hat, a blanket for warmth, or pillows to pad outdoor seating.

- Another option is to provide the massage near a window.

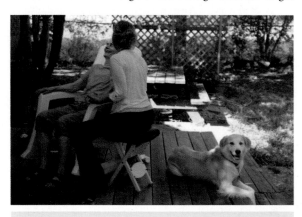

Figure 10.9
Whether massage is provided in a private home, group home, or inpatient setting, an outdoor session can boost patient spirits. A portable stool such as the one pictured makes it an easy option when the weather is nice.

(Photo by Candice White.)

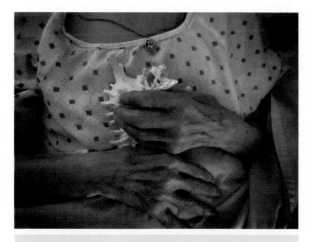

Figure 10.10
When patients can no longer access the outdoors, nature can sometimes be brought to the bedside.

(Photo by author.)

- Bringing nature indoors can be as simple as a flower from the garden in a jar of water, a sprig of fresh mint or other herb, a rock, a shell, or a photograph of a preferred nature setting such as the beach or mountains.

- Nature soundtracks are available online and can be used during massage, including ocean waves, waterfalls, the rain, and birdsong. As always, patients or loved ones can assist in selecting sounds that are personally appealing.

Touching story 10.1. Bringing the ocean to a nursing home

At my first meeting with a 94-year-old patient in the nursing home, I admired several small seashells perched on her windowsill. Her eyes lit up when she spoke of her love of the ocean. She shared her sadness that she would likely never hear the sound of waves again.

Several weeks later, I traveled to Galveston Island, where I visited a shop that I remembered from my childhood. The shop was filled with shells, and I spent some time picking out a large conch, which was filled with the sound of the ocean. I brought the shell home with great excitement. But upon arriving home, I was dismayed to find that the sound of the ocean was gone. My research revealed that shells resonate with ambient sound, and given the distance from the ocean, there were no waves in close enough proximity to make the shell sing. I wrapped the shell in tissue paper and held it briefly between my palms, hoping that it might nevertheless bring joy to the recipient.

The following week, I took the shell to my patient. I told her I was not sure if she would be able to hear the ocean in the shell, but that I wanted her to know I'd been thinking of her on my trip. She smiled and took the shell and held it to her ear. Her eyes became wide,

and she said repeatedly, "I hear it! I hear it!" As I massaged her feet, she kept the shell at her ear, weeping and laughing intermittently.

When we live in awareness, miracles are everywhere. Even between the dingy walls of an understaffed nursing home. Even amidst the smell of urine and the daily indignity of dependence on others. There is much that we cannot change in the face of suffering. But we can keep showing up, bearing imperfect gifts that sometimes turn out to be enough.

Conclusion

Touch therapists can play a role in helping people access a variety of experiences that bring them comfort and joy. With an open mind and deference to the patient's needs and preferences, each massage session can be customized with the inclusion of other therapies, including aroma, music, energy, movement, and nature. These additions can be subtle and presented as choices that recognize and embrace individuality while allowing the patient to have control. Therapies to complement massage are a way to celebrate the wholeness of life, and the wholeness of each person we touch. Patients and we ourselves will benefit from this expanded approach.

References

Baldwin, A., 2020. *Reiki in clinical practice: a science-based guide*. Edinburgh: Handspring Publishing.

Fearrington, M. A. et al., 2019. Essential oils to reduce postoperative nausea and vomiting. *Journal of Peri Anesthesia Nursing*, [e-journal] (34)5, pp. 1057–1053. Available at: <https://doi.org/10.1016/j.jopan.2019.01.010>.

Gallagher, L. M. et al., 2017. Outcomes of music therapy interventions on symptom management in palliative medicine patients. *American Journal of Hospice and*

Palliative Medicine, [e-journal] 35(2), pp. 250–257. Available at: <https://doi.org/10.1177/1049909117696723>.

Godfrey, H., 2018. *Essential oils for mindfulness and meditation.* Rochester, VT: Healing Arts Press.

Hartman, V., 2012. *Aromatherapy in hospice: the connection to biblical oils.* [online] Available at: <https://hrhshospice.wordpress.com/2012/09/06/aromatherapy-in-hospice-the-connection-to-biblical-oils>.

Kerkhof, M., 2015. *Complementary nursing in end-of-life care: integrative care in palliative care.* Wernhout: Kicozo.

Kerkhof, M., 2019. Fusion aromatherapy in palliative care. Handouts from a three-day training course in Atlanta, GA.

Kerkhof, M., 2022. Updated information on aromacare. [email] (Personal communication, 2 March).

Lakhan, S. E. et al., 2016. The effectiveness of aromatherapy in reducing pain: a systematic review and meta-analysis. *Pain Research and Treatment,* [e-journal] 7(1), pp. 1–13. Available at: <https://doi.org/10.1155/2016/8158693>.

Louis, M. and Kowalski, S. D., 2002. Use of aromatherapy with hospice patients to decrease pain, anxiety, and depression and to promote an increased sense of well-being. *American Journal of Hospice and Palliative Medicine,* [e-journal] 19(6), pp. 381–386. Available at: <https://doi.org/10.1177/104990910201900607>.

Mendoza, 2019. *The power of music at the end of life: when words are not enough.* [online] Available at: <https://www.psychologytoday.com/us/blog/understanding-grief/201908/the-power-music-the-end-life>.

Montes, K., 2021. Discussion of music therapy. [conversation] (Personal communication, 21 May 2021).

Moore, R., 2012. Body Sphere Interview on massage therapy. Interviewed by Amanda Smith. [radio] ABC Radio, 12 August 2012, 17:35. Available at: <https://www.abc.net.au/radionational/programs/archived/bodysphere/touch3a-massage-therapy/4179788>.

Rossi, B. and Arnold, R., 2015. *Music therapy.* [online] Available at: <mypcnow.org/fast-fact/music-therapy>.

Santiago-Palma, J. and Payne, R., 2001. Palliative care and rehabilitation. *American Cancer Society Journals,* [e-journal] 94(4), pp. 1049–1052. Available at: <https://pubmed.ncbi.nlm.nih.gov/11519032>.

Secretan, A., 2021. Beyond touch: aromatherapy massage sessions in health care. In: MacDonald G. and Tague, C. *Hands in health care: massage therapy for the adult hospital patient.* Edinburgh: Handspring Publishing. Ch. 13.

Sinclair, M., 2020. *Hydrotherapy for bodyworkers: improving outcomes with water therapies.* Edinburgh: Handspring Publishing.

Warner, F., 2018. *Sacred oils.* London: Hay House UK Ltd.

Providing inclusive care

We all have different gifts, so we all have different ways of saying to the world who we are.
–Fred Rogers

Caring for others is an opportunity to encounter one another in the fullness of our differences and our similarities. Both ends of this spectrum – differences *and* similarities – can feel magnified in intensity at the end of life. As therapists, our work is to embrace a range of diverse human experiences, just as they are expressed in each person we touch. With thoughtful awareness and the "humility of consistent self-examination," says Rabbi Ariel Burger, such encounters can push us to explore our limiting beliefs, our biases, and our capacity to grow our minds and our hearts (Burger, 2021).

Chapter 11 is an exploration of some of the ways that culture, race, religion, gender identity, sexual orientation, socioeconomic status, body size, physical and cognitive differences, and other varieties of experience can impact disease, dying, and caregiving. These are complex subjects, and these few pages can aim, at best, to scratch the surface. My goal is not to provide solid answers, but to encourage reflection, dialogue, and action as tools to provide more equitable and compassionate care. Examples related to specific groups are included *not* to promote the very kinds of assumptions this chapter hopes to challenge, but merely to suggest a range of issues that might come to the foreground during the dying process.

Efforts to be inclusive require that we slow down and resist shortcuts. We may need to learn new ways of speaking to one another, new ways of listening, and new ways of being that help others feel safe and valued in our company. There will likely be discomfort, and times when we fall short or even doubt that our efforts can make a difference. In these moments, we must summon our courage and link arms with the countless other people striving to

make the world a better place, not just for some of us, but for *all* of us.

Bias and being human

The human brain has a natural tendency to notice patterns and make associations. This ability allows us to process, store, and apply information necessary to our daily survival. To simplify the vast amount of data it receives, the brain often takes the shortest route to a conclusion. As "story-telling devices," our brains create stories to fill gaps in information (Jordan, 2021). The risk is that we become attached to these stories, regardless of whether they are true or kind, and even without the awareness that we have created them.

Unconscious bias, also known as implicit bias, is a subconscious association, belief, or attitude toward any group of people. The bias may involve favoritism (positive bias) or prejudice (negative bias). Bias is influenced by many factors, including social conditioning and the media, experiences which palliative care physician Kimberly Curseen refers to as "the hidden curriculum" (Curseen, 2019). While we are often unaware of our biases, we can, with practice, start to notice thoughts that distort our perceptions of others and impact the care we provide. The only way to begin this process is to become aware of the judgments that lurk beneath the surface of our best intentions.

Recent conversations on this topic with my hospice colleagues, all compassionate caregivers, revealed that many of us are biased about the medical interventions that people choose or decline. We might feel strongly that we would never choose a feeding tube, or that we would not allow a loved one to suffer out of ignorance about the "appropriate" use of opioids. Several of us admitted biases for or against a person's politics or religion, presumptions based on the television channel on in a patient's room, or the apparel worn by the patient or the patient's visitors. Most of us have made assumptions about family members who were absent from the bedside, insisting we could never leave a loved one to die alone. When family *are* at the bedside, we are prone to biases regarding how they should behave: how large the group should be, how loud, how emotive, how long they should stay, and how they should treat the patient and each other. Labeling patients and families as noncompliant, demanding, or difficult reveals biases about how deferential we think they should be to our care plan and our workload.

Kimberly Acquaviva, author of the book *LGBTQ-Inclusive Hospice and Palliative Care*, is reassuring that these thoughts and feelings do not make us bad people; they simply make us human. Our task, she says, is to become aware of these feelings when we experience them and then to "make a conscious choice" not to allow them to interfere with providing the best care possible (Acquaviva, 2017). But this can be easier said than done. Bias is often insidious, creeping into our caregiving in subtle ways, such as when we avoid or shorten encounters with patients who are different from us while allocating more time to encounters that are "likely to go well" (Cates, 2020). Noticing and holding ourselves accountable for these disparities are the first steps toward mitigating their impact.

The scars of exclusion and how they impact healthcare

Many people have experienced the devastating effects of discrimination, including but not limited to people of color; the LGBTQ community; indigenous or First Nations cultures; immigrants, refugees, and newcomers; people living in poverty; people without insurance; people who are older; people living in large bodies; people with physical, intellectual, and cognitive differences; and people with stigmatized conditions such as mental illness, substance misuse, and HIV. The harm inflicted on these and other groups ranges from a vague sense of being unwelcome to overt harassment and even violence. The US Department of Justice reported 7,759 hate crimes

involving 10,528 victims in 2020, primarily related to race, ethnicity, ancestry, or sexual orientation. A smaller percentage of these crimes pertained to religion, gender identity, and disability, with crimes related to gender identity trending upward compared to 2019 (USDJ, 2020).

While these are US statistics, evidence suggests that other countries have their own accounts of exclusion and oppression of some groups by others. According to the Organization for Security and Co-operation in Europe (OSCE), hate crimes, or "bias crimes," occur all over the world (OSCE, 2009). Healthcare settings are sadly not immune to discrimination. Abuse of research subjects and other medical atrocities have left indelible marks on the histories of numerous countries, compounded by inequities that remain familiar to many. These can include refusal of care, substandard care, inability to access care, and countless other service failures both glaring and subtle. Specific examples that I am personally aware of include the following:

- A loving same-sex partner of a dying man was denied access to the bedside when the patient's estranged family insisted the partner be placed on the restricted visitor list. No one had thought to support the couple in developing a written plan to protect the partner's rights.

- A home health aide providing care to a hospitalized Muslim patient shaved off the patient's beard, not knowing that it was a sign of his obedience to Allah. The man's family was horrified. There were no Muslims on staff to help avoid or mitigate the situation.

- An uninsured African–American man in his twenties arrived at a local emergency department in severe pain from a sickle cell crisis. The staff thought that he was drug seeking and refused to treat him, resulting in a devastating stroke from which he died two weeks later. The man's distraught mother kept saying, "I just don't understand."

These kinds of experiences, accumulated over time, are extremely damaging to the trust between patients, families, and healthcare providers. Studies consistently confirm that certain groups are less likely to seek preventive care and early treatment for curable diseases, less likely to use palliative care or hospice, and more likely to endure the trauma of futile interventions at the end of life (Elk and Felder, 2018; Shahid et al., 2018). When palliative care *is* utilized, these same groups are more likely to experience undertreatment of pain and other symptoms (Hagarty et al., 2020; Hoffman et al., 2016). Added to this distress are countless microaggressions, described as "brief, everyday exchanges that send denigrating messages to certain individuals" (Sue, 2021). Microaggressions include verbal, behavioral, and environmental indignities such as interruptions, speaking of the patient in the third person when the patient is present, and failure to provide medical equipment to accommodate people over a certain size.

Bias and exclusion can also impact our relationships with colleagues. One of my favorite teammates recently shared that he often feels ostracized in our female-dominated work culture. He recounted that whenever a conversation between coworkers stops as he approaches, he feels as if he is an intruder. In return for his honest sharing, I confessed that my first impression upon meeting him had nothing to do with him being male or Black. *My* bias was that he seemed too young to be a hospice chaplain. My assumption that he could not possibly relate to the depth of suffering our patients endure was completely unfounded, and quickly debunked.

Heads up 11.1. Advance directives

Advanced care planning, or an advanced directive, is a term for a legal document that indicates how you wish to be cared for at the end of life. This document takes different forms and is governed by different laws, depending on location. It typically defines your wishes regarding life-sustaining medical treatment and who you wish to speak on your behalf when you can no longer speak for yourself. The document is legally binding, but can be amended over time if your preferences change.

Advance directives are important for everyone, but especially for people and partnerships that are particularly vulnerable: those with cognitive differences, for example, and people in nontraditional relationships. As the COVID pandemic has illustrated, none of us knows when a catastrophic event could occur that would render us unable to direct our own care. Designating a trusted person who knows what you want and *don't* want under these circumstances can help to ensure that your wishes will be honored, and that the person of your choosing will be empowered to act on your behalf.

Varieties of experience at the end of life

The United Nations defines culture as a "set of distinctive spiritual, material, intellectual, and emotional features of a social group" (UNESCO, 2001). Groups may be united by race, ethnicity, religion, age, social class, gender identity, sexual orientation, neurotype, or any other shared characteristics or experiences. Outward expressions of these connections may include how people dress, the language they speak, the food they eat, the music they enjoy, the holidays they observe, and the symbols they treasure. Other cultural constructs may include notions of time, etiquette, and roles related to age, gender, class, and family. Families, by birth or by choice, can represent a culture within a culture, adopting variations of their own traditions and patterns of behavior.

Individuals bring all the above to the experience of advanced illness, influencing decision making, problem solving, and privacy preferences. Some groups prefer a direct approach to dying while others prefer less direct.

An example would be a family who does not want the patient to know they are in hospice. Preferences regarding modesty may require that certain body parts remain covered, or that contact between genders be restricted. There may be observances that require support from staff in care settings such as the presence of certain objects at the bedside, a need for privacy to pray at certain hours, or a desire for the hospital bed to face a certain direction. Foods and medications containing animal products may be prohibited. There is hardly an aspect of patient care, the dying process, after-death care, or mourning that is not affected by a person's beliefs and socially conditioned behaviors.

Many aspects of culture are fluid and dynamic. Changes may occur over time within groups, with some individuals adhering to old traditions while others adopt new ways. An example is the wide range of practices within a single religion such as Judaism, which includes ultra-orthodox, orthodox, conservative, reformed, and secular subgroups. Within groups and subgroups, the extent to which any individual identifies with their culture is variable. An individual may also identify with more than

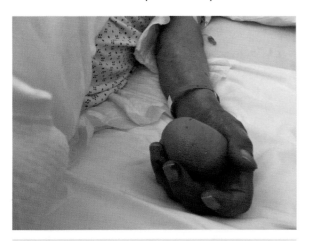

Figure 11.1
The family of a Buddhist patient placed this mandarin orange in his hand while he was actively dying, as food for the afterlife.

(Photo by author.)

one group (a Haitian immigrant who is transgender, for example). Such rich and ever-evolving layers of human identity make the goal of cultural *competence* unrealistic. Cultural *humility* is a more helpful objective, beginning with the understanding that assumptions should never be made about any individual, regardless of the group(s) they belong to. Cultural humility is not a fixed objective. It is an ongoing, lifelong process of reflection and discovery, in an effort to build "honest and trustworthy relationships" (Yeager and Bauer-Wu, 2013).

One aspect of cultural humility is the recognition that beliefs and practices that differ from our own can be beneficial, providing a sense of meaning, belonging, comfort, and resilience. Group affiliations can strengthen these assets and should be supported by the care team whenever possible. Encounters that are nonjudgmental, open, and curious can lead to new appreciation for different ways of being in the world. On the other hand, we may encounter beliefs and behaviors that collide with the values we hold most dear. In these instances, we are called to make space for multiple views to be held in tension with one another (Baugher, 2019). Compassion, says Baugher, does not require that we agree with everyone. It only asks that we recognize our common humanity and that we respond to the suffering of others with unconditional respect and caring. Those who provide healthcare for others have an ethical imperative to uphold this ideal.

Varieties of communication

Many of the misunderstandings that occur between patients, families, and healthcare providers (indeed, between any two human beings) are due to mishaps in communication. This challenge is most obvious when the language of the care provider differs from the language of the patient. In these cases, professional interpreters are preferred, whether in person or via video or phone. In practice, however, families at the bedside often bear this burden, including young children (Green and Nze, 2017). When placed in this position, family members may misinterpret medical information, censor delicate topics, or summarize medical information in a way that distorts meaning (Howard, 2015). Translation apps can likewise be problematic. The Google translation of the term palliative care in Chinese means "do nothing care," an unfortunate and grossly inaccurate rewording (Pan, 2019).

Even when two parties speak the same language, there is no guarantee that communication will go smoothly. In her poem "Professional Spanish Knocks on the Door," Elisabet Velasquez shares the perception that Spanish spoken by a person of authority is "the kind of Spanish that comes to take things away from you . . . the kind of Spanish that looks at your Spanish like it needs help" (Velasquez, 2021). Trust and respect can likewise be undermined by assumptions about the language a person speaks or does not speak. Dr. Derald Wing Sue, a Columbia University professor and second-generation Asian–American, writes that people frequently compliment his "good English." The implication, he says, is that he and other people of color will forever be perceived as foreigners in their own country (Sue, 2021). The phenomenon of "elderspeak" is another common example of disparaging communication, in which older adults are addressed in exaggerated prosody resembling baby talk (Shaw and Gordon, 2021).

Language is only part of communication, of course. Other aspects include eye contact, personal space, touching, and expression of emotion. These behaviors can be cultural or extremely personal. Heads up 11.2 below describes examples of potential preferences of Islamic individuals, some of which could also apply to non-Muslim individuals. People on the autism spectrum, for example, can feel uncomfortable with a handshake or direct eye contact. As always, preferences must be clarified with each patient and family.

Heads up 11.2. End-of-life care and Islam

- Modesty is valued by many Muslim patients. Pause when entering a patient room, as women may want time to cover themselves (Habib et al., 2021).

- Modesty extends to touching, which may include handshakes. An alternative to shaking hands is to place your right hand over your heart, bow, and say hello (Khan, 2019).

- Direct eye contact may be considered disrespectful. Follow the patient's lead (Khan, 2019).

- While touch between unrelated people of opposite genders may be discouraged, touch between family members is valued. It can be nice to invite family to be involved in the massage. Explain the benefit of massage, and that massage can be provided over clothing or with lotion on the skin. Ask the patient and family what would be most helpful to them (Khan, 2019).

The words we use

Part of inclusivity and respect for others is learning new vocabulary as the process of naming evolves. This is a more nuanced and challenging endeavor than simply avoiding blatantly hurtful language. Subtle offenses can also be stigmatizing, even words that are commonly used in the medical community. Levels of function are often used to describe people with cognitive conditions, for example, but many consider these labels to be dismissive or insulting. People described as "high-functioning" may feel their struggles are minimized, while the term "low-functioning" discounts a person's actual abilities. The label "obese" has been cited by activist Amelia Mitchell as demeaning to people with large bodies who are much more than a medical condition to be pathologized and corrected (Mitchell, 2021). And many people who use wheelchairs prefer not to be described as "wheelchair-bound," a term which reduces a person to a relationship with a piece of equipment (NCDJ, 2021).

Sometimes preferences are local or personal. People-first language is favored by some individuals (a woman who is deaf, for example), while others take pride in identity-first language (a deaf woman). Some people who have had a limb amputation might refer to their "stump," while others prefer the term "residual limb," or simply "my leg." A growing number of groups, including the Centers for Disease Control and Prevention (CDC), maintain updated lists of preferred terms. But it must be acknowledged that there is no universal consensus on the use of these words, both between *and within* groups of people. Sometimes members of a particular community refer to themselves and each other in ways that would not be welcome from outsiders. A few disability activists have reclaimed the word "cripple," for example. Mitchell refers to herself as "a fat woman." It is important to err on the side of caution in avoiding the pitfall of cultural appropriation, defined by the *Cambridge Dictionary* as taking or using things from another culture, especially without showing due regard or understanding.

We must do the best we can to educate ourselves, deferring to individuals to let us know their preferences, but not expecting patients and families to assume the burden of our diversity training. A growing number of advocacy groups offer online courses and resources to enhance our knowledge and sensitivity; a list of these resources appears on p. 218. Training and support are also needed for healthcare providers who are on the receiving end of bias. A survey revealed that 70% of African–American physicians and 69% of Asian physicians have endured derogatory remarks from a patient or caregiver in the past five years (Cajigal and Scudder, 2017). A female Muslim doctor reports that she made the painful decision to forego wearing hijab in the interest of "building rapport" after three years of negative comments from patients, caregivers, and colleagues (WebMD, 2017).

Ideas to cultivate inclusive practices

Palliative care is formally recognized by the World Health Organization as a universal human right, to be provided through integrated, person-centered health services that support the needs and preferences of the individual

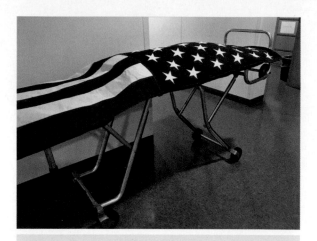

Figure 11.2
The day that a 106-year-old African–American World War II veteran died at our inpatient unit, staff lined the halls and saluted his body as it was taken out of the building on this flag-draped gurney. While we could not undo the racism this man likely endured in his life, we were able to provide respectful care for him at the end. Veterans are another group that has experienced stigma and barriers to healthcare.

(Photo by author.)

(WHO, 2020). A good foundation for inclusive practices is to genuinely believe in the right of every individual to be treated with such care. As part of the human family, we are called to advocate for inclusivity whenever and wherever possible. Some of us are in positions to effect change at societal or institutional levels. *All* of us are compelled to comport ourselves at a personal level with respect for each person we touch. Below are some practical ideas to facilitate inclusive interactions.

Lobby for inclusive intake and infrastructure

An inclusive intake process is a first step toward helping patients and their loved ones feel acknowledged and comfortable. The use of inclusive pronouns, recognition of important relationships, and availability of materials and services in a person's preferred language all convey a sense of reassurance that one's identity will be honored. This information should be shared with the care team so that all staff are apprised and appropriate resources can be brought to bear. The family should not have to orient every provider who steps through the door.

Mindful infrastructure is also needed to ensure that care settings are welcoming to people of all sizes and abilities. Environments should be accessible with diverse seating options, bariatric hospital beds and wheelchairs, assorted gown sizes, and equipment designed to assist with the care of people who have large bodies or small bodies, and everyone in between. "Those with power and privilege," says Mitchell, "need to advocate for those without" (Mitchell, 2019).

Slow down and be mindful

Rushed encounters are more likely to result in unintended blunders. Slowing down allows us to engage tools of mindfulness, which can simultaneously foster compassion for self and others (return to Chapter 2 as needed for tools to foster mindfulness). As we become more observant of our bodies, emotions, and thoughts, we can develop better sensitivity for noticing and naming implicit bias when it comes up for us. We are then able to challenge this thinking and choose more constructive alternatives. Mindful presence also increases our powers of clinical observation, making it less likely that we will miss something important.

Heads up 11.3. Taking off our blinders

Health disparities can occur anytime we get blinded by the "usual" presentation of a sign or symptom. Skin cancer is rare in people of color, for example, but the mortality rate is much higher. While melanoma occurs on sun-exposed areas in fair-skinned people, it is often missed on darker-skinned people, where it tends to present on areas that are rarely exposed to sun, including the soles of the feet, oral mucosa, groin, and perianal area (Ezenwa and Buster, 2019). Likewise, colon cancer in young people (NCI, 2020) and breast cancer in men (CDC, 2020) are diagnosed at later stages when these diseases are more fatal; in both cases, Black people are affected at higher rates than white people.

Address the dynamics of power and control

Therapists working in end-of-life care must be mindful that patients and their families often feel a loss of control and agency, especially when dying occurs in settings other than home. We can empower them by entering the room with deference to their needs, communicating at eye level rather than standing over them, offering choices, and supporting preferences regarding as many aspects of the session as possible. These may include where and when to have the massage, whether others participate in providing massage, whether to work over clothing or skin, what lubricant to use, positioning and propping, whether to have music (and if so, what kind), and the areas of the body that are to be touched or avoided. Obtaining informed consent for massage is paramount, as discussed on p. 52.

Address each person as they wish to be addressed

One of the first things I like to determine in an encounter with someone new is what name they wish to be called. If the patient is alert and verbal, we can ask them directly: "What name would you like me to call you?" If the patient is nonverbal, we can ask their representative: "What name would your parent/sibling/partner like me to use?" In the absence of this information, use neutral language, preferably the second person "you" to address the patient directly. Terms of endearment ("honey," "sweetheart," etc.) are perceived by many people to be patronizing and disrespectful.

Resist assumptions

Irshad Manji, founder of the Moral Courage Project, shares in her book *Don't Label Me* that the word "respect" comes from Latin, meaning *to see someone in a new light*, "to be curious about that person's experience and to spend time finding out about them" (Manji, 2019). Autism expert Dr. Stephen Shore famously said, "When you meet one person with Autism, you've met *one* person with Autism" (Shore, 2018). This wisdom can be applied to everyone we meet. Simply put, the person in front of us is a unique, one-of-a-kind human being, likely far more interesting than the stories our brain might create about them.

Heads up 11.4. Assumptions to avoid

- Never attempt to make a visual determination of a person's sex, gender identity, gender orientation, or preferred pronouns.

- Never make assumptions about a person's race, ethnicity, or where they are "from."

- It is impossible to tell what language a person might speak based on how they look.

- Avoid assumptions about religion and religious practice, as these are highly variable.

- Avoid assumptions about a person's abilities or disabilities. Allow them to reveal the vocabulary they use to describe these aspects of themselves.

- Do not make assumptions about how sick someone might be based on how they look or act. They may or may not appear gaunt or frail. Their suffering may be visible or invisible, and their dying process may or may not resemble the norms described in Chapter 5.

- Refrain from making guesses about relationships between people.

- Don't assume that people know they are dying, or that they understand or remember the specifics of their medical condition. Meet them where they are.

- Beware of judgments related to a person's diagnosis, including opinions about what they could or should have done differently. Their journey is not ours to evaluate.

Keep the words brief but get them as right as you can

It is often the case, especially at the end of life when patients may be losing verbal capacity, that very few words are needed by touch therapists. Our smiles, our silence, and our gentle hands can communicate respect and caring that are often more eloquent than words. Unless relevant to the care we are providing, it will likely be unnecessary to refer to a person's disability or any other aspect of their identity beyond their preferred name. When words are needed, it is likely that getting them right will primarily depend on having "large ears" (Baugher, 2019), as we listen for the language each person uses to describe themselves, their bodies, their needs, and their relationships. Until preferences are revealed to us, it is best to default to neutral language.

Get to know the person's people

As described in Chapter 1, family is defined by the patient. Given the endless variations of traditional, nontraditional, and blended families, therapists should refrain from assumptions regarding relationships. Acquaviva recommends that we direct our questions and take our cues from the patient, while "warmly" acknowledging the presence of significant others (Acquaviva, 2017). If the patient is verbal, we might ask, "Who do you have with you today?" If the patient is nonverbal, visitors can be asked, "How do you know this beautiful person?" The answers can be quite illuminating.

What if we slip?

Inclusivity is not a topic for a single chapter at the end of a book. It must begin on page one. There are no pronouns assumed anywhere in this book, only those that were stated preferences of specific people in photo captions and stories. The importance of allowing people to tell us how they wish to be addressed and who is important to them was described in Chapter 4. Chapter 7 addresses support for people with limb differences, mental health concerns, and substance use issues. Chapter 9 offers suggestions for working with individuals who have sight, hearing, or mobility challenges. But for all of our earnest intentions, we will undoubtedly fall short at times in our efforts to be inclusive. What do we do when this happens?

According to Clare Madrigal, we admit when we are wrong, we apologize, and we move on. A prolonged expression of embarrassment or self-reproach, says Madrigal, shifts the focus to our own experience of discomfort, in which the injured party may feel a need to make us feel better (Madrigal and Sturgeon, 2021). If we slip, as we likely will, we must learn from our mistakes and allow our missteps to be part of the dance.

Embracing the reciprocity of caring

Therapists working in end-of-life care will have the opportunity to experience deep connections with people of different backgrounds whom they might otherwise be unlikely to meet. Normal social boundaries become permeable when others sense that our only agenda is to honor their dignity and ease their suffering. A humble spirit and friendly, calm presence can convey our loving intentions when words fall short.

Touching story 11.1. The reciprocity of care

One of our home-based patients was a Pakistani Muslim woman who spoke minimal English. She was referred to the massage therapy team for symptom management, general discomfort, and anxiety. I was greeted at the door by three men of varying ages wearing shalwar kameez and slippers rather than shoes. I put on my shoe covers, one of our standard pieces of equipment, as many of our clients are accustomed to not wearing shoes in the home. I was ushered into a nearby room. A woman lay swathed in cloth, rigidly hunched in a very low bed, surrounded by a group of male family members with closed, troubled faces. They looked formidable but nodded a welcome.

I was offered tea and small cakes on an exquisite dish, while we carefully negotiated a plan for the massage session. The men then seated themselves around the bed to watch over proceedings. As I gently applied my hands to their wife and mother, the men all leaned forward to observe my every move, inches away from me. I paused to introduce soft Arabic music (via my phone) and the men began to relax, as did my client, murmuring with relief as I moved my hands slowly across her clothed back. Two of the younger men held each other, heads touching, as they leaned against the wall and watched their mother's body soften and surrender. By the end of the session, all the men had quietly smiled at me and crept away. The woman slept with deep and regular breathing. On departure, more tea and cakes were shared, and we all beamed at each other in a way that felt like mutual gratitude.

RMT Ronna Moore, Australia

Compassion is not about a relationship between the healer and the wounded, says Roman Catholic priest Gregory Boyle; it is about shifting into an "expansive place of fellowship," in which we stand in awe at what people have

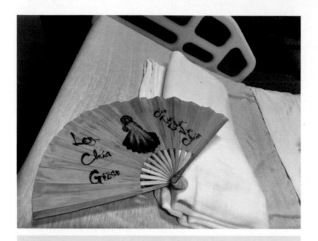

Figure 11.3
This fan belonged to a patient with a large Vietnamese family who spoke very little English. When it was admired by the therapist (who pointed, smiled, and said "so pretty!"), the family insisted on giving it to her as a thank you gift for the massage.

(Photo by author.)

to carry, "rather than judgment at how they carry it" (Boyle, 2010). Such interactions are only possible through the generosity of dying people and their loved ones who trust us to enter their world, just when their world may be falling apart. John Baugher reminds us that it is a profound gift when patients extend this invitation to us (Baugher, 2019). Each moment that we share with these fellow humans presents an opening to transcend the painful experiences and stories that might separate us under different circumstances. This is the true gift of this work: that despite our human flaws and limitations, we have recurring opportunities to rise above them.

One of the most moving examples of the transformative power of this work is described in a growing number of hospice prison programs, where individuals who are incarcerated volunteer to care for their fellow inmates at the end of their lives. In bleak, restrictive, and often hostile prison environments, stories of great tenderness are unfolding. Award-winning photographer Lori Waselchuk captured images of these stories at a maximum-security prison in a

book titled *Grace Before Dying*, in which she suggests that the recognition of our shared humanity might be "the core of all social problems" (Waselchuk, 2010). The volunteers provide hands-on care, including bathing and massage. At the time of death, they wrap the body in a quilt that they themselves have sewn, customized to honor the unique heritage and personality of the deceased. Out of respect, the guards allow the volunteers to carry the body to the morgue. As palliative care expert Ira Byock says, "We all have something to learn from that" (Byock, 2002).

Conclusion

Bias and exclusion of people we perceive to be "other" are universal problems that have likely been with us since humans first roamed the planet. In 1138, a man named Moses Maimonides was born in Spain under Muslim rule. Known as Maimonides to English speakers and Rambam to Hebrew speakers, Maimonides was one of many Jews at the time who were forced out of Spain to seek asylum in Egypt. A philosopher–physician whose writings in Arabic and Hebrew achieved both fame and controversy, Maimonides was no stranger to discrimination. Yet the words of his oath have surprising relevance for us today: "In the sufferer," he said, "let me see only the human being" (Seeskin, 2021).

Caring for people at the end of life puts us in touch with the vulnerability we all share and invites us to learn to love more deeply. Massage can be a bridge between our differences, a chance to connect with one another in a profoundly intimate way. If we truly care about inclusivity, we must focus on the individual we are touching, rather than the groups to which we think they might belong. The goal is not to be "color blind," but to take off our blinders so that we don't miss the chance to truly see, hear, and care for one another, in all our wondrous complexity. Inclusion means we embrace it all: the challenge, our blunders, our pain, and the potential for healing connection.

References

Acquaviva, K. D., 2017. *LGBTQ-inclusive hospice and palliative care: a practical guide to transforming professional practice*. New York: Harrington Park Press.

Baugher, J., 2019. *Contemplative caregiving: finding healing, compassion, and spiritual growth through end-of-life care*. Boulder, CO: Shambhala.

Boyle, G., 2010. *Tattoos on the heart: the power of boundless compassion*. New York: Free Press.

Burger, A., 2021. *Learning and teaching from the heart in troubled times*. [online] Available at: <https://gratefulness.org/resource/learning-and-teaching-from-the-heart-in-troubled-times>.

Byock, I. R., 2002. Dying well in corrections: why should we care? *Correctcare,* [e-journal] 16(4), p. 18. Available at: <https://pubmed.ncbi.nlm.nih.gov/12705265>.

Cajigal, S. and Scudder, L., 2017. Patient prejudice: when credentials aren't enough. [online] Available at: <https://www.medscape.com/slideshow/2017-patient-prejudice-report-6009134>.

Cates, C., 2020. Mind the gap. *It's getting real in here,* [blog] 21 December. Available at: <https://www.calcates.com/post/mind-the-gap>.

Centers for Disease Control and Prevention (CDC), 2020. *Male breast cancer incidence and mortality*. Available at: <https://www.cdc.gov/cancer/uscs/about/data-briefs/no19-male-breast-cancer-incidence-mortality-United-States-2013-2017.htm>.

Curseen, K., 2019. *Implicit bias and its impact on palliative care*. [online] Available at: <https://www.capc.org/blog/palliative-pulse-palliative-pulse-july-2017-overcome-implicit-bias-palliative-care>.

Elk, R. and Felder, T. M., 2018. Social inequalities in palliative care for cancer patients in the US: a structured review. *Seminars in Oncology Nursing,* [e-journal] 34(3), pp. 303–315. Available at: <https://doi.org/10.1016/j.soncn.2018.06.011>.

Ezenwa, E. and Buster, K., 2019. *Health disparities and skin cancer in people of color*. [online] Available at: <https://practicaldermatology.com/articles/2019-apr/health-disparities-and-skin-cancer-in-people-of-color>.

Green, A. R. and Nze, C., 2017. Language-based inequity in health care: who is the "poor historian"? *AMA Journal of Ethics,* [e-journal] (19)3, pp. 263–271. Available at: <https://journalofethics.ama-assn.org/article/language-based-inequity-health-care-who-poor-historian/2017-03>.

Habib, M. H., et al., 2021. *End-of-life care considerations for Muslim patients*. [online] Available at: <https://www.mypcnow.org/fast-fact/end-of-life-care-considerations-for-muslim-patients>.

Hagarty, A. M. et al., 2020. Severe pain at the end of life: a population-level observational study. *BMC Palliative Care,* [e-journal] 19(60). https://doi.org/10.1186/s12904-020-00569-2.

Hoffman, K. M. et al., 2016. Racial bias in pain assessment and treatment recommendations, and false beliefs about biological differences between blacks and whites. *PNAS,* [e-journal] 113(16), pp. 4296–4301. Available at: <www.pnas.org/cgi/doi/10.1073/pnas.1516047113>.

Howard, S., 2015. *Use of interpreters in palliative care*. [online] Available at: <https://www.mypcnow.org/fast-fact/use-of-interpreters-in-palliative-care>.

Jordan, K., 2021. Implicit bias: interrupting the stories that prevent us from delivering optimal care. [online training via Healwell] Available at: <https://online.healwell.org/courses/unconscious-bias>.

Khan, Y., 2019. End-of-life care and Islam. Handouts from a presentation provided at T. Boone Pickens in Dallas, Texas.

Madrigal, C. and Sturgeon, R. 2021. Creating an affirming and inclusive practice. [online training via Healwell] Available at: <https://online.healwell.org/courses/creating-an-affirming-and-inclusive-practice>.

Manji, I., 2019. *Don't label me: an incredible conversation for divided times*. New York: St. Martin's Press.

Mitchell, A., 2019. Clothing the fat body 101. *Aunt Amelia: your queer fat auntie experiencing cancer,* [blog] 24 October. Available at: <https://aunt-amelia.com/clothing-the-fat-body-101>.

Mitchell, A., 2021. What are we going to do about the weight? [online training via Healwell] Available at: <https://online.healwell.org/courses/weight-stigma>.

National Center on Disability and Journalism (NCDJ), 2021. *Style guide.* [online] Available at: <https://ncdj.org/style-guide>.

National Cancer Institute (NCI), 2020. *Why is colorectal cancer rising rapidly among young adults?* [online] Available at: <https://www.cancer.gov/news-events/cancer-currents-blog/2020/colorectal-cancer-rising-younger-adults>.

Organization for Security and Co-operation in Europe (OSCE), 2009. *Preventing and responding to hate crimes: a resource guide for NGOs in the OSCE region.* [pdf] Available at: <https://www.osce.org/files/f/documents/8/a/39821.pdf>.

Pan, C. X., 2019. *Lost in translation: Google's translation of palliative care to "do-nothing care".* [online] Available at: <https://www.geripal.org/2019/05/lost-in-translation-googles-translation-of-palliative-care.html>.

Seeskin, K., 2021. *Maimonides.* [online] Available at: <https://plato.stanford.edu/archives/spr2021/entries/maimonides>.

Shahid, S. et al., 2018. Key features of palliative care service delivery to Indigenous peoples in Australia, New Zealand, Canada, and the United States: a comprehensive review. *BMC Palliative Care*, [e-journal] 17(72). Available at: <https://doi.org/10.1186/s12904-018-0325-1>.

Shaw, C. A. and Gordon, J. K., 2021. Understanding Elderspeak: an evolutionary concept analysis. *Innovation in Aging*, [e-journal] 5(3), pp. 1–18. Available at: <https://doi.org/10.1093/geroni/igab023>.

Shore, S., 2018. *Leading perspectives on disability: a Q&A with Dr. Stephen Shore.* [online] Available at: <https://www.limeconnect.com/opportunities_news/detail/leading-perspectives-on-disability-a-qa-with-dr-stephen-shore>.

Sue, D. W., 2021. *Microaggressions: death by a thousand cuts.* [online] Available at: <https://www.scientificamerican.com/article/microaggressions-death-by-a-thousand-cuts>.

The United Nations Educational, Scientific and Cultural Organization (UNESCO), 2001. *Universal declaration on cultural diversity.* [pdf] Available at: <http://www.unesco.org/new/fileadmin/MULTIMEDIA/HQ/CLT/pdf/5_Cultural_Diversity_EN.pdf>.

The United States Department of Justice (USDJ), 2020. *Hate Crime Statistics.* [online] Available at: <https://www.justice.gov/hatecrimes/hate-crime-statistics>.

Velasquez, E., 2021. *Professional Spanish knocks on the door.* [online] Available at: <https://poets.org/poem/professional-spanish-knocks-door>.

Waselchuk, L., 2010. *Grace before dying.* New York: Umbrage Editions, Inc.

WebMD, 2017. Patient prejudice: doctors share their stories. [online] Available at: <https://www.webmd.com/a-to-z-guides/video/video-patient-bias>.

World Health Organization (WHO), 2020. *Palliative care fact sheet.* [online] Available at: <https://www.who.int/news-room/fact-sheets/detail/palliative-care>.

Yeager, K. A. and Bauer-Wu, S., 2013. Cultural humility: essential foundation for clinical researchers. *Applied Nursing Research*, [e-journal] 26(4), pp. 251–256. Available at: <https://doi.org/10.1016/j.apnr.2013.06.008>.

Additional resources

Angelou, M., 2011. On the power of words, Oprah's Master Class, aired on 1/16/2011, CCTV-14. Available at: <https://www.oprah.com/own-master-class/dr-maya-angelou-on-the-power-of-words-video>.

Australian Institute of Health and Welfare (AIHW), 2020. *Culturally-safe healthcare for Indigenous Australians.* [online] Available at: <https://www.aihw.gov.au/reports/australias-health/culturally-safe-healthcare-indigenous-australians>.

Autism Toolbox, 2019. *What does neurodiversity mean?* [online] Available at: <http://www.autismtoolbox.co.uk/what-does-neurodiversity-mean>.

Autistic Self-Advocacy Network, 2011. *Identity-first language.* [online] Available at: <https://autisticadvocacy.org/about-asan/identity-first-language>.

Charter for Compassion: https://charterforcompassion.org.

Grassman, D., 2021. *Hospice care for veterans: hope and healing webinar.* [online] Available at: <https://www.wehonorveterans.org/event/hospice-care-for-veterans-hope-and-healing-webinar>.

Kairuz, C. A. et al., 2020. Impact of racism and discrimination on the physical and mental health among Aboriginal and Torres Strait Islander peoples living in Australia: a protocol for a scoping review. *Systematic Reviews*, [e-journal] 9(1), p. 223. Available at: <https://doi.org/10.1186/s13643-020-01480-w>.

Kumagai, A. K. and Lypson, M. L., 2009. Beyond cultural competence: critical consciousness, social justice, and multicultural education. *Academic Medicine*, [e-journal] 84(6), pp. 782–787. Available at: <https://www.williamjames.edu/about/welcome/upload/beyond-cultural-competence-critical-33.pdf>.

Moral Courage College: https://moralcourage.com/.

Phelan, S. M. et al., 2015. Impact of weight bias and stigma on quality of care and outcomes for patients with obesity. *Obesity Reviews*, [e-journal] 16(4), pp. 319–326. Available at: <https://www.ncbi.nlm.nih.gov/pmc/articles/PMC4381543/pdf/obr0016-0319.pdf>

Public Health England, 2017. *Chapter 5: inequality in health.* [online] Available at: <https://www.gov.uk/government/publications/health-profile-for-england/chapter-5-inequality-in-health>.

Racial Equity Tools: https://www.racialequitytools.org/.

Rising, M. L. et al., 2019. Hispanic hospice utilization: integrative review and meta-analysis. *Journal of Health Care for the Poor and Underserved*, [e-journal] 30(2), pp. 468–494. Available at: <https://pubmed.ncbi.nlm.nih.gov/31130531>.

The United Nations Educational, Scientific and Cultural Organization (UNESCO), 2001. *Universal declaration on cultural diversity.* [pdf] Available at: <http://www.unesco.org/new/fileadmin/MULTIMEDIA/HQ/CLT/pdf/5_Cultural_Diversity_EN.pdf>.

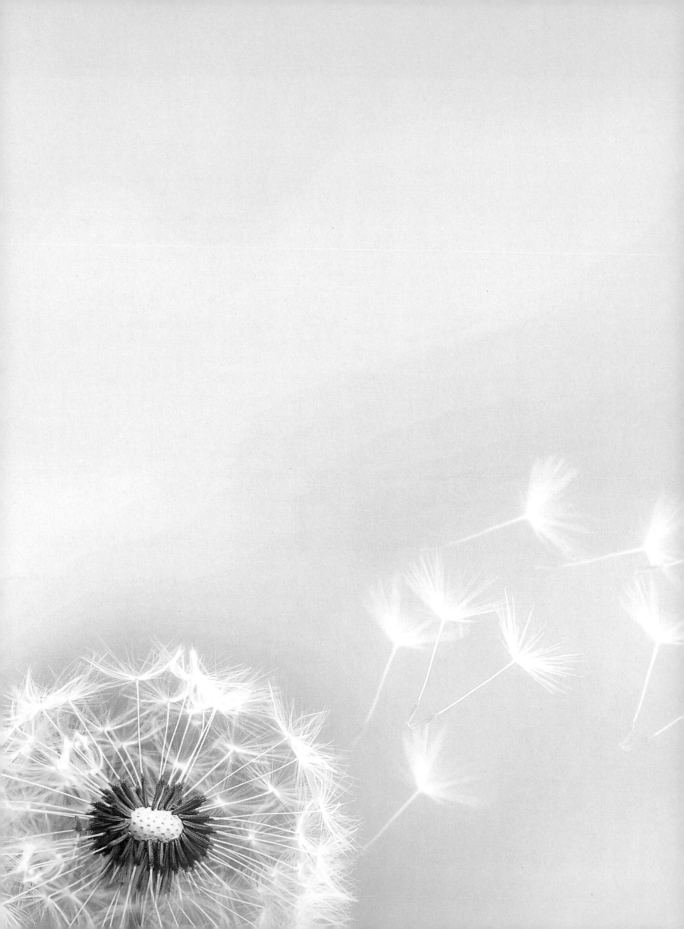

Epilogue Parting lessons

We need, in love, to practice only this: letting each other go.

–Rainer Maria Rilke

The first massage I ever provided for my father was nine days before he died, when he asked me to rub Bengay on his legs. He was confined to his recliner at that point, and his hope was that the Bengay would improve his circulation so that he might walk again. He had also ordered an electric massager from Amazon, which he kept referring to as his "vibrator," sending my sister and me into fits of suppressed giggles. I am certain that my dad had never received nor ever once considered receiving a professional massage.

We settled into a routine in which I massaged Bengay on Dad's legs every few hours. He said several times, "That feels good," and once told me my hands were soft. I incorporated some passive range of motion, pointing and flexing his feet, slowly circling his ankles. Dad often closed his eyes and sometimes slept.

I began opening our sessions with warm, damp washcloths, gently wiping his face, neck, arms, and hands. Reheating the cloths, I wrapped them around his feet as compresses, holding them in place with binder clips from his desk drawer. The moist warmth and texture of the terrycloth served to exfoliate his peeling skin and Dad seemed to love this. It was as if he was shedding his old skin, and a new improved skin was emerging from underneath.

On the fifth day, he declined the Bengay, but did allow me to apply lotion to his skin. I used the lotion provided by hospice, carefully warming it in the microwave. I applied the lotion liberally to all of Dad's skin that I could reach: his face, neck, shoulders, arms, hands, legs, and feet. I brushed his fine, white hair.

On two occasions, we managed to turn my father onto his side, and I was able to massage his back. He enjoyed this but could not tolerate side-lying position for more than a few minutes. A lot of what my sister and I did for comfort during his last days involved the rotation of five pillows to provide small changes in his position.

On the ninth day, I realized my father was letting go. It was a Saturday, and I was alone with him. I propped and cushioned him as best I could and told him I loved him and that it was okay to go if he needed to. In my Dad's understated way, he simply said, "okay." I pulled a chair to his bedside and held his right hand, reading aloud to him from his self-published autobiography. His breathing began to slow, and I put the book down. Holding one of my father's hands, my other hand over his heart, I leaned in close to him. We inhaled and exhaled together as Dad's respirations grew farther apart. His eyes were partly open, staring into a different world. Time seemed suspended and extraordinarily quiet. Very gently and without struggle, Dad's breathing diminished. And then it stopped. It was the shortest and easiest death I've ever witnessed.

What I learned from those extraordinary nine days with my father is that all the information in this book can be boiled down to a few simple things.

#1. Hospice offers unparalleled support

We found hospice to be indispensable for a home death, even a quick one. The equipment they provided, including a hospital bed and supplemental oxygen, made caregiving easier for us, and dying easier for my father. He did not end up needing medication, but I was more relaxed knowing we had comfort meds onsite. The aides who came to bathe and shave Dad were wonderful.

In the middle of what turned out to be my father's last night, I called hospice when he realized he was unable to urinate. He asked for a catheter and a nurse arrived at dawn as requested, driving an hour to get to Dad's house. The catheter took less than a minute to insert and she also increased his oxygen from 2 to 4 liters. I'm convinced that both of those measures were necessary to achieve the peaceful death that he experienced just a few hours later.

#2. Supplies don't have to be fancy

Our supplies included four pillows from the Dollar General Store, one slim decorative pillow from Dad's sofa which we covered with a pillowcase, a stack of cheap washcloths from the hardware store, and the lotion provided by hospice, which I referred to as an "inferior" product in Chapter 3. Warming the lotion and the washcloths made all the difference. We likely could have used vegetable oil from his kitchen pantry.

#3. Self-care can also be very simple

For us that week in the Texas Hill Country, there was no access to yoga classes or fancy coffee. But we managed to feed and water our souls. For my sister, that meant leaving the house each morning to buy herself an iced tea. We both took occasional walks. One day we opened the door to Dad's apartment to let in some fresh air and watched a patch of sun creep across the floor all morning, marveling at an occasional hummingbird. We stayed in touch with supportive family and friends via text. We laughed at random absurdities when we could and cried when we needed to. We took turns sleeping. We kept breathing. It was enough.

#4. Skills matter, but they're not what matter most

I'd like to think that the skills and knowledge I've developed over a 22-year career have value. But I believe the greatest asset I brought to my father's bedside was not clinical expertise, but simply a confidence born of preparation. In short, I did not feel afraid to touch and *be* with him. My lack of fear created a space that we could share, and when the time came, that allowed him to leave in peace.

In the end, massage for my father was my love language. It helped him feel more comfortable, cherished, and cared for, and it helped me feel more connected to him, even as I was losing him. My father was a man of few words, but we didn't need many words at the end.

I hope, someday, when I come to the end of my life, that I'm able to summon a fraction of my father's grace for the experience of dying. I hope to say "okay" and to gradually let go of the need for breath so that I can step across the threshold of whatever comes next. And I hope that one of you reading this might be there, to gently hold my hand.

Name of patient	
Name of therapist	
Date of assessment	

Check, circle, or underline all that apply

Position

- [ ] supine in bed/hospital bed, left leaning/right leaning
- [ ] Fowler's, HOB slightly elevated
- [ ] high Fowler's, HOB nearly upright
- [ ] side lying, left/right
- [ ] in geri chair
- [ ] in wheelchair
- [ ] regular chair or sofa
- [ ] seated upright on edge of bed

Level of arousal

- [ ] awake
- [ ] alert
- [ ] confused, mild/moderate/severe
- [ ] lethargic/weak
- [ ] fatigued/sleepy/groggy
- [ ] opens eyes but minimally responsive
- [ ] eyes partially open, no tracking
- [ ] eyes closed, unresponsive to verbal stimuli

Ability to communicate

- [ ] able to make needs known
- [ ] hearing impaired
- [ ] slow thought process/difficulty finding words
- [ ] slurred speech or mumbling
- [ ] word salad
- [ ] nonverbal

Breathing

- [ ] unlabored, steady
- [ ] deep, relaxed
- [ ] shallow
- [ ] rapid
- [ ] labored, use of accessory muscles
- [ ] audible snoring
- [ ] secretions, gurgling
- [ ] periods of apnea, lasting ____seconds
- [ ] room air
- [ ] O_2 cannula
- [ ] BiPap or tracheostomy

Skin

- [ ] color, jaundiced/cyanotic/pale
- [ ] temperature, febrile/sweating/warm/cool
- [ ] skin intact
- [ ] dry skin, surface peeling/scaling
- [ ] complaint of itching
- [ ] wounds: skin tears/lacerations/blisters/bandages, locations
- [ ] pressure injuries, locations
- [ ] areas of risk, skin touching skin/red/pink, locations
- [ ] constrictions of jewelry, hospital band, socks, elastic, locations

Abdomen and torso

- [ ] distended (ascites)
- [ ] port-a-cath/catheters/devices
- [ ] surgical or radiation sites

Extremities

- [ ] peripheral neuropathy
- [ ] nonfunctioning limbs/spasm/R lower/L lower/R upper/L upper
- [ ] fungal infection
- [ ] edema, R lower/L lower/R upper/L upper
- [ ] lymphedema, R lower/L lower/R upper/L upper
- [ ] amputation(s), R lower, L lower/R upper/L upper
- [ ] mottling, knees/feet/toes

Face

- [ ] soft, relaxed
- [ ] facial grimace, furrowed brow
- [ ] swelling
- [ ] bruising
- [ ] laceration

Psychosocial

- [ ] quiet, calm, accepting
- [ ] quiet, subdued, resigned
- [ ] pleasant affect, conversational
- [ ] distressed, anxious
- [ ] withdrawn/depressed
- [ ] tearful
- [ ] caregiver present, family/professional
- [ ] caregiver not present
- [ ] caregiver supportive, engaged with patient
- [ ] caregiver tearful
- [ ] caregiver tension, anger, or dissatisfaction with care

Response to massage

- [ ] fell asleep
- [ ] became relaxed, sigh, deeper breathing
- [ ] positive verbal feedback
- [ ] no change observed
- [ ] adverse response, increased agitation or patient asked to stop

The mnemonic **ABCDE** can help therapists make observations during the patient assessment and be used afterward to recall these observations for charting or sharing with the palliative care team.

A Alertness or Arousal

What do you notice about the patient's level of alertness? Are they able to engage with you? Are they sleeping lightly such that they arouse easily when you speak to or touch them? Or are they sleeping deeply? How does level of arousal compare to your previous visits if this is not your first? Level of arousal can indicate progression of the dying process or may be a temporary response to medication or fatigue.

B Breathing

What do you notice about the patient's respirations? Are they fast or slow? Shallow or deep? Does there appear to be effort involved in breathing? Are they short of breath? Are they on mechanical ventilation or using oxygen?

C Comfort

What do you observe about the patient's comfort? Are the face and body relaxed, or is there a facial expression or body movement that suggests pain or other distress? Do they appear to be in a comfortable position with good pillow support?

D Dermis

What do you observe about the patient's skin? Do you see any cracking or peeling to indicate that the skin is dry? Is any broken skin visible? Any bruises? What do you observe about the color of the skin? Is it pale, jaundiced (yellow), or cyanotic (blue)? Are there any red areas or rashes?

E Edema

Do you observe any swelling in the face, torso, body, or limbs?

Recommended listening

A Network for Grateful Living (available at www.gratefulliving.org) – a library of blogs, videos, audios, and other resources. Described as an "online sanctuary" created by Brother David Steindl-Rast. Topics include loss and grief, peace and justice, nature, and living more simply. Free newsletter.

Healwell (available at www.healwell.org) – podcasts and online training on topics of equity and inclusion for massage therapists and other caregiving disciplines.

On Being (available at www.onbeing.org) – a podcast and public radio show hosted by Krista Tippet, devoted to "civil conversations and social healing," as well as topics related to the body, mind, and spirit, including death and dying.

Sounds True (available at soundstrue. com) – podcasts hosted by Tami Simon on a wide range of subjects including self-compassion, spirituality, mindfulness, health, and healing.

Recommended reading

Top 10 List

At home with dying: a zen hospice approach. Merrill Collett, 1999. Boston, MA: Shambhala Publications, Inc.

Awake at the bedside: contemplative teachings on palliative and end-of-life care. Koshin Palex Ellison and Matt Weingast, eds, 2016. Somerville, MA: Wisdom Publishers.

Being mortal: medicine and what matters in the end. Atul Gawande, 2014. New York: Picador.

Being with dying: cultivating compassion and fearlessness in the presence of death. Joan Halifax, 2009. Boston, MA: Shambhala.

Contemplative caregiving: finding healing, compassion & spiritual growth through end-of-life care. John Baugher, 2019. Boulder, CO: Shambhala Classic.

Final Gifts: Understanding the Special Awareness, Needs, and Communications of the Dying. Maggie Callanan and Patricia Kelley, 1992. New York: Simon & Schuster reprint, 2012.

Hard choices for loving people: CPR, feeding tubes, palliative care, comfort measures, and the patient with serious illness. Hank Dunn, 2016. Naples, FL: Quality of Life Publishing Co.

Preparing to die: practical advice and spiritual wisdom from the Tibetan Buddhist tradition. Andrew Holecek, 2013. Boston, MA: Snow Lion.

Soul midwives' handbook: the holistic and spiritual care of the dying. Felicity Warner, 2013. London: Hay House UK Ltd.

What does it feel like to die? Inspiring new insights into the experience of dying. Jennie Dear, 2019. New York: Citadel Press-Kensington Publishing Corp.

General life, death, and dying

Advice for future corpses and those who love them: a practical perspective on death and dying. Sally Tisdale, 2018. New York: Touchstone.

A path with heart. Jack Kornfield, 1994. London: Random House Group.

Handbook for mortals: guidance for people facing serious illness. Joanne Lynn, Joan Harrold, and Janice Lynch Schuster, 2011, 2nd ed. New York: Oxford University Press.

Kitchen table wisdom: stories that heal. Rachel Naomi Remen, 1994, 2006. New York: Riverhead, Penguin Group.

Midwife for souls: spiritual care for the dying. Kathy Kalina, 2007. Boston, MA: Pauline Books and Media.

The best care possible: a physician's quest to transform care through the end of life. Ira Byock, 2013. New York: Penguin Group.

The etiquette of illness: what to say when you can't find the words. Susan P. Halpern, 2004. New York: Bloomsbury, Holtzbrinck Publishers.

The five invitations: discovering what death can teach us about living fully. Frank Ostaseski, 2017. New York: Flatiron Books.

Using the power of hope to cope with dying: the four stages of hope. Cathleen Fanslow-Brunjes, 2008. Sanger, CA: Quill Driver Books-Word Dancer Press, Inc.

Massage

Comfort touch: massage for the elderly and the ill. Mary Kathleen Rose, 2010. Philadelphia: Wolters Kluwer Health-Lippincott Williams & Williams.

From the heart through the hands: the power of touch in caregiving. Dawn Nelson, 2006. Forres, Scotland: Findhorn Press.

Hands in health care: massage therapy for the adult hospital patient. Gayle MacDonald and Carolyn Tague, 2021. Edinburgh: Handspring Publishing Ltd.

Massage in hospice care: an everflowing approach. Irene Smith, 2014. Text, video and audio format. Available at: <https://books.apple.com/us/book/massage-in-hospice-care/id915933540>.

Medicine hands: massage therapy for people with cancer. Gayle MacDonald, 2014. Forres, Scotland: Findhorn Press.

Oncology massage: an integrative approach to cancer care. Janet Penny and Rebecca L. Sturgeon, 2021. Edinburgh: Handspring Publishing Limited.

Touch, caring and cancer: simple instruction for family and friends. William Collinge and the National Cancer Institute. Text, video and audio format. Available at: <www.touchcaringand cancer.com>.

Other complementary therapies

A touching goodbye: the gentle use of Jin Shin Jyutsu at times of critical illness. Judith B. Andry, 2008. Chicago: Ampersand, Inc.

Complementary nursing in end-of-life care: handbook for nurses and health care professionals. Madeleine Kerkhof-Knapp Hayes, 2015. Wernhout, Netherlands: Kicozo.

Hydrotherapy for bodyworkers: improving outcomes with water therapies. MaryBetts Sinclair, Edinburgh: Handspring Publishing.

Namaste care: the end-of-life program for people with dementia. Joyce Simard, 2018. Baltimore: Health Professions Press.

Reiki energy medicine: bringing healing touch into home, hospital, and hospice. Libby Barnett and Maggie Babb, 1996. Rochester, VT: Healing Arts Press.

Reiki in clinical practice: a science-based guide. Ann Baldwin, 2020. Edinburgh: Handspring Publishing.

Doula perspectives

Accompanying the dying: practical, heart-centered wisdom for the end-of-life doula and health care advocate. Deanna Cochran, 2019. Sacred Life Publishers.

Finding peace at the end of life: a death doula's guide for families and caregivers. Henry Fersko-Weiss, 2020. Newburyport, MA: Red Wheel-Weiser, LLC.

The doula business guide: how to succeed as a birth, postpartum or end-of-life doula, 3rd ed. Patty Brennan, 2019. Ann Arbor, MI: DreamStreet Press.

Self-care

Anchored: how to befriend your nervous system. Deb Dana, 2021. Boulder, CO: Sounds True.

Help for the helper: self-care strategies for managing burnout and stress. Babette Rothschild, 2006. New York: W. W. Norton & Company.

My grandmother's hands: racialized trauma and the pathway to mending our hearts and bodies. Resmaa Menakem, 2017. Las Vegas: Central Recovery Press.

Polyvagal exercises for safety and connection: 50 client-centered practices. Deb Dana, 2020. New York: W.W. Norton & Company.

Resilient: how to grow an unshakeable core of calm, strength and happiness. Rick Hanson, 2018. New York: Harmony Books-Penguin Random House LLC.

The mindful brain: reflection and attunement in the cultivation of wellbeing. Daniel Siegel, 2007. New York: W.W. Norton.

Trauma stewardship: everyday guide to caring for self while caring for others. Laura vanDernoot Lipsky with Connie Burk, 2009. San Francisco: Berrett-Koehler Publishers, Inc.

Inclusivity

Don't label me: how to do diversity without inflaming the culture wars. Irshad Manji, 2019. New York: St. Martin's Griffin.

LGBTQ-inclusive hospice and palliative care: a practical guide to transforming professional practice. Kimberly Acquaviva, 2017. New York: Harrington Park Press.

Racial Equity Tools is an online compendium including links to a newsletter, research, films, diversity training, a glossary, tips, and other resources related to racism and social justice. Available at www.racialequitytools.org.

Rituals

Sacred dying: creating rituals for embracing the end of life. Megory Anderson, 2003. New York: Marlowe & Company-Avalon Publishing Group Incorporated.

The power of ritual: turning everyday activities into soulful practices. Casper Ter Kuile, 2020. New York: Harper One–Harper Collins Publishing.

The wild edge of sorrow: rituals of renewal and the sacred work of grief. Francis Weller, 2015. Berkeley, CA: North Atlantic Books.

Clinical and reference

A massage therapist's guide to pathology. Ruth Werner, 7th ed, 2019. Boulder, CO: Books of Discovery.

End-of-life care: a practical guide. Barry M. Kinzbrunner and Joel S. Policzer, 2nd ed, 2011.

New York: McGraw Hill Medical-McGraw Hill Companies, Inc.

End-of-life issues, grief, and bereavement: what clinicians need to know. Sara H. Qualls and Julia E. Kasl-Godley, 2011. Hoboken, NJ: John Wiley & Sons, Inc.

Professional organizations

National End-of-Life Doula Alliance – professional group in the US for EOL doulas, with information on doula training and resources for NEDA members. Doula locator link and networking opportunities.

National Hospice and Palliative Care Organization – largest professional group in the US for hospice and palliative care providers, including integrative therapists. Free online resources and job postings. Available at: <https://www.nhpco.org>.

Society for Oncology Massage – a worldwide organization for all things related to oncology massage, including training, networking opportunities, and more. Resources for members, nonmembers, and clients seeking to locate oncology-trained therapists. Available at: <https://www.s4om.org>.

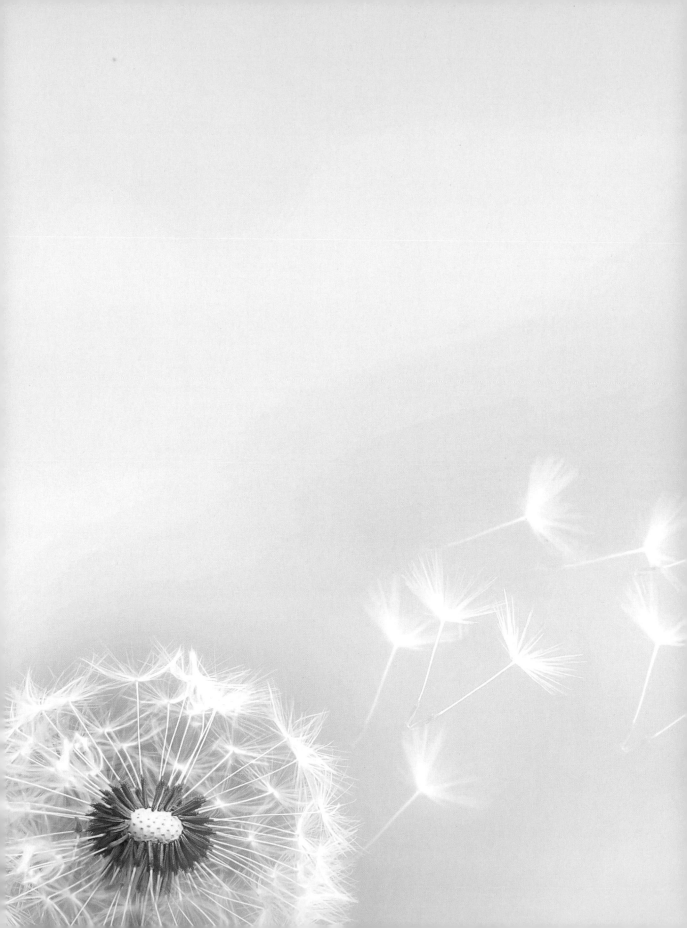

INDEX

Note: Page numbers in *italics* denote figures and **bold** denote tables.

A

abdominal massage 100, *101*
abdominal swelling 56
above-the-elbow amputation (AEA) 140
above-the-knee amputation (AKA) 140
acquired brain injury (ABI) 133
active dying 84–6
    comfort care 84
    Daniel's case 87–8
    death rattle 86
    electrolyte disturbances 86
    last surge of energy 85
    massage session for 86
    physical changes 86
    timing of death 85
adapting to massage session
    for ascites 98–9
    brain disorders and injuries 134
    during cachexia 96
    cardiovascular disease 120
    for confusion, delirium, and terminal
        restlessness 100
    for constipation 101–2
    dementia 127–8
    for depression 102
    for diarrhea 102
    dying process 77, 80, 82
    dyspnea (shortness of breath) 102–3, *103*
    edema and lymphedema 104, *104*
    for end-of-life apnea 98
    falls 105
    fatigue 105–6, *106*
    fever 106
    fractures 107
    hiccups 107
    HIV/AIDS 138–9
    kidney disease 131
    liver disease 132–3
    lung disease 129
    massage precautions 35–8
    nausea with or without vomiting 107
    neurodegenerative diseases 136–7
    oncology massage 121, 124
    pain 109–10
    peripheral neuropathy (PN) 110
    pruritus (itching) 111
    to reduce anxiety 97–8
    secretions 111
    seizures 111–12
    skin changes 112–13
    tremors and myoclonus 113
    wounds 114
addiction 139
advanced care planning 201
altruism 18
Alzheimer's disease 125
American Academy of Neurology 156
amputation and limb differences 139
amyotrophic lateral sclerosis (ALS) 135–6
anorexia 95–6
anoxic brain injury 133
anticholinergic drugs 148
anticholinergic properties 148
anticoagulants 148
    aspirin 157
    warfarin 157
antihypertensives 148
antiretroviral therapy (ART) 137
anxiety at end-of-life 96–7
apnea 98
aromatherapy 186
arrhythmias, life-threatening 148
artificial nutrition and hydration 171
aspiration pneumonia 140
assessment of patient
    extremities 56
    face, head, and neck 55–6
    skin 56–7, *57*
    symptoms 58
    torso 56
atherosclerotic cardiovascular disease
    (ASCVD) 119
automatic implanted cardiovertor defibrillator
    (AICD) 169

B

Baugher, John 23
bed-based massage 62–5
    Fowler's position 64–6, *65*
    home beds 62–3, *62–3*
    hospital beds 63–5, *63–5*
    pillows needed 65
    repositioning 66, *66*
    side-lying massage 62–5, *63–5*
Beers list 148
Beers warnings 149
below-the-elbow amputation (BEA) 140
below-the-knee amputation (BKA) 140
blood pressure medications 148
body fluid principle 38
boundary awareness 19–20
bowel and urinary tract devices 172–4

C

cachexia 95–6
calciphylaxis 130–1
Campbell, Robert Chodo 88
cancer, end-stage 120–4, *121*
    bleeding and clotting issues 121
    complications 123
    hypercalcemia in 122
    lymphedema in 122
    obstructions in 122–3
    pathological fractures in 122
Cannabis indica 156
capsaicin 110
cardiac devices 169
cardiac patients, end-stage 119–20
cardiomyopathy 119
cardiopulmonary resuscitation 177
cardiovascular disease (CVD) 118–19
caregivers
    massage for 70
    providing massage 70–1, *71*
caring, nature of 17–18
carrier oils 186
Catholic Sisters of Charity 4
Centers for Disease Control and Prevention
    (CDC) 204
cerebrovascular accident (CVA) 133
certified nursing assistant (CNA) 7
Cheyne–Stokes breathing 98
cholesterol medications 148
chronic disease trajectories 146
chronic kidney disease (CKD) 130
chronic obstructive pulmonary disease
    (COPD) 128
cirrhosis 132
cold packs 190
cold therapy 190
combined decongestive therapy (CDT) 122
comfort kit 150
communication
    with dying person 54–5
    varieties of 202
    and visual devices 168–9
compassionate extubation 178
compressions 30

brain disorders and injuries 133–4
    common symptoms 134
breakthrough pain 109
breathing and grounding exercises 22, *22*
breathing treatments 175–6

confusion 99
congestive heart failure (CHF) 119
constipation 100
contentment 23
continuous care 8
contusion 112–13
cooling techniques 190
coronary artery bypass grafting (CABG) 118
coronary artery disease (CAD) 119
coronary heart disease (CHD) 119
cultural constructs 201
cultural humility 202

D

day-to-day caretaking 8
death doula programs 12
death rattle 86
decubitus ulcers 114
deep vein thrombosis (DVT) 36, 106, 120
delirium 99
delivery systems and dosing 151
dementia 125–8
    common symptoms 126
    medications 148
    pain assessment in people with 126–7
depression 102
destination therapy 169
devices for nutrition and hydration 171–2
dialysis 175
dialyzer 175
diarrhea 102
diazepam (valium) 155
doula business guide, The 12
*Drugs Most Commonly Used at St.
    Christopher's Hospice* 145
durable medical equipment (DME) 165
    types of 166
dying process 75
    active 84–6
    adapting to massage session 77, 80, 82
    beginning of 76
    care while dying 88
    concept of good death 76–7
    Daniel's decline stages, case 78–81, 83–4,
        87–8
    emotional and psychosocial adjustments
        76–7, *78*, 79–80, 82
    last breath and beyond 88
    late decline 79–81
    near death awareness (NDA) 80
    physical changes 76, 79, 81–2
    pre-active dying 81–2
    see also active dying
dyspnea (shortness of breath) 102–3

E

ecchymoses 113
edema *57*, 104, *104*
Edmonton scale 58
effleurage 30, *30*
electric blankets and heating pads 189
eleventh hour volunteers 13
emotional contagion 18
emotional demands of work 18–20
empathy 18
end-of-life care 4, 20
    being with work 21–3
    location of care at 7–8
    preparing to do 20–1
    professional and personal development 24
    spectrum of 3–4
    staying with work 23–6
    supervision 24
    touch therapists in 11
end-of-life (EOL) doula programs 14, 24
end-stage renal disease (ESRD) 117, 130–1
    see also specific entries
engaged in life *118*
equanimity 23
ergonomics 8
erythema 113
esophageal varices 132
essential oils 187

F

family
    defined 11
    in end-of-life care 11
fatigue 105–6, *106*
Felicia, Dr *125*
fever 106
fistulas 113–14
folded washcloth *45*
Fowler's position 64–6, *65*, 97, 103, 107, 141
fractures 106–7
freestanding inpatient unit (IPU) 10
frontotemporal dementia 125
Functional Assessment Staging Scale (FAST)
    126
fungating tumors 113
furosemide (Lasix) 155, 161

G

general inpatient care (GIP) 8
geriatric massage 12

geri chair 62
gloves and gloving practices 40–1
good death concept 76–7
goodness of fit 20–1
gout 140
Grace Before Dying 208

H

Halifax, Joan 24, 77, 84
haloperidol (Haldol) 154
Hanson, Rick 23
healthcare power of attorney (HPOA) 11
heat therapy 188–90
hepatic encephalopathy 132
herpes simplex 40
hiccups 107
HIV/AIDS 137–9
    common symptoms 138
    impact of 138
hospice
    agencies 13
    as continuum 6
    focus of 5
    houses 4
    present times 5
hospital beds 9, *11*, 63–5, *64*
Huntington's Disease 11, 125, 136
Huntsman Cancer Institute 146
hyperkalemia 131

I

implanted defibrillators 169, 178
incontinence 172
intake process 48–9
International Association for Hospice and
    Palliative Care (IAHPC) 145
intracerebral hemorrhage (ICH) 133
intubation 170–1
ischemic heart disease 119
ischemic stroke 134

J

jugular vein distention (JVD) 123

K

Karnofsky Performance Scale 76
kidney disease, end-stage 130–1
    common symptoms 131
    complications 130–1
Kornfield, Jack 17

L

left ventricular assist devices (LVADs) 118, 169
levetiracetam (Keppra) 155
lewy body dementia 125
LGBTQ community 200
LGBTQ-Inclusive Hospice and Palliative Care 200
licensed massage therapist (LMT) 13
life expectancy 5
liver disease, end-stage 131–3
   common causes 132
   common symptoms 132
   complications 132
London hospice 4
lorazepam (Ativan) 155
lower-extremity ulcers 113
lung disease, end-stage 128–9
   common symptoms 128–9
LVAD deactivation 178
lymphedema *37,* 37–8

M

MacDonald, Gayle 7, 9
manual lymphatic drainage (MLD) 12, 125
marijuana use 156–7
massage 6–7, *7*
   in bed 62–5
   benefits of 6–7, 12
   centering of hands 66–7
   dose 31
   in facilities 9
   geriatric 12
   home visits 8, *9*
   in hospice inpatient setting 9, *10*
   oncology 12
   power of holding 67
   pressure 31–5
   sequencing of 67–8
   tables 58–9, *59*
   teamwork 9
   techniques 29–30, *30*
   using cloth 68
   for Veterans 12
   wrapping up 69
massage precautions 35–42
   adapting session 35–8
   airborne 39
   against clotting and bleeding 36
   contact 39–40
   contraindications 40
   droplet 39
   gloves and gloving practices 40–1
   hand hygiene 38–9
   impaired sensation and feedback 35, *35*

   against loss of bone strength 37
   against loss of skin integrity 35
   lymphedema and lymphedema risk *37,* 37–8
   oxygen safety 41–2
   risk for DVT and PE 36
   standard 38–9
   transmission-based 39–41
   use of personal care products 42
   use of personal protective equipment (PPE) and sanitizer 38–9
massage therapist
   agency and facility work 12–14
   carry-in items 45–6
   car stock 44–5
   clothing and accessories 42–3
   contract work 13
   dual role of 14
   employment via agencies 13–14
   licensed massage therapist (LMT) 13
   odor management 46
   private practice 12
   referral and intake 48–9
   volunteering 13
mattress options 167
mechanical ventilation 178
medical charts 99
medical power of attorney (MPOA) 11
medications
   antibiotics 156
   approaches to prescribing 149–51
   for anxiety and agitation 154
   Beers list 148–9
   common in palliative care 152–6, **158–60**
   for constipation 154
   delivery systems 151–2
   for depression 154–5
   discontinued 147–8
   dosing 151–2
   essential and common 152–6
   for fluid retention 155
   for itching and hiccups 155
   for nausea and vomiting 155
   oral 151
   for oral secretions 155–6
   for pain 152–4
   for seizures 155
   for shortness of breath 155
   for wounds 156
meeting and communicating with patients and families
   assessment 55–8
   conditions affecting communications 54–5
   introductions and consent 52–4
   patient's environment 51–2

Menakem, Resmaa 22, 24
mental illness 140–1
methicillin-resistant *Staphylococcus aureus* (MRSA) 40
metronidazole (Flagyl) 156
Michael, Sister Mary *127*
mindful infrastructure 205
mobility devices 166
Moore, Ronna 69
morphine 109
mottling *87*
Mount, Balfour 5
multiple sclerosis (MS) 136
music thanatology 191
myocardial infarction (MI) 119
myoclonus 130

N

nasal cannulas and nasal pillows 170
nausea 107, *108*
near death awareness (NDA) 80, 99
nephrostomies 172
neurodegenerative diseases 135–7
neuropathic pain 109
Newton, Nanci 66
nicotine and caffeine withdrawal 139
noninvasive ventilation (NIV) 170

O

odor management 46, 114
oncology massage 12
opioid doses 146
oral medications 151
Organization for Security and Co-operation in Europe (OSCE) 200
orthostatic hypotension 160

P

pacemakers and implanted defibrillators 169
pain *108,* 108–10
   control devices 174
palliative approach 146
palliative care 5, 7–8, 10–14, 17–19, 24, 38, 76, 115, 117, 120, 128, 135, 204
   community 146
   as continuum 6
palliative or hospice care team 12, 133
palliative performance scale (PPS) 76
"pampered patient" program 12
paracentesis and thoracentesis 176
Parkinson's disease 125, 135, 148

pathological altruism 18
peripheral artery disease (PAD) 119
peripheral neuropathy 110
petrissage 30, *30*
phantom limb pain 140
pitting edema 104
pleasure feeding 96
pleural effusions 141
positioning and propping of patient 58–66, 140
  to reduce anxiety 97
post-mortem care 89
post-traumatic stress disorder (PTSD) 142
pre-active dying 81–2
  emotional and psychosocial adjustments 82
  massage during 83
  physical changes 81–2
  see also dying process
prescriptive music 191
pressure injury (bedsores) 36, 114
pressure ulcers 114
primary caregiver (PCG) 11
Princess Leia scroll 66
private practice 12
"Professional Spanish Knocks on the Door" 203
pruritus (itching), 110–11
pulmonary effusions 141
pulmonary embolism (PE) 36, 106
purpura 113

R

range of motion 193–4
reclining massage 62, *62*
referrals 48–9
Reiki 24, 70, 142
Remen, Rachel Naomi 18
renal osteodystrophy 131
repositioning 66, *66*, 111
resilience 23
respiratory devices 170
responses to massage
  adverse 69
  positive 68
rituals 25–6

S

sacred oils 186
saliva substitutes 114
sanctuary 24–5, *25*

Saunders, Dame Cicely 4, 95
scope of practice 10
seated massage 60, *60–2*
  in seated forward fold *61–2*
  upright *60–1*
secretions 111
seizures 111–12
self-acceptance 17
self-awareness 18–19, 21–4, 26
self-care 17–18
  anchoring heart technique 22
  breathing and grounding exercises 22, *22*
  questions related to awareness 21–2
  recognizing and responding to discomfort 22–3
  recommendations 21–2
  taking in the good 23
self-compassion 18–21, 24
self-expansion 24
self-preservation 24
self-reflective journaling 24
self-regulation 18–21, 24
sepsis 141–2
shoulder massage 70
skin tears 113
Slocum, Erika 66
Smith, Irene 51
spinal cord compression 123
statins 148
Stay Close and Do Nothing (Merrill Collett) 75
stomas
  types of 172
strokes 30
subarachnoid hemorrhage (SAH) 134
substance use disorder 139
suctioning 111
suggestions for providing massage
  in group homes 72
  at home 71–2
  in hospital or IPU 72
superior vena cava syndrome (SVCS) 122
supervision 24
supplies
  bulk 46
  carry-in items for home and group home visits 45–6
  clothing and accessories 42–3
  in inpatient setting 46–7
  lubricants 43–4
  management of 44–5
  for self-care 47–8
  in self-care bag 48
  suggested car stock 45

T

tapotement 129
terminal agitation *see* terminal restlessness
terminal care 5
terminal restlessness 99
therapeutic touch 24
Tisdale, Sallie 77
topical products
  gels 151
  lotions 151
  ointments 151
total suffering 95
touch therapists 145, 168, 185, 192, 194, 197
  in clinical settings 145
transdermal patches 151
transitional objects *98*
trauma-informed care 142
traumatic brain injury (TBI) 134
tremors and myoclonus 113
triage 8

U

urinary retention 173
urinary tract infections (UTIs) 126

V

vancomycin-resistant enterococcus (VRE) 39–40
vascular dementia 125
vitamins 148
volunteering 13

W

Wald, Florence 5
Walton, Tracy 38
Weil, Andrew 24
World Health Organization (WHO) 152, 165
wounded healers 18
wounds 113–14
wrapping up session 69

X

xerostomia (dry mouth) 114